Current Techniques and Materials in Dentistry

Current Techniques and Materials in Dentistry

Editor

Mitsuru Motoyoshi

MDPI • Basel • Beijing • Wuhan • Barcelona • Belgrade • Manchester • Tokyo • Cluj • Tianjin

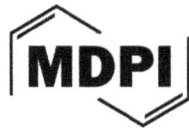

Editor
Mitsuru Motoyoshi
Nihon University School of Dentistry
Japan

Editorial Office
MDPI
St. Alban-Anlage 66
4052 Basel, Switzerland

This is a reprint of articles from the Special Issue published online in the open access journal *Applied Sciences* (ISSN 2076-3417) (available at: https://www.mdpi.com/journal/applsci/special_issues/dental_adhesives).

For citation purposes, cite each article independently as indicated on the article page online and as indicated below:

LastName, A.A.; LastName, B.B.; LastName, C.C. Article Title. *Journal Name* **Year**, *Volume Number*, Page Range.

ISBN 978-3-0365-4413-7 (Hbk)
ISBN 978-3-0365-4414-4 (PDF)

© 2022 by the authors. Articles in this book are Open Access and distributed under the Creative Commons Attribution (CC BY) license, which allows users to download, copy and build upon published articles, as long as the author and publisher are properly credited, which ensures maximum dissemination and a wider impact of our publications.

The book as a whole is distributed by MDPI under the terms and conditions of the Creative Commons license CC BY-NC-ND.

Contents

About the Editor vii

Mitsuru Motoyoshi
Special Issue on Current Techniques and Materials in Dentistry
Reprinted from: *Appl. Sci.* **2022**, *12*, 4439, doi:10.3390/app12094439 1

**Sorana Maria Bucur, Laszlo Barna Iantovics, Anamaria Bud, Eugen Silviu Bud,
Dorin Ioan Cocoș and Alexandru Vlasa**
Retrospective Study Regarding Orthodontic Retention Complications in Clinical Practice
Reprinted from: *Appl. Sci.* **2022**, *12*, 273, doi:10.3390/app12010273 5

Chie Tachiki, Yasushi Nishii, Masae Yamamoto and Takashi Takaki
Treatment Option Criteria for Open Bite with Receiver Operating Characteristic Analysis—A
Retrospective Study
Reprinted from: *Appl. Sci.* **2021**, *11*, 8736, doi:10.3390/app11188736 21

Shinichi Negishi, Kota Sato and Kazutaka Kasai
The Effects of Chewing Exercises on Masticatory Function after Surgical Orthodontic Treatment
Reprinted from: *Appl. Sci.* **2021**, *11*, 8488, doi:10.3390/app11188488 31

**Yuriko Tezuka, Yasuhiro Namura, Akihisa Utsu, Kiyotaka Wake, Yasuki Uchida,
Mizuki Inaba, Toshiki Takamizawa and Mitsuru Motoyoshi**
Influence of Pre-Etched Area and Functional Monomers on the Enamel Bond Strength of
Orthodontic Adhesive Pastes
Reprinted from: *Appl. Sci.* **2021**, *11*, 8251, doi:10.3390/app11178251 43

Ibrahim Barrak, Gábor Braunitzer, József Piffkó and Emil Segatto
Heat Generation and Temperature Control during Bone Drilling for Orthodontic Mini-Implants:
An In Vitro Study
Reprinted from: *Appl. Sci.* **2021**, *11*, 7689, doi:10.3390/app11167689 53

**Toshiki Takamizawa, Munenori Yokoyama, Keiichi Sai, Sho Shibasaki,
Wayne W. Barkmeier, Mark A. Latta, Akimasa Tsujimoto and Masashi Miyazaki**
Effect of Adhesive Application Method on the Enamel Bond Durability of a Two-Step Adhesive
System Utilizing a Universal Adhesive-Derived Primer
Reprinted from: *Appl. Sci.* **2021**, *11*, 7675, doi:10.3390/app11167675 63

Janine Tiu, Renan Belli and Ulrich Lohbauer
Characterization of Heat-Polymerized Monomer Formulations for Dental Infiltrated Ceramic
Networks
Reprinted from: *Appl. Sci.* **2021**, *11*, 7370, doi:10.3390/app11167370 81

**Alexandru Vlasa, Eugen Silviu Bud, Mariana Păcurar, Luminița Lazăr, Laura Streiche,
Sorana Maria Bucur, Dorin Ioan Cocoș and Anamaria Bud**
Effects of Composite Resin on the Enamel after Debonding: An In Vitro Study—Metal Brackets
vs. Ceramic Brackets
Reprinted from: *Appl. Sci.* **2021**, *11*, 7353, doi:10.3390/app11167353 95

Bálint Nemes, Dorottya Frank, Andreu Puigdollers and Domingo Martín
Occlusal Splint Therapy Followed by Orthodontic Molar Intrusion as an Effective Treatment
Method to Treat Patients with Temporomandibular Disorder: A Retrospective Study
Reprinted from: *Appl. Sci.* **2021**, *11*, 7249, doi:10.3390/app11167249 107

Amit Wolfoviz-Zilberman, Yael Houri-Haddad and Nurit Beyth
A Novel Dental Caries Model Replacing, Refining, and Reducing Animal Sacrifice
Reprinted from: *Appl. Sci.* **2021**, *11*, 7141, doi:10.3390/app11157141 . . . . **119**

Monika Bjelopavlovic, Michael Weyhrauch, Christina Erbe, Franziska Burkard, Katja Petrowski and Karl Martin Lehmann
Influencing Factors on Aesthetics: Highly Controlled Study Based on Eye Movement and the Forensic Aspects in Computer-Based Assessment of Visual Appeal in Upper Front Teeth
Reprinted from: *Appl. Sci.* **2021**, *11*, 6797, doi:10.3390/app11156797 . . . . **133**

Cindy Batisse and Emmanuel Nicolas
Comparison of CAD/CAM and Conventional Denture Base Resins: A Systematic Review
Reprinted from: *Appl. Sci.* **2021**, *11*, 5990, doi:10.3390/app11135990 . . . . **143**

About the Editor

Mitsuru Motoyoshi

Mitsuru Motoyoshi, DDS, PhD, is a research scientist at the Division of Clinical Research of the Nihon University School of Dentistry's Dental Research Center, and a Professor at as well as Chair of the Department of Orthodontics at the Nihon University School of Dentistry. He plays a leading part in clinical education as a director of education management. He received his DDS at the Nihon University School of Dentistry at Matsudo, and his PhD in orthodontics at the Nihon University School of Dentistry (1990). He was an expert advisor of the Pharmaceutical and Medical Devices Agency, an Independent Administrative Corporation in Japan (2014–2016). His research interests relate to biomechanics in the areas of orthodontics and dentofacial orthopedics. His research is widely cited, has received several awards, and has appeared in many leading academic journals, both in the USA and in Europe. He was a member of the committee appointed to consider ethical and medical issues in the Japanese Orthodontic Society, and greatly contributed to the pharmaceutical approval of orthodontic anchor screws in Japan. He is also a clinician with much experience, who has performed placements exceeding thousands cases of orthodontic anchor screws and skeletal anchorage plates. He is engaged in the development of a system of effective orthodontics using the orthodontic anchor screw, supported by the Nihon University Business, Research and Intellectual Property Center.

Editorial

Special Issue on Current Techniques and Materials in Dentistry

Mitsuru Motoyoshi [1,2]

1 Department of Orthodontics, Nihon University School of Dentistry, Tokyo 101-8310, Japan; motoyoshi.mitsuru@nihon-u.ac.jp; Tel.: +81-33219-8000
2 Division of Clinical Research, Dental Research Center, Nihon University School of Dentistry, Tokyo 101-8310, Japan

1. Introduction

In the field of dentistry, the use of regenerative therapy, as well as biocompatible and biomimetic materials, is well-established. Biocompatible and biomimetic materials have advanced, as have methods for maximizing the effectiveness of their applications and the associated technology. The application of polymer compounds, such as composite resins and dentin adhesives, in crown restoration is an extremely interesting topic, along with techniques for implanting jawbones and digital dentistry. Advances therein over time have led to innovations.

2. Innovations in Dental Materials and Technology

Composite resins, which are among the most innovative dental materials, are composed of organic polymers, inorganic fillers, and silane coupling agents [1,2]. Composite resins imitate the tooth structure and require a lot of attention; they form cured products via the polymerization of monomers, and the polymerization reaction affects their properties.

For photo-polymerized resins under ambient temperatures, the double bond conversion is rapid [3]. As the resin turns glassy and vitrifies, mobility is reduced, monomer conversion is hindered, and the reaction rate slows [4,5]. Mobility is reduced to the extent that photo-polymerization always leads to incomplete conversion. For photo-polymerized composites, there are guiding principles to maximize conversion, where insufficient conversion can lead to color instability and material degradation [6–10]. It has been suggested that heat polymerization, as used in polymer-infiltrated ceramic network (PICN) materials, may provide a more consistent source of energy for the reaction, leading to a higher degree of conversion.

The bond between the resin composite and tooth surface has also been subject to many innovations. Functional monomers with hydrophilic groups, which form chemical bonds with the tooth surface, have been used in various resin-based materials, such as self-adhesive resin cements, universal adhesives, self-adhesive flowable restorative materials, and orthodontic adhesive pastes. These adherent materials can simply be applied to the tooth substance. However, they have weaker etching capabilities than previous adhesive systems, leading to concerns about their low elastic modulus and marginal gap formation when used on enamel without any pre-treatment [11,12]. The effect of the application method on adhesiveness is also of concern.

Dental implants are one of the most interesting types of dental materials. For dental implant materials, inorganic materials such as titanium, titanium alloys, alumina oxide-based ceramics, hydroxyapatite and zirconia have been presented along with various applications. PEEK (polyetheretherketone) has recently been reported as a further innovation in polymer implant materials [13], although it has not yet met biomechanical requirements. In orthodontics, mini-implants are crucial to the success of treatment and are used in various clinical situations. Mini-implants, composed of titanium, titanium alloys, or other materials, are implanted into the bone, and the implant success rate is an important clinical endpoint.

Microcracks caused by over-torquing in thick and hard bone [14], and the consequent heat production, may lower the success rate.

Digital technology is also revolutionizing the field of dentistry. Computer-aided design/computer-aided manufacturing (CAD/CAM) techniques are becoming increasingly popular. In the field of prosthodontics, 30 years after the first report on digital removable prostheses, many systems now exist to reduce the number of patient appointments and laboratory time [15–18]. The process of manufacturing complete dentures using computer-assisted technology involves the acquisition of clinical information and designing the prostheses using computer software. Complete dentures can be produced using an additive (3D printing) or subtractive (milling) process. Thus, CAD/CAM techniques for denture fabrication have many clinical and laboratory advantages [19–22].

Treatment planning and diagnosis are also expected to improve greatly with innovations in materials and technology. Although this Special Issue is now closed, innovative and detailed research on dental material technology is expected in the future. We encourage the integration and upgrading of clinical practice applications.

Institutional Review Board Statement: Not applicable.

Informed Consent Statement: Not applicable.

Data Availability Statement: Not applicable.

Acknowledgments: This issue would not have been possible without the contributions of the talented authors and dedicated reviewers. We would like to take this opportunity to express our heartfelt gratitude to all those involved.

Conflicts of Interest: The authors declare no conflict of interest.

References

1. Cramer, N.; Stansbury, J.; Bowman, C. Recent advances and developments in composite dental restorative materials. *J. Dent. Res.* **2010**, *90*, 402–416. [CrossRef] [PubMed]
2. Ferracane, J.L. Resin composite-State of the art. *Dent. Mater.* **2011**, *27*, 29–38. [CrossRef] [PubMed]
3. Stansbury, J.W.; Dickens, S.H. Network formation and compositional drift during photo-initiated copolymerization of dimethacrylate monomers. *Polymer* **2001**, *42*, 6363–6369. [CrossRef]
4. Lovell, L.G.; Berchtold, K.A.; Elliott, J.E.; Lu, H.; Bowman, C.N. Understanding the kinetics and network formation of dimethacrylate dental resins. *Polym. Adv. Technol.* **2001**, *12*, 335–345. [CrossRef]
5. Dickens, S.H.; Stansbury, J.; Choi, K.; Floyd, C. Photopolymerization kinetics of methacrylate dental resins. *Macromolecules* **2003**, *36*, 6043–6053. [CrossRef]
6. Tanaka, K.; Taira, M.; Shintani, H.; Wakasa, K.; Yamaki, M. Residual monomers (TEGDMA and Bis-GMA) of a set visible-light-cured dental composite resin when immersed in water. *J. Oral Rehabil.* **1991**, *18*, 353–362. [CrossRef]
7. Rathbun, M.A.; Craig, R.G.; Hanks, C.T.; Filisko, F.E. Cytotoxicity of a BIS-GMA dental composite before and after leaching in organic solvents. *J. Biomed. Mater. Res.* **1991**, *25*, 443–457. [CrossRef]
8. Mohsen, N.; Craig, R.G.; Hanks, C. Cytotoxicity of urethane dimethacrylate composites before and after aging and leaching. *J. Biomed. Mater. Res.* **1998**, *39*, 252–260. [CrossRef]
9. Söderholm, K.-J.; Mariotti, A. BIS-GMA–based resins in dentistry: Are they safe? *J. Am. Dent. Assoc.* **1999**, *130*, 201–209. [CrossRef]
10. Van Landuyt, K.L.; Nawrot, T.; Geebelen, B.; De Munck, J.; Snauwaert, J.; Yoshihara, K.; Scheers, H.; Godderis, L.; Hoet, P.; Van Meerbeek, B.; et al. How much do resin-based dental materials release? A meta-analytical approach. *Dent. Mater.* **2011**, *27*, 723–747. [CrossRef]
11. Takamizawa, T.; Barkmeier, W.W.; Latta, M.A.; Berry, T.P.; Tsujimoto, A.; Miyazaki, M. Simulated wear of self-adhesive resin cements. *Oper. Dent.* **2016**, *41*, 327–338. [CrossRef] [PubMed]
12. Imai, A.; Takamizawa, T.; Sugimura, R.; Tsujimoto, A.; Ishii, R.; Kawazu, M.; Saito, T.; Miyazaki, M. Interrelation among the handling, mechanical, and wear properties of the newly developed flowable resin composites. *J. Mech. Behav. Biomed. Mater.* **2019**, *89*, 72–80. [CrossRef] [PubMed]
13. Ghazal-Maghras, R.; Vilaplana-Vivo, J.; Camacho-Alonso, F.; Martínez-Beneyto, Y. Properties of polyetheretherketone (PEEK) implant abutments: A systematic review. *J. Clin. Exp. Dent.* **2022**, *14*, e349–e358. [CrossRef]
14. Tachibana, R.; Motoyoshi, M.; Shinohara, A.; Shigeeda, T.; Shimizu, N. Safe placement techniques for self-drilling orthodontic mini-implants. *Int. J. Oral Maxillofac. Surg.* **2012**, *41*, 1439–1444. [CrossRef]
15. Kattadiyil, M.T.; Goodacre, C.J.; Baba, N.Z. CAD/CAM complete dentures: A review of two commercial fabrication systems. *J. Calif. Dent. Assoc.* **2013**, *41*, 407–416.

16. Schwindling, F.S.; Stober, T. A comparison of two digital techniques for the fabrication of complete removable dental prostheses: A pilot clinical study. *J. Prosthet. Dent.* **2016**, *116*, 756–763. [CrossRef] [PubMed]
17. Steinmassl, P.-A.; Klaunzer, F.; Steinmassl, O.; Dumfahrt, H.; Grunert, I. Evaluation of currently available CAD/CAM denture systems. *Int. J. Prosthodont.* **2017**, *30*, 116–122. [CrossRef] [PubMed]
18. Kattadiyil, M.T.; AlHelal, A. An update on computer-engineered complete dentures: A systematic review on clinical outcomes. *J. Prosthet. Dent.* **2017**, *117*, 478–485. [CrossRef]
19. Goodacre, C.J.; Garbacea, A.; Naylor, W.P.; Daher, T.; Marchack, C.B.; Lowry, J. CAD/CAM fabricated complete dentures: Concepts and clinical methods of obtaining required morphological data. *J. Prosthet. Dent.* **2012**, *107*, 34–46. [CrossRef]
20. Bidra, A.S.; Taylor, T.D.; Agar, J.R. Computer-aided technology for fabricating complete dentures: Systematic review of historical background, current status, and future perspectives. *J. Prosthet. Dent.* **2013**, *109*, 361–366. [CrossRef]
21. Infante, L.; Yilmaz, B.; McGlumphy, E.; Finger, I. Fabricating complete dentures with CAD/CAM technology. *J. Prosthet. Dent.* **2014**, *111*, 351–355. [CrossRef] [PubMed]
22. Saponaro, P.C.; Yilmaz, B.; Heshmati, R.H.; McGlumphy, E.A. Clinical performance of CAD-CAM-fabricated complete dentures: A cross-sectional study. *J. Prosthet. Dent.* **2016**, *116*, 431–435. [CrossRef] [PubMed]

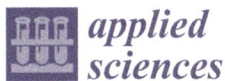

Article

Retrospective Study Regarding Orthodontic Retention Complications in Clinical Practice

Sorana Maria Bucur [1], Laszlo Barna Iantovics [2], Anamaria Bud [3,*], Eugen Silviu Bud [3,*], Dorin Ioan Cocoș [1,*] and Alexandru Vlasa [3]

1. Faculty of Medicine, Dimitrie Cantemir University, 3-5 Bodoni Sandor Str., 540545 Targu Mures, Romania; bucursoranamaria@gmail.com
2. Faculty of Engineering and Information Technology, George Emil Palade University of Medicine, Pharmacy, Science and Technology, 38 Gheorghe Marinescu Str., 540139 Targu Mures, Romania; barna.iantovics@umfst.ro
3. Faculty of Dental Medicine, George Emil Palade University of Medicine, Pharmacy, Science and Technology, 38 Gheorghe Marinescu Str., 540139 Targu Mures, Romania; alexandru.vlasa@umfst.ro
* Correspondence: anamaria.bud@umfst.ro (A.B.); eugen.bud@umfst.ro (E.S.B.); cdorin1123@gmail.com (D.I.C.)

Abstract: At the end of any orthodontic treatment, retention is a necessary phase. Unfortunately, the current retention devices and the lack of proper oral hygiene on the part of patients lead to the accumulation of dental plaque, periodontal inflammation, and gingival retraction. Our retrospective study included 116 adult patients wearing various types of orthodontic retainers. To quantitatively determine the accumulation of dental plaque, we used the Quigley–Hein plaque index modified by Turesky and the Navy plaque index modified by Rustogi. Another studied parameter was related to the gingival recession associated with retention devices. We had investigated the correctness of patients' dental hygiene, their preferences for auxiliary means of oral hygiene, the consistency with which they wear the mobile retainers, and respect the orthodontist's instructions; we also investigated the inconveniences and the accidents that may occur during the retention period. Statistical analysis showed that plaque accumulation is significantly lower in the case of mobile retainer than fixed retainer wearers; the exception was the Hawley plate, where the interdental plaque was more than in all the other studied retainers. Periodontal recessions were more frequent in the case of fixed retainer wearing. Flossing was the most commonly used auxiliary mean for oral hygiene. The compliance of women in wearing vacuum-formed retainers was better than that of men. Patients with a class III history had more plaque accumulation, and class II/1 had the most problems related to detachment/damage of fixed retainers. Mobile retainers proved better results for oral hygiene, but fixed retainers cannot be waved.

Keywords: orthodontic retainer; oral hygiene; gingival recession; patient compliance

1. Introduction

Periodontal disease is one of the oldest pathologies as it occurs in most people examined from the past to the present day, regardless of geographical location and age [1–3]. Periodontitis is an inflammatory condition that starts with the formation of dental plaque at the gingival margin. The microbial load of the dental plaque generates an inflammatory response that initially affects only the gingival margin; in conditions such as individual susceptibility, behavioral factors, or general pathologies, the supporting tissues are affected [4]. The loss of periodontal tissue is closely linked to inflammation and is influenced by infections and interactions between bacterial microorganisms like *Fusobacterium nucleatum*, *Porphyromonas gingivalis*, *Tannerella forsythia*, *Filifactor alocis*, *Treponema denticola*, and *Aggregatibacter actinomycetemcomitans* [4,5]; nowadays, the determining role of the microbial factor and the immune response in the etiology of periodontal disease is supported [3].

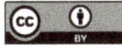

In literature, there are controversial opinions on the effect of orthodontic retainers on the periodontium. Some authors found no significant difference between stainless steel fixed retainers bonded to the anterior teeth and canines only in terms of periodontal outcomes, at 12-month and 3-year follow-ups [6,7]. Periodontal damages caused by mandibular Hawley retainers comparatively with mandibular stainless steel fixed retainers proved no significant difference in a 3-year follow-up [7]. No significant difference in the survival rate of multistrand stainless steel fixed retainers and esthetic retainers made of polyethylene woven ribbon or polyethylene fiber-reinforced resin composite was found [8]. Orthodontic fixed retainers seem to be compatible with periodontal health or at least not related to severe detrimental effects on the periodontium. Other authors [8] found increased plaque accumulation, gingival recession, increase in periodontal pockets' depth, marginal gingival recession, and calculus accumulation in fixed retainers wearers. The adherent microorganisms of the biofilm are different from the free planktonic bacteria because they could not be affected by antibiotics, disinfectants, and the body's defense agents [9]. Other aggressive factors for periodontal tissues are tartar, incorrectly adapted fillings, inadequate prosthetic works, orthodontic braces, rings, and retainers [10–12].

Gingival recession is the movement of the free gingival margin in the apical direction from the enamel-cement junction. The etiology is multifactorial still, periodontal disease and mechanical trauma are causes for gingival recessions. Orthodontic treatment can help develop gingival recession [11]. One possible mechanism is the displacement of the teeth' roots closer or even outside the alveolar cortex, leading finally to bone dehiscence; gingival margin without proper bone support migrates apically, and roots are exposed [8,12]. In addition, a fixed orthodontic appliance creates retentive areas for the bacterial plaque. Inadequate removal of bacterial plaque and gingival inflammation leads to periodontal degradation [11,13].

Mlinek et al. (1973) [14] quantified results came across, as in two types of gingival recession:

- smaller than 3 mm in both shallow and narrow dimensions;
- larger than 3 mm in both deep and wide dimensions.

Retention is an important treatment phase since the periodontal tissues are affected by the modified position of the teeth, and they need time to reorganize and settle after the active treatment [15]. The teeth may be in an unstable position which is vulnerable to the action of the soft tissues. Other reasons for recurrence are the continuous increase and constant change of occlusion ratios throughout a lifetime [16]. For artificial retention are used Hawley retainers (HRs), removable vacuum-formed retainers (VFRs), fixed oral retainers, and various functional orthodontic devices [16–19].

The Hawley retainer designed by Charles Hawley in 1920 (Figure 1) has proven its effectiveness for more than a century. Along with the retention, it can also be an active orthodontic instrument which, through the action of mechanical forces, produces small changes such as the closure of the remaining interdental spaces due to the anchoring by the orthodontic rings [18].

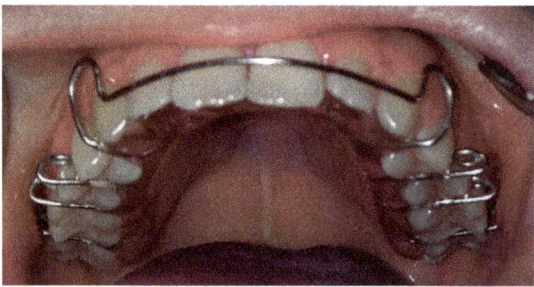

Figure 1. Hawley retainer used in the study.

However, in an attempt to achieve a more aesthetic retention method in 1971 a transparent retainer was designed [20] (Figure 2). Vacuum-formed retainers (VFRs) are easier to make and cheaper than the Hawley retainers (HRs). The VFRs are easy to replace if they deteriorate or fracture. Patients' compliance is much better when wearing VFRs because they do not interfere with the palate and cause vomiting reflex. Their occlusal thickness prevents vertical movements that are possible in the case of HRs [16–20].

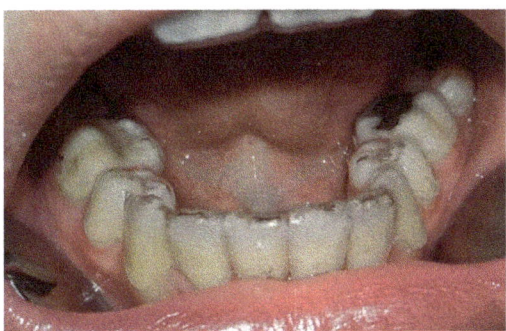

Figure 2. Inferior vacuum-formed retainer used in the study.

Fixed retainers (Figure 3) were introduced into clinical practice in the 1970s to prevent recurrences in the lower inter-canine zone are now commonly used [8,12]. Their advantages are aesthetics, effectiveness, the long-lasting, and the character of being fixed by which their behavior does not depend on the patient's cooperation. The disadvantages are fragility, the vulnerable bonding technique, and the possibility of causing periodontal pathology due to a more difficult oral hygiene [8,12].

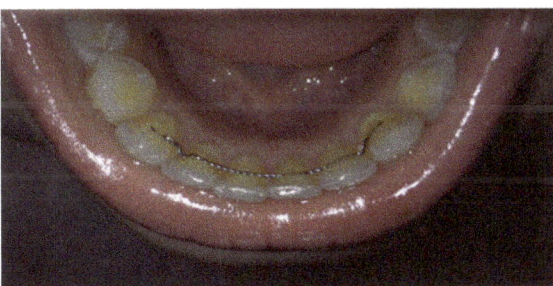

Figure 3. Inferior fixed retainer used in the study.

Our retrospective study aimed to determine and quantify the impact of the most common orthodontic retainers on dental hygiene and periodontal tissues by the following variables:

- the patient's sex;
- Tureski Modified Quigley–Hein Plaque Index (TMQHPI);
- Rustogi Modification of the Navy Plaque Index (RMNPI);
- gingival recession;
- retainer's type
- initial orthodontic diagnosis

The studied hypotheses were:

- orthodontic retainers negatively influence periodontal health;
- patients with fixed retainers face more periodontal problems than those with mobile retainers;

- periodontal pathology of orthodontic retention wearers differs depending on gender;

2. Material and Method

The Rustogi Modification of the Navy Plaque Index (RMNPI) [21] has been proved a very high precision in determining the dental hygiene status because of the detailed examination of the vestibular and oral surfaces of the teeth, divided into nine areas, 18 in total. The score is 0 if the bacterial plaque is not present; if BP exists, the score of the affected area is denoted by 1. The index per tooth = sum of all areas marked with 1. The third molars are not in the calculation. The index value is determined by dividing the sum of the indices calculated for every present tooth by the number of teeth. The value of RMNPI could be between 0 and 1, 0 signifying excellent dental hygiene, and 1 a lack of hygiene.

Turesky Modified Quigley–Hein Plaque Index (TMQHPI) is very sensitive to changes in dental hygiene [22]. To determine this index all the present teeth except the third molars are taken into account. The presence of bacterial plaque is determined by the examination of the vestibular and oral surfaces of the teeth, so the maximum number of investigated surfaces will be 56. The amount of bacterial plaque (BP) will be quantified as follows: 0 = absence of BP; 1 = BP as a discontinuous line at the gingival margin; 2 = BP as a continuous line less than 1 mm width at the cervical level; 3 = continuous BP greater than 1 mm in width but not reaching 1/3 of the surface; 4 = BP covering between 1/3 and 2/3 of the surface; 5 = BP surpassing more than 2/3 of the surface [22]. The average TMQHPI will be the total number of points for each tooth/total number of examined areas Index interpretation: <0–1—excellent hygiene; <1–2—good hygiene; <2–3—moderate hygiene; <3–4—poor hygiene; <4–5—absent hygiene.

We chose to use these two indices in determining the dental plaque because they are easy to evaluate, and their accuracy is high [21,22].

The recessions were determined on all the teeth included in retention systems as the shortest distance from the cementoenamel junction to the deepest curvature of the gingival margin by using a standard periodontal probe.

Our study included a group of 116 patients aged between 18.3 and 27.6 years, with a mean age of 23.8. The patients were from our town, Târgu Mureș, and its surroundings. The inclusion criteria were as follows:

- the absence of gingival recessions before the orthodontic treatment;
- fixed orthodontic appliance placed for at least one year;
- patients who wearing a fixed or mobile restraint device at the time of the examination;
- fixed retentions performed with multistranded wires. The balanced study group consisted of 45 men (38.79% of the total) and 71 women (61.21% of the total). The selected patients were asked to complete an 11-question questionnaire regarding their oral health status (Appendix A). The questionnaire aims to investigate the oral hygiene habits, to collect information about the retention type and the compliance of the patients wearing them. The questionnaire was designed according to our clinical experience and theoretical knowledge.

After the patient filled up the questionnaire, we performed the clinical examination using the dental mirrors, the Williams periodontal probes, and the plaque-revealing tablets. During the clinical examination the following indices were determined:

- the Quigley–Hein plate index modified by Turesky
- the Navy plaque index was modified by Rustogi. For determining the RMNPI we used the following strategy: the gumline areas were divided into subgroups A, B, C, and the interproximal tooth areas were assigned to subgroups D, F.

Based on a comprehensive study of the state-of-the-art power analysis research [23–25] and the supposed data distribution on other similar research (verified after we have already obtained the data) we established 100 as a minimal sample size. Finally, we have performed the study on a sample of 116 in case some data fail to pass the quality assessments (missing data, for instance).

For the verification of the normal distribution of percentages regarding the choice of an appropriate study design [26], we used the Shapiro–Wilk test (SW test) [27]. The selection of the SW test instead of the One-sample Kolmogorov–Smirnov test or the Lilliefors test was because Shapiro–Wilk test has the highest statistical power and works well with few data [28]. Even if it can be applied at different significance levels (e.g., 0.01, 0.1), we chose the significance level α_{sw} = 0.05 considering it the most appropriate. As a good practice, we recommend the SW test together with the visual interpretation of the normality by using the QQ plot. We do not want to overcomplicate the statistics because the paper regards the medical staff, so we do not present the QQ plots [29] associated with the data. For detecting a significant difference between the values (extremely high and extremely low ones), it was applied the two-sided Grubbs outliers detection test [30] with the significance level α_{gr} = 0.5 (considered the most appropriate value for the significance level). The choosing of the Grubbs test was based on the requirement of data normality, being for our data the most appropriate outliers detection test. The Grubbs test can detect a single extreme (low or high value) at one application; if the test detects an extreme value or a value statistically furthest from the rest at the first application, it could be repeated until no extremes are found. The minimal sample size requirement for the application of the test is 3.

The Pearson correlation coefficient [31] was used instead of Spearman Correlation Coefficient that we recommend for the nonparametric cases when the normal assumption fails.

3. Results

According to our analysis (Figure 4), male patients of the study group wore: inferior fixed retainer 39%, superior and inferior VFRs 18%, superior fixed retainer 13%, Hawley retainer 13%, inferior together with superior fixed retainers 9%, inferior fixed retainer together with superior VRF 4%, and only superior VFR 4%. Applying the SW test on data from Figure 4, the p-value = 0.06 was obtained; 0.06 > α_{sw} indicated the passing of the normality assumption. The Grubbs test results indicate 39% as a statistically significantly higher value than the rest. Since the data passed the normality assumption, the mean was chosen as the central tendency indicator. The mean of the values is 14.29%, with a standard deviation (SD) = 12.02 and variance = 144.48.

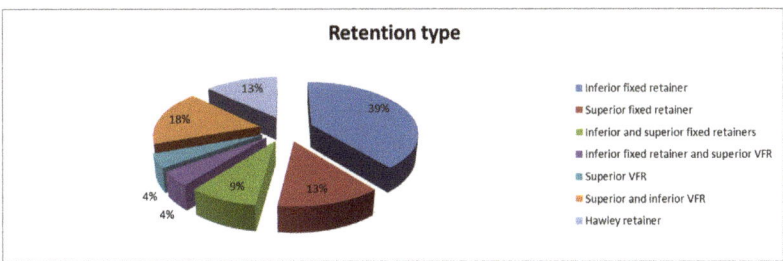

Figure 4. Male patients' distribution according to retention type.

For the study group involving male patients, the fixed lower retainer was present in the highest percentage of 39% while the lowest percentage values of 4% were observed in the upper VFR and in using the lower fixed retainer and the upper VFR together.

83% of male patients have had at least one descaling since retention. 57% of male patients stated that they used dental floss as an auxiliary means for oral hygiene; 30% used interdental brushes; 26% used oral mouthwash; 26% used the water flosser. 9% stated that they did not use any auxiliary method of oral hygiene but only regular toothbrushing.

In this group, 39 patients (87%) felt the need for a scaling procedure during retention time; 77% of them wore fixed retainers, 13% wore VRFs, and 10% were patients with Hawley retainers.

Figure 5 data passed the normality assumption, with SW test *p*-value = 0.74, α_{sw} = 0.05 significance level, where 0.74 > α_{sw}. In the case of the Navy plaque index modified by Rustogi, the male study group, for detecting values that are statistically significantly higher or lower than the rest of the values it was applied the two-sided Grubbs test since the data passed the normality assumption.

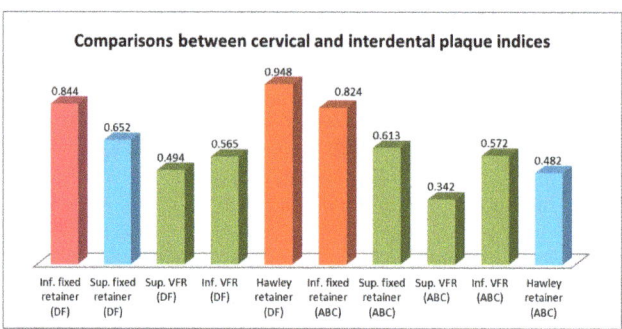

Figure 5. Navy plaque index modified by Rustogi, male study group. DF = interproximal areas ABC = gumline areas.

At the first application of the test, it was not detected any extremely high or low-value just only a value, 0.948 (corresponding to Hawley retainer–DF) that was statistically furthest (higher) from the rest. After removing 0.948, applying the Grubbs test again it was detected 0.342 (Superior VFR–ABC) as a statistically furthest (lower) value from the rest. By consecutive application of the test were detected the following values in the order: 0.844 (Inferior fixed retainer-DF), 0.824 (Inferior fixed retainer-ABC), 0.652 (Superior fixed retainer-DF), 0.613 (Superior fixed retainer-ABC), 0.482 (Hawley retainer-ABC), and finally 0.494 (Superior VFR-DF). Regarding the Navy plaque index modified by Rustogi applied for the male study group, the statistically highest value was obtained when examining patients wearing Hawley retainer (DF). The statistically lowest value was obtained for Superior VFR–ABC.

Figure 6 data passed the normality assumption, with SW test *p*-value = 0.123 (0.123 > α_{sw}; αsw = 0.05). Based on this result it was applied the Grubbs test and the following values were statistically furthest from the rest: 1st application identified 1.244 (Inferior and superior VFR), followed by 1.373 (Superior fixed retainer), 1.422 (Superior VFR), 1.482 (Hawley retainer) and finally 1.881 (Inferior and superior fixed retainers). Regarding the Quigley–Hein plaque index modified by Turesky applied for the male study group, the highest value was obtained when examining patients wearing inferior and superior fixed retainers (it is the highest, but not statistically significantly higher than those others). The statistically lowest value was of Inf. and sup. VFR.

Regarding the gingival recessions (Figure 7) associated with retention devices in the group of male patients, 28 (62.2%) had gingival recessions of 1–3 mm in the lower arch, and 17 (37.7%) of them had recessions of 1–2.5 mm in the upper; 15 patients (33%) had gingival recessions in both dental arches at clinical examination.

According to our analysis, female patients of the study group wore (Figure 8): inferior fixed retainer 35%, superior VFRs 21%, both inferior and superior VFRs 21%, Hawley retainer 7%, superior fixed retainer 6%, both inferior and superior fixed retainers 6%, and only 4% wore inferior fixed retainer together with superior VFR. The SW test with the significance level α_{sw} = 0.05 was applied for the data presented in Figure 8; we get the *p*-value = 0.076, 0.76 > α_{sw} indicated the passing of the normality assumption. The two-sided Grubbs outliers test indicated that no value is extremely high or low, just the value of 35% is furthest from the rest. The calculated mean was 14.29, SD = 11.66, and variance = 136.96.

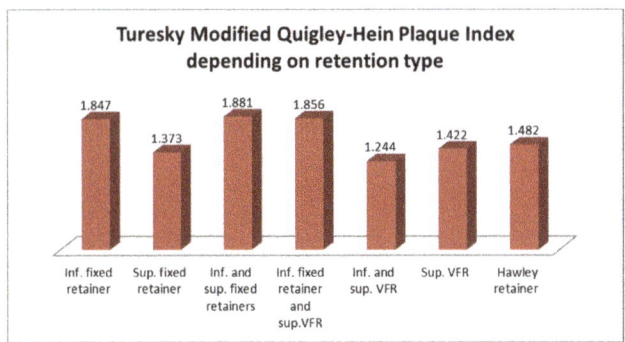

Figure 6. Turesky Modified Quigley–Hein Plaque Index, male study group.

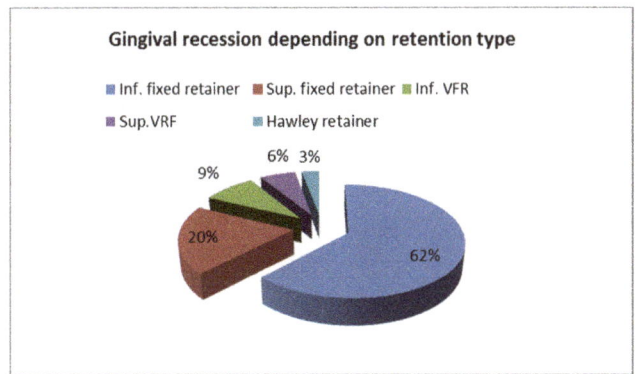

Figure 7. Gingival recession, male group.

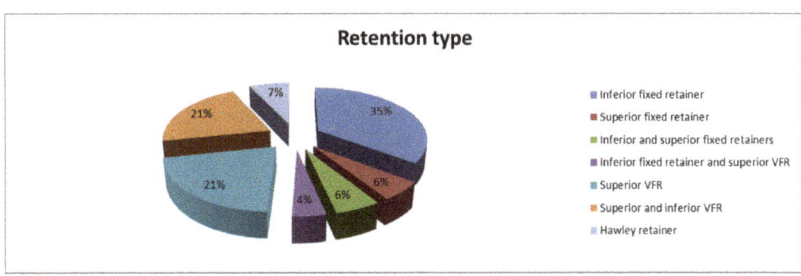

Figure 8. Female patients' distribution according to retention type.

62% of female patients stated that they use dental floss as an auxiliary mean for oral hygiene; 35% used interdental brushes; 28% used an oral mouthwash; 19% used the water flosser. 2% stated that they do not use any auxiliary method of oral hygiene but only regular toothbrushing.

In this study group, 51 patients (72%) needed at least one scaling procedure during retention time; 80% of them wore fixed retainers, 12% wore VRFs, and 8% were patients with Hawley retainers (Figures 9 and 10).

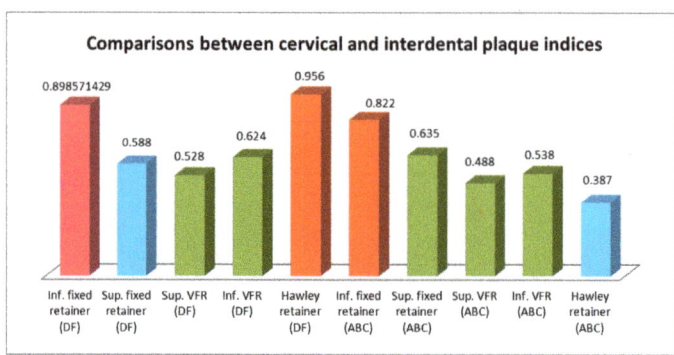

Figure 9. Navy plaque index modified by Rustogi, female study group. DF = interproximal areas ABC = gumline areas.

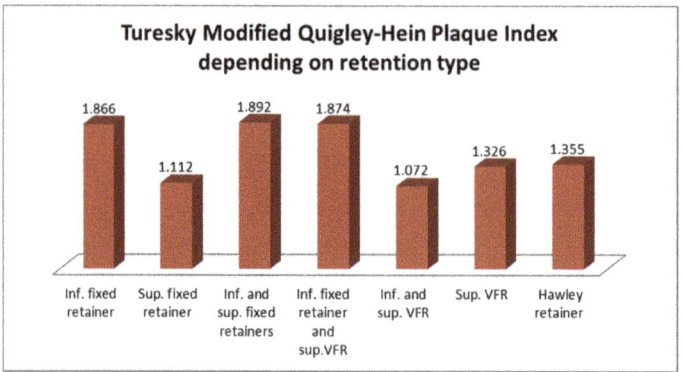

Figure 10. Turesky Modified Quigley-Hein Plaque Index, female study group.

Figure 9 data passed the normality assumption, with SW test p-value = 0.41 (0.41 > α_{sw}; α_{sw} = 0.05). Based on this result it was applied the two-sided Grubbs test with α_{gr} = 0.05 consecutively identifying the following values as statistically furthest from the rest. 1st application identified 0.956 (Hawley retainer-DF), followed by 0.898 (Inferior fixed retainer-DF), 0.822 (Inferior fixed retainer-ABC), 0.387 (Hawley retainer -ABC), 0.488 (Superior VFR-ABC), 0.528 (Superior VFR-DF), and finally 0.588 (Superior fixed retainer -DF). Regarding the Navy plaque index modified by Rustogi applied for the female study group, the statistically highest value was obtained when examining patients wearing Hawley retainer (DF). The statistically lowest value was obtained for the Hawley retainer (ABC).

Figure 10 data passed the normality assumption, with SW test p-value = 0.7 (0.7 > α_{sw}; α_{sw} = 0.05). Based on this result it was applied the two-sided Grubbs test with α_{gr} = 0.05 consecutively identifying the following values as statistically furthest from the rest. 1st application identified 1.072 (Inferior and superior VFR), followed by 1.112 (Superior fixed retainer), 1.326 (Superior VFR), 1.355 (Hawley retainer), and finally 1.892 (Inferior fixed retainer). Regarding the Turesky Modified Quigley-Hein Plaque Index applied for the female study group, the statistically highest value was obtained when examining patients wearing an Inferior fixed retainer. The statistically lowest value was obtained for the Inferior and superior VFR.

Regarding the gingival recessions (Figure 11) associated with retention devices of female patients, 41 (57.7%) had gingival recessions of 1–3 mm in the lower arch, and 21 (29.5%) of them had gingival recessions of 1–2.5 mm in the upper arch; 19 patients (26%) had gingival recessions in both dental arches at clinical examination.

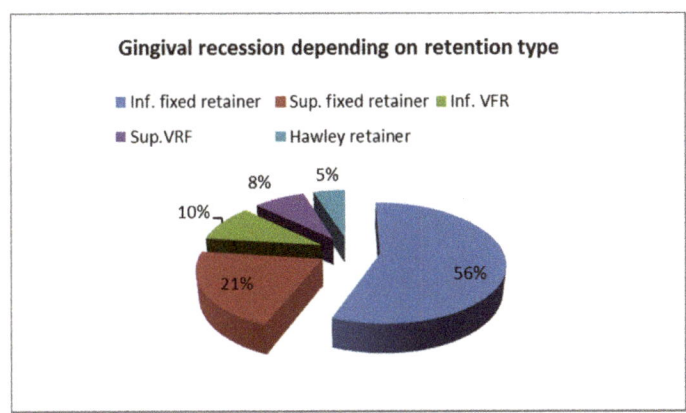

Figure 11. Gingival recession, female group.

The existence of a linear correlation between Figures 5 and 9 data of the RMNPI in male and female study groups was checked. Figure 12 presents the plotted regression line with the 95% confidence interval. Applying the Pearson correlation coefficient we get r = 0.93, with the 95% confidence interval, [0.74, 0.98]. Since r > 0 and 0.74 > 0, it can be concluded that exists a positive correlation; r indicates a very strong correlation (the visual interpretation of Figure 12 leads to the same conclusion). Table 1 illustrates the two indices' values in the male and female groups.

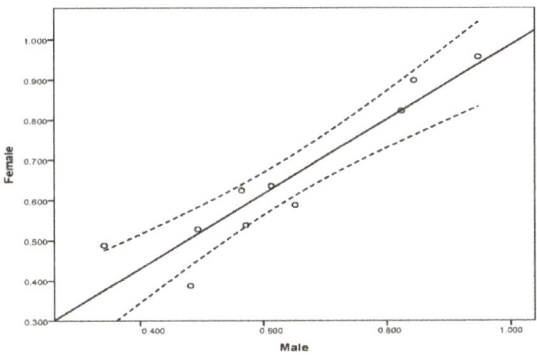

Figure 12. The regression line for male and female study group, applying the Navy plaque index modified by Rustogi.

Table 1. RMNPI and TMQHPI in male and female groups.

RMNPI	IFR(DF)	SFR(DF)	SVFR(DF)	IVFR(DF)	HR(DF)	IFR(ABC)	SFR(ABC)	SVFR(ABC)	IVFR(ABC)	HR(ABC)
Males	0.844	0.652	0.494	0.565	0.948	0.824	0.613	0.342	0.572	0.482
Females	0.898	0.588	0.528	0.624	0.956	0.822	0.635	0.488	0.538	0.387
TMQHPI	IFR	SFR	I&S FR	IFR&SVFR	I&S VFR	SVFR	HR			
Males	1.847	1.373	1.881	1.856	1.244	1.422	1.482			
Females	1.866	1.112	1.892	1.874	1.072	1.326	1.355			

It was analyzed the existence of a linear correlation between Figures 6 and 10 data of the TMQHPI in male and female study groups. Figure 13 presents the plotted regression line with the 95% confidence interval (dotted line). As a next step based on data normality it was decided for the calculus of the Pearson correlation coefficient, r = 0.99, with the 95% confidence interval, [0.94, 0.998]. As r > 0 and 0.94 > 0 it can be concluded that exists a positive correlation. r ∈ [0.9,1] indicates the existence of a very strong correlation (the visual interpretation of Figure 13 lead to the same conclusion).

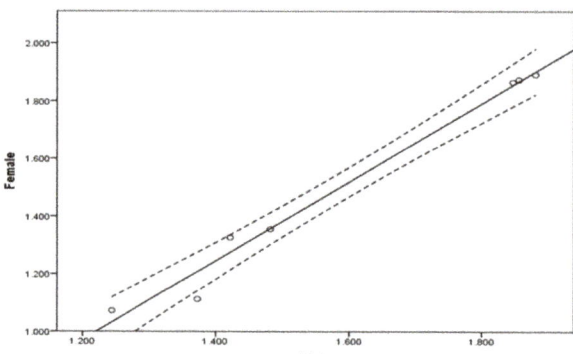

Figure 13. The regression line male and female study group, Turesky Modified Quigley–Hein Plaque Index.

33% of men declare that they wear VFRs every night, 22% once every two nights, 17% once a week, and 28% do not wear them at all; the most common reason men wear them for less time than have been indicated is that they forget (48%). 45% of women said they wear VFRs every night, 18% once every two nights, 15% once a week, and 22% do not wear them at all; the common reasons for wearing less than indicated time are: they forgot (36%), or they did not like how it (them) felt (30%).

The questionnaire's results indicated that most damages/detachments/fractures (75%) occurred in patients with lower retainers, 10% in upper retainers, 10% in VFRs, and only 5% in HRs wearers. Regarding the VFRs wear, 33% of men confess that they wear them every night, 22% once every two nights, 17% once a week, and 28% do not wear them at all; the most common reason men wear them for less time than have been indicated is that they forget (48%). 45% of women say they wear VFRs every night, 18% once every two nights, 15% once a week, and 22% do not wear them at all; the common reasons for wearing less than indicated time are: they forgot (36%), or they did not like how it (them) felt (30%).

Patients with a history of class III have more plaque accumulation (66%), and class II/1 had the most problems related to detachment/damage of fixed retainers (20%)

4. Discussions

In our detailed study, we examined the possible effects of the most commonly used orthodontic retainers on dental hygiene and marginal periodontium. We intended to identify the least harmful way of orthodontic retention for the periodontium. The most important effect of orthodontic retainers is to favor bacterial plaque deposits that maintain a chronic inflammatory periodontal condition which leads to gradual bone loss, gingival retractions, and tooth sensitivity [32,33].

Fixed orthodontic retainers were used for cases that need a long-term and recurrent contention in an arch. They include anterior mandibular or maxillary teeth; the cementation of the retainer on teeth is with modern adhesive techniques. The purposes of fixed retention are to keep the curvature of the frontal arch and maintain the teeth in the new and correct position established by the orthodontic treatment [33].

Our results showed that in the male group, the lower fixed retainers are the most harmful for the periodontium; they favor a massive accumulation of interdental and cervical BP. The value of BP in the cervical area ABC was 0.824 out of 1, the maximum score of RMNPI; the value of BP in the interdental areas DF was even bigger (0.844) and surpassed only by the value for the same tooth zones observed in the case of using the Hawley retainer (0.948). In the same group, the lowest values of cervical and interdental BP were found in upper VFR's wearers (0.342, respectively 0.494). Investigate comparatively the plaque indices in cervical and interdental zones for each retainer type, the biggest difference was in the Hawley retainer wearers; the reason could be that the HRs' wire anchoring system facilitates the BP accumulation at the interdental areas whilst the cervical areas are more accessible for self-cleaning.

In the case of male patients, the subjective need for descaling and professional hygiene was the highest (77%) for those who wore fixed retentions and the lowest (10%) for the Hawley retainer wearers.

For the female group, the highest values of cervical plaque in ABC areas were determined in the case of lower fixed retainer wearers (0.822), and the lowest in the case of Hawley retainer wearers (0.387). The highest values of interdental plaque (DF) were demonstrated, similar with the male group by the Hawley retainer's wearers (0.956) and the lowest by those with upper VFRs (0.488). Superior VFRs cause less cervical and interdental plaque accumulation in both male and female groups.

By statistical means, it was found a very strong correlation between the values of the Navy plaque index modified by Rustogi in male and female study groups.

In the case of the Quigley–Hein plaque index modified by Turesky (TMQHPI) the highest value for the male group was demonstrated by patients wearing inferior and superior fixed retainers (1.881). TMQHPI values are also high when the lower retainer is used as a single element (1.847) or in combination with the upper VFR (1.856). However, TMQHPI values demonstrate the presence of good dental hygiene at the limit. The highest value of TMQHPI in female patients was also found in those with lower fixed retainers (1.866) and combinations of this with the upper retainer (1.892) and upper VFR (1.874). By analyzing the values of this index we can even support the positive effect of VFR in combating dental plaque formation because the lowest values of the averages (1.244 in the male group and 1.072 in the female group) were demonstrated by patients with both lower and upper VFRs.

In the case of female patients, the subjective need for descaling and professional hygiene was the highest (80%) for those who wore fixed retentions and the lowest (8%) for the Hawley retainer wearers.

A very strong correlation was found between the values of the Quigley–Hein plaque index modified by Turesky (TMQHPI) in male and female study groups.

Flossing is the most commonly used auxiliary means for oral hygiene in both male and female groups (57%, respectively 62%), followed by interdental brushes (30%, respectively 35%), mouthwash (26%, respectively 28%), and water flosser (26%, respectively 19%). 9% of the male group and 2% from the female group stated that they did not use any auxiliary method of oral hygiene but only regular tooth brushing.

According to the latest studies, it would be desirable to recommend to our patients with orthodontic retainers the use of electric and sonic toothbrushes [34–36]. The use of both rotating-oscillating heads and sonic action heads powered toothbrushes proved to be better than manual toothbrushes in managing oral hygiene, without causing damages to periodontal structures. It is still difficult to determine which one of these has more efficacity [34]. Better long-term results were in favor of sonic toothbrushes for both the gingival and bleeding indices [34,36]. The possibility of using kinds of toothpaste for home use with hyaluronic acid, vitamins E, lactoferrin, and paraprobiotics may help the hygiene of soft tissues along the edge of the retainers [37].

Levin et al. [38] had also demonstrated that lower retainers increased plaque accumulation, gingival recession, and gingival inflammation gingival revealed by bleeding on probing. Pandis et al. [39] highlighted the negative effects of long-term fixed retention in the lower arch: periodontal irritation, marginal gingival recession, plaque accumulation. Their results were related to the long-term wearing of fixed retainers rather than the bonding materials used [40]. As in our study, Butler and Dowling [41] found large accumulations of dental plaque in interproximal areas that are more difficult to clean. Multistranded wire retainers are bonded to each tooth separately, being effective for the prevention of individual dental rotations caused by the residual tension of the periodontal ligaments that tend to return the teeth to their original position. Their great advantage is the flexibility which allows the physiological movement of the bonded teeth [39].

If the occlusion is not stable at the end of the orthodontic treatment, later changes in the position of the anterior teeth can lead to altered aesthetics of the frontal area that cause dissatisfaction for both doctor and patient. Fixed contention in the anterior frontal arch ensures the stability over time of the results of the active orthodontic treatment [39].

Our study showed that gingival recessions for 62% of male patients and 56% of female patients occur while wearing the lower fixed retainer. A study [42] performed by the "Third National Health, Nutrition Examination Survey" found similar results: men had higher gingival recessions and much more tartar accumulation compared to women, mainly due to a much larger size of their teeth [43]. The lowest values of gingival recessions in both male and female groups were in patients wearing Hawley retainers (3% for males and 5% for women). There are still many studies that contradict the opinion that long-term fixed retainers cause gingival retractions and periodontal damages [6,12,44].

Other issues are related to damage/detachment/fracture in orthodontic retainers. These accidents make the periodontal tissue reorganize to the status before wearing the orthodontic appliance, with harmful effects on periodontium: gingival recessions, bone resorptions, etc. We found that most damages/detachments/fractures (75%) occurred in patients with fixed lower retainers and only 5% in HRs wearers. A similar study showed that these accidents lead to additional costs for the patients; the authors proposed that all the responsibility for retention should be transferred to the patient by applying a mobile retention device, or that the fixed retainers should be removed after a few years [45].

Al-Nimri et al. [6] demonstrated that multistranded wire retainers fractured more frequently than the round wire retainers, even if the difference was not statistically significant ($p = 0.352$). The same authors also concluded that using multistrand wire retainer, the distal surfaces of the lower anterior teeth have more plaque accumulations than using round wire retainers, even if they were more efficient for incisor alignment. The reasons for the failure of fixed retainers are separations between the wire and the bonding material used or between the tooth's enamel and the bonding material [12], the wire's breakage, or the inadvertent tooth movement with fixed lingual retainers [46].

Moshkelgosha et al. [47] demonstrated that polyethylene VFRs are not indicated in clinical situations when greater wear resistance is needed; in such conditions, it is better to use polymethyl-methacrylate-based devices like Hawley retainers that are more resistant to wear and breakage. Their results support the results of our study.

The patient's non-compliance in case of VFRs will also lead to unfavorable consequences for the periodontium, relapse of orthodontic treatments. Only a third of men declare that they wear them every night, and the common reason men wear them lesser is that they forget. Women, on the other hand, seem to have a greater sense of responsibility, almost a half say they wear VFRs every night, and the common reasons for wearing less are they forgot or did not like how it (them) felt.

Pratt et al. [48] found in a comparative study between VRFs and HRs better compliance with VFRs for the first two years after debonding. Compliance with VFRs decreased much faster than with HRs; at any time longer than two years after debonding, the patient's compliance was greater with HRs, and overall compliance was better with Hawley retainers. These results discourage orthodontists who recommend VFRs instead of Hawley retainers. The preference to recommend VRFs for esthetic reasons was not justified because most patients were not concerned about the esthetic aspect of the retainer, or even if so, the perceptions of VFRs and HRs were equal [48].

In another study, Almuqbil and Banabilh found that 15% of patients with VFRs who did not comply reported the loss of the retainers. For those who did not comply with mobile retainers, the majority said it affected their eating (84.3%), speech (56.9%), comfort

(47.1%), and breath odor (43.1%) [49]. The compliance decreased with increasing the time since the fixed orthodontic appliance was de-bonded [49]. The participants were more compliant with HRs than with VFRs. However, VFRs provide better relapse prevention of incisor irregularity than HRs in both arches so, they are more useful in orthodontic practice [50].

The results proved strong correlations between male and female groups regarding the two investigated plaque indices. Another study comparatively investigates the prevalence of dental plaque in adults by using the TMQHPI and Löe–Silness gingivitis index found no significant differences for dental plaque and gingivitis scores irrespective of gender [51]. Our results are different from other findings of a review article published in 2021 that concluded men are more likely to ignore oral health, have poorer oral hygiene habits than women, and have higher rates of periodontal disease [52]. Women demonstrate better oral health behaviors than men. Men and women disproportionately develop periodontal diseases because of biological and gender-related reasons that include immune system factors, hormone differences, and poorer oral hygiene habits of men [52].

According to the initial orthodontic anomaly, those with a history of class III have more plaque accumulation, and class II/1 had the most problems related to detachment/damage of fixed retainers.

Comparing the two types of orthodontic retainers, both mobile and fixed ones have advantages and disadvantages. The great advantage of fixed retainers is that being bonded, the patient wears them; the weak spot is that the accumulation of dental plaque is much more than in mobile retainers. The vacuum-formed retainers used together have the lowest plaque index score of all retention devices, but the main disadvantage is the non-compliance of patients who forget to wear them.

The present study contributes to the increase in reference data in the literature, supporting future research in this field. The limitation of our study is the small number of subjects due to pandemic conditions that restricted the clinic activity because of the high infection rate with the COVID-19 virus.

5. Conclusions

Plaque accumulation was more, and gingival recessions occurred most often in the case of patients wearing fixed inferior retainers. Oral hygiene of the group with fixed orthodontic retainers was compromised, while the hygiene of the group with mobile orthodontic retainers was better. Investigated plaque indices showed a higher score in the case of fixed retainers. Usage of the Hawley plate resulted in the highest accumulation of interdental plaque of all studied retainers. Mobile retainers are superior for maintaining oral hygiene, but the benefits of fixed retainers are not to be ignored.

Flossing was the most commonly used auxiliary means for oral hygiene. Compliance of women in wearing vacuum-formed retainers is better than that of men. Patients with a class III history had more plaque accumulation, and class II/1 had the most problems related to detachment/damage of fixed retainers.

Author Contributions: Conceptualization, S.M.B. and A.V.; methodology, S.M.B., A.B. and E.S.B.; software, L.B.I. and D.I.C.; validation, S.M.B. and A.V.; formal analysis, L.B.I.; investigation, S.M.B., E.S.B. and D.I.C.; resources, A.B.; data curation, L.B.I.; writing—original draft preparation, A.B.; writing—review and editing, E.S.B.; visualization, S.M.B. and L.B.I.; supervision, S.M.B. and A.V. All authors have read and agreed to the published version of the manuscript.

Funding: This research received no external funding.

Institutional Review Board Statement: The study was conducted according to the guidelines of the Declaration of Helsinki and approved by the Ethics Committee of SC Algocalm SRL, Târgu-Mureș, Romania, 899/1 February 2021.

Informed Consent Statement: Informed consent was obtained from all subjects involved in the study.

Data Availability Statement: Data supporting reported results can be found by contacting Anamaria Bud, anamaria.bud@umfst.ro.

Conflicts of Interest: The authors declare that they have no conflict of interest regarding this manuscript.

Appendix A

Name Age Sex

1. What kind of retainer do you have?
    - A. Hawley retainer
    - B. Fixed retainer
    - C. VFR
2. How long have you had the retainer?
3. Have you had any dental scaling while wearing the retainer?
4. If yes, specify the number of scalings performed:
5. What auxiliary means of oral hygiene do you use?
    - A. Dental floss
    - B. Mouthwash
    - C. Water irrigator
    - D. Interdental brushes
6. Have you noticed a greater accumulation of dental plaque after applying the retainer?
    - A. Yes
    - B. No
7. Does the retainer make you brush/clean your teeth more often than you usually do?
    - A. Yes
    - B. No
8. How much time do you spend cleaning, brushing the area where the retainer is applied?
    - A. As much as for the other dental areas
    - B. 1–2 min more because it is a food retention area
9. Have you had problems since you wear your retainer?
    - A. No.
    - B. Yes, the retainer came off my teeth
    - C. Yes, it has deteriorated/fractured
    - D. Yes, it was not effective, the teeth returned partially/totally to the initial position
10. How often do you wear the retainer(s) at night?
    - A. Never: if so, how long have you given up wearing them? ....
    - B. Once a month
    - C. Once a week
    - D. Every night
    - E. Every two nights
    - F. Another answer ....
11. If you do not wear the retainer(s) as often as you have been trained, which is the reason?
    - A. I don't like the way it looks (they look)
    - B. I don't like how it feels (they feel)
    - C. I forgot to wear it/them
    - D. It's (there are) a headache, a waste of time
    - E. I lost it/them
    - F. Retainer(s) no longer fit

G. It affects (they affect) my speech
H. Another answer ....

References

1. Nazir, M.A. Prevalence of periodontal disease, its association with systemic diseases and prevention. *Int. J. Health Sci.* **2017**, *11*, 72–80.
2. Raitapuro-Murray, T.; Molleson, T.I.; Hughes, F.J. The prevalence of periodontal disease in a Romano-British population c. 200–400 AD. *Br. Dent. J.* **2014**, *217*, 459–466. [CrossRef] [PubMed]
3. Locker, D.; Slade, G.D.; Murray, H. Epidemiology of periodontal disease among older adults: A review. *Periodontology* **1998**, *16*, 16–33. [CrossRef] [PubMed]
4. Könönen, E.; Gursoy, M.; Gursoy, U.K. Periodontitis: A Multifaceted Disease of Tooth-Supporting Tissues. *J. Clin. Med.* **2019**, *8*, 1135. [CrossRef] [PubMed]
5. Gibertoni, F.; Sommer, M.E.L.; Esquisatto, M.A.M.; Amaral, M.E.C.D.; Oliveira, C.A.; Andrade, T.A.M.; Mendonça, F.A.S.; Santamaria, M., Jr.; Felonato, M. Evolution of Periodontal Disease: Immune Response and RANK/RANKL/OPG System. *Braz. Dent. J.* **2017**, *28*, 679–687. [CrossRef]
6. Al-Nimri, K.; Al Habashneh, R.; Obeidat, M. Gingival health and relapse tendency: A prospective study of two types of lower fixed retainers. *Aust. Orthod. J.* **2009**, *25*, 142–146.
7. Artun, J.; Spadafora, A.T.; Shapiro, P.A. A 3-year follow-up study of various types of orthodontic canine-to-canine retainers. *Eur. J. Orthod.* **1997**, *19*, 501–509. [CrossRef]
8. Kartal, Y.; Kaya, B. Fixed Orthodontic Retainers: A Review. *Turk. J. Orthod.* **2019**, *32*, 110–114. [CrossRef]
9. Jain, K.; Parida, S.; Mangwani, N.; Dash, H.R.; Das, S. Isolation and characterization of biofilm-forming bacteria and associated extracellular polymeric substances from oral cavity. *Ann. Microbiol.* **2013**, *63*, 1553–1562. [CrossRef]
10. Sirajuddin, S.; Narasappa, K.M.; Gundapaneni, V.; Chungkham, S.; Walikar, A.S. Iatrogenic Damage to Periodontium by Restorative Treatment Procedures: An Overview. *Open Dent. J.* **2015**, *9*, 217–222. [CrossRef]
11. Talic, N.F. Adverse effects of orthodontic treatment: A clinical perspective. *Saudi Dent. J.* **2011**, *23*, 55–59. [CrossRef] [PubMed]
12. Bucur, S.M.; Chiarati, C.R.; Avino, P.; Migliorino, I.; Kartal, Y.; Cocoș, D.I.; Bud, E.S.; Bud, A.; Vlasa, A. Retrospective study regarding the status of the superficial marginal periodontium in adult patients wearing orthodontic retainers. *Rom. J. Oral Rehabil.* **2021**, *13*, 194–201.
13. Hănțoiu, T.; Monea, A.; Lazăr, L.; Hănțoiu, L. Clinical evaluation of periodontal health during orthodontic treatment with fixed appliances. *Acta Med. Marisiensis* **2015**, *60*, 265–268. [CrossRef]
14. Mlinek, A.; Smukler, H.; Buchner, A. The use of free gingival grafts for the coverage of denuded roots. *J. Periodontol.* **1974**, *44*, 248–254. [CrossRef] [PubMed]
15. Riedel, R.A. A review of the retention problem. *Angle Orthod.* **1960**, *30*, 179–199. [CrossRef] [PubMed]
16. Alassiry, A.M. Orthodontic Retainers: A Contemporary Overview. *J. Contemp. Dent. Pract.* **2019**, *20*, 857–862.
17. Mai, W.; He, J.; Meng, H.; Jiang, Y.; Huang, C.; Li, M.; Yuan, K.; Kang, N. Comparison of vacuum-formed and Hawley retainers: A systematic review. *Am. J. Orthod. Dentofac. Orthop.* **2014**, *145*, 720–727. [CrossRef]
18. Sun, J.; Yu, Y.C.; Liu, M.Y.; Chen, L.; Li, H.W.; Zhang, L.; Zhou, Y.; Ao, D.; Tao, R.; Lai, W.L. Survival time comparison between Hawley and clear overlay retainers: A randomized trial. *J. Dent. Res.* **2011**, *90*, 1197–1201. [CrossRef]
19. Kalha, A.S. Hawley or vacuum-formed retainers following orthodontic treatment? *Evid. Based Dent.* **2014**, *15*, 110–111. [CrossRef]
20. Vaida, L.L.; Bud, E.S.; Halitchi, L.G.; Cavalu, S.; Todor, B.I.; Negrutiu, B.M.; Moca, A.E.; Bodog, F.D. The Behavior of Two Types of Upper Removable Retainers-Our Clinical Experience. *Children* **2020**, *7*, 295. [CrossRef]
21. Rustogi, K.N.; Curtis, J.P.; Volpe, A.R.; Kemp, J.H.; McCool, J.J.; Korn, L.R. Refinement of the Modified Navy Plaque Index to increase plaque scoring efficiency in gumline and interproximal tooth areas. *J. Clin. Dent.* **1992**, *3* (Suppl. C), C9–C12. [PubMed]
22. Deinzer, R.; Jahns, S.; Harnacke, D. Establishment of a new marginal plaque index with high sensitivity for changes in oral hygiene. *J. Periodontol.* **2014**, *85*, 1730–1738. [CrossRef] [PubMed]
23. Vasileiou, K.; Barnett, J.; Thorpe, S.; Young, T. Characterizing and justifying sample size sufficiency in interview-based studies: Systematic analysis of qualitative health research over a 15-year period. *BMC Med. Res. Methodol.* **2018**, *18*, 148. [CrossRef] [PubMed]
24. Krejcie, R.V.; Morgan, D.W. Determining Sample Size for Research Activities. *Educ. Psychol. Meas.* **1970**, *30*, 607–610. [CrossRef]
25. Smeden, M.; Moons, K.G.M.; Groot, J.A.H.; Collins, G.S.; Altman, D.G.; Eijkemans, M.J.C.; Reitsma, J.B. Sample size for binary logistic prediction models: Beyond events per variable criteria. *Stat. Methods Med. Res.* **2019**, *28*, 2455–2474. [CrossRef]
26. Iantovics, L.B.; Rotar, C.; Morar, F. Survey on establishing the optimal number of factors in exploratory factor analysis applied to data mining. *Wiley Interdiscip. Rev. Data Min. Knowl. Discov.* **2019**, *9*, e1294. [CrossRef]
27. Shapiro, S.S.; Wilk, M.B. An analysis of variance test for normality (complete samples). *Biometrika* **1965**, *52*, 591–611. [CrossRef]
28. Razali, N.; Wah, Y.B. Power comparisons of Shapiro-Wilk, Kolmogorov-Smirnov, Lilliefors and Anderson-Darling tests. *J. Stat. Model. Anal.* **2011**, *2*, 21–33.
29. Makkonen, L. Bringing closure to the plotting position controversy. *Commun. Stat.–Theory Methods* **2008**, *37*, 460–467. [CrossRef]
30. Barnett, V.; Lewis, T. *Outliers in Statistical Data*, 3rd ed.; Wiley: New York, NY, USA, 1994.
31. Stigler, S.M. Francis Galton's Account of the Invention of Correlation. *Stat. Sci.* **1989**, *4*, 73–79. [CrossRef]

32. Jati, A.S.; Furquim, L.Z.; Consolaro, A. Gingival recession: Its causes and types, and the importance of orthodontic treatment. *Dental Press J. Orthod.* **2016**, *21*, 18–29. [CrossRef]
33. Juloski, J.; Glisic, B.; Vandevska-Radunovic, V. Long-term influence of fixed lingual retainers on the development of gingival recession: A retrospective, longitudinal cohort study. *Angle Orthod.* **2017**, *87*, 658–664. [CrossRef]
34. Preda, C.; Butera, A.; Pelle, S.; Pautasso, E.; Chiesa, A.; Esposito, F.; Oldoini, G.; Scribante, A.; Genovesi, A.M.; Cosola, S. The Efficacy of Powered Oscillating Heads vs. Powered Sonic Action Heads Toothbrushes to Maintain Periodontal and Peri-Implant Health: A Narrative Review. *Int. J. Environ. Res. Public Health* **2021**, *18*, 1468. [CrossRef] [PubMed]
35. Petker, W.; Weik, U.; Margraf-Stiksrud, J.; Deinzer, R. Oral cleanliness in daily users of powered vs. manual toothbrushes—A cross-sectional study. *BMC Oral. Health* **2019**, *19*, 96. [CrossRef] [PubMed]
36. Digel, I.; Kern, I.; Geenen, E.M.; Akimbekov, N. Dental Plaque Removal by Ultrasonic Toothbrushes. *Dent. J.* **2020**, *8*, 28. [CrossRef]
37. Butera, A.; Gallo, S.; Maiorani, C.; Preda, C.; Chiesa, A.; Esposito, F.; Pascadopoli, M.; Scribante, A. Management of Gingival Bleeding in Periodontal Patients with Domiciliary Use of Toothpastes Containing Hyaluronic Acid, Lactoferrin, or Paraprobiotics: A Randomized Controlled Clinical Trial. *Appl. Sci.* **2021**, *11*, 8586. [CrossRef]
38. Levin, L.; Samorodnitzky-Naveh, G.R.; Machtei, E.E. The association of orthodontic treatment and fixed retainers with gingival health. *J. Periodontol.* **2008**, *79*, 2087–2092. [CrossRef]
39. Pandis, N.; Vlahopoulos, K.; Madianos, P.; Eliades, T. Long-term periodontal status of patients with mandibular lingual fixed retention. *Eur. J. Orthod.* **2007**, *29*, 471–476. [CrossRef]
40. Artun, J.; Zachrisson, B. Improving the handling properties of a composite resin for direct bonding. *Am. J. Orthod.* **1982**, *81*, 269–276. [CrossRef]
41. Butler, J.; Dowling, P. Orthodontic bonded retainers. *J. Ir. Dent. Assoc.* **2005**, *51*, 29–32.
42. Albandar, J.M.; Kingman, A. Gingival recession, gingival bleeding, and dental calculus in adults 30 years of age and older in the United States, 1988–1994. *J. Periodontol.* **1999**, *70*, 30–43. [CrossRef]
43. Chu, S.J. Range and mean distribution frequency of individual tooth width of the maxillary anterior dentition. *Pract. Proced. Aesthet. Dent.* **2007**, *19*, 209–215.
44. Booth, F.A.; Edelman, J.M.; Proffit, W.R. Twenty-year follow-up of patients with permanently bonded mandibular canine-to-canine retainers. *Am. J. Orthod. Dentofac. Orthop.* **2008**, *133*, 70–76. [CrossRef]
45. Westerlund, A.; Daxberg, E.L.; Liljegren, A.; Oikonomou, C.; Ransjö, M.; Samuelsson, O.; Sjögren, P. Stability and Side Effects of Orthodontic Retainers—A Systematic Review. *Dentistry* **2014**, *4*, 258. [CrossRef]
46. Shaughnessy, T.G.; Proffit, W.R.; Samara, S.A. Inadvertent tooth movement with fixed lingual retainers. *Am. J. Orthod. Dentofac. Orthop.* **2016**, *149*, 277–286. [CrossRef]
47. Moshkelgosha, V.; Shomali, M.; Momeni, M. Comparison of Wear Resistance of Hawley and Vacuum Formed Retainers: An in-vitro Study. *J. Dent. Biomater.* **2016**, *3*, 248–253.
48. Pratt, M.C.; Kluemper, T.; Lindstrom, A.F. Patient compliance with orthodontic retainers in the postretention phase. *Am. J. Orthod. Dentofac. Orthop.* **2011**, *140*, 196–201. [CrossRef]
49. Almuqbil, S.; Banabilh, S. Postretention phase: Patients' compliance and reasons for noncompliance with removable retainers. *Int. J. Orthod. Rehabil.* **2019**, *10*, 18–22.
50. Outhaisavanh, S.; Liu, Y.; Song, J. The origin and evolution of the Hawley retainer for the effectiveness to maintain tooth position after fixed orthodontic treatment compare to vacuum-formed retainer: A systematic review of RCTs. *Int. Orthod.* **2020**, *18*, 225–236. [CrossRef] [PubMed]
51. Handelman, C.S.; Eltink, A.P.; BeGole, E. Quantitative measures of gingival recession and the influence of gender, race, and attrition. *Prog. Orthod.* **2018**, *19*, 5. [CrossRef] [PubMed]
52. Lipsky, M.S.; Su, S.; Crespo, C.J.; Hung, M. Men and Oral Health: A Review of Sex and Gender Differences. *Am. J. Mens. Health* **2021**, *15*, 15579883211016361. [CrossRef] [PubMed]

Article

Treatment Option Criteria for Open Bite with Receiver Operating Characteristic Analysis—A Retrospective Study

Chie Tachiki [1,*], Yasushi Nishii [1], Masae Yamamoto [2] and Takashi Takaki [3]

1 Department of Orthodontics, Tokyo Dental College, 2-9-18, Kandamisaki-cho, Chiyoda-ku, Tokyo 101-0061, Japan; nishii@tdc.ac.jp
2 Department of Oral Pathobiological Science and Surgery, Tokyo Dental College, 5-11-13, Sugano, Ichikawa-shi, Chiba 272-8513, Japan; yamamotomasae@tdc.ac.jp
3 Department of Oral and Maxillofacial Surgery, Tokyo Dental College, 1-2-2, Mihama-ku, Chiba-shi, Chiba 261-8502, Japan; ttakaki@tdc.ac.jp
* Correspondence: tachikichie@tdc.ac.jp; Tel.: +81-3-6380-9240

Abstract: Temporary anchorage devices (TADs) allow molar intrusion as an additional treatment option to conventional treatment for open bite cases. We investigated the treatment option criteria for open bite treatment. A total of 33 patients with skeletal Class I to Class II open bite who had stable occlusion one year after treatment were enrolled in the study, including 15 patients who had undergone surgical orthodontic treatment, 8 patients who had undergone treatment with molar intrusion, and 10 patients who had undergone treatment with anterior teeth extrusion. Pre-treatment cephalometric analysis of these patients was used for comparison. Furthermore, receiver operating characteristic (ROC) curve analysis was employed to examine the measurement parameters that would be valid as treatment criteria. In the results, FMA showed that patients treated with molar intrusion had a moderately high angle, while those treated with surgical orthodontic treatment had a severe high angle. The area under the curve (AUC) of the ROC curve indicated that FMA is the most appropriate parameter for treatment option criteria. In addition, the cutoff value indicated that the borderline between molar intrusion and surgical orthodontic treatment was 37.5° for FMA. In this study, we suggested criteria for the treatment of open bite with molar intrusion.

Keywords: open bite; molar intrusion; TADs; cephalometric analysis; treatment option criteria; ROC analysis

Citation: Tachiki, C.; Nishii, Y.; Yamamoto, M.; Takaki, T. Treatment Option Criteria for Open Bite with Receiver Operating Characteristic Analysis—A Retrospective Study. *Appl. Sci.* **2021**, *11*, 8736. https://doi.org/10.3390/app11188736

Academic Editor: Mitsuru Motoyoshi

Received: 20 August 2021
Accepted: 16 September 2021
Published: 19 September 2021

Publisher's Note: MDPI stays neutral with regard to jurisdictional claims in published maps and institutional affiliations.

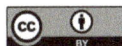

Copyright: © 2021 by the authors. Licensee MDPI, Basel, Switzerland. This article is an open access article distributed under the terms and conditions of the Creative Commons Attribution (CC BY) license (https://creativecommons.org/licenses/by/4.0/).

1. Introduction

Open bite is considered to be one of the most difficult malocclusions in orthodontic treatment; therefore, in open bite cases, decision of treatment method, mechanics, and maintenance have been the topic of focus [1–5]. This is due to the fact that open bite can be associated with many complex problems such as TMD and tongue habits, which make treatment and maintenance difficult. In addition, the approach to open bite varies depending on skeletal type and dental type [6].

Conventionally, skeletal open bite has been corrected by surgically repositioning the maxilla or mandible [7] (Figure 1), and dental open bite by extruding the anterior teeth [8,9] (Figure 2). In recent years, however, the use of temporary anchorage devices (TADs) in orthodontics has changed the treatment of open bite cases—specifically, intruding the molars using TADs to rotate the mandible counterclockwise and improving open bite [10–12] (Figure 3). This treatment method has been reported in many cases and has shown good results and long-term stability [1,13,14]. Therefore, molar intrusion has been established as one of the treatment methods for open bite cases.

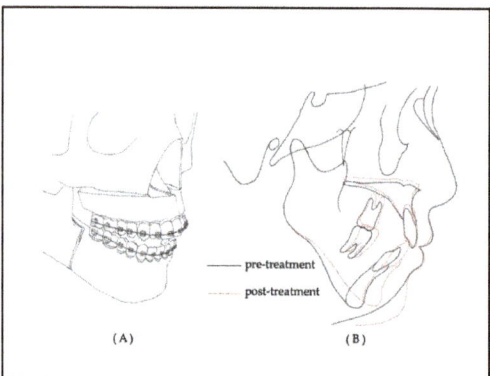

Figure 1. A schema of surgical orthodontic treatment. (**A**) Orthognathic surgery; Le Fort 1 osteotomy and sagittal split ramus osteotomy. (**B**) Superimposition of cephalometric trace changes pre- and post-treatment.

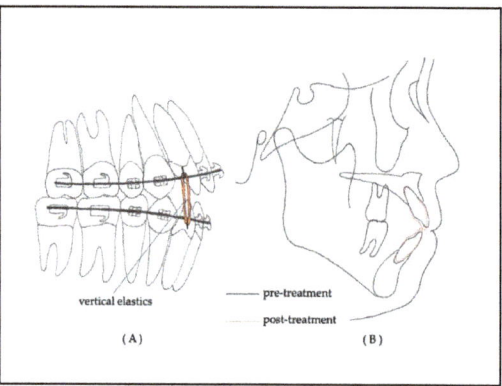

Figure 2. (**A**) A schema of orthodontic treatment of open bite with extruding anterior teeth using a multi-bracket appliance system and vertical elastics. (**B**) Superimposition of cephalometric trace pre- and post-treatment.

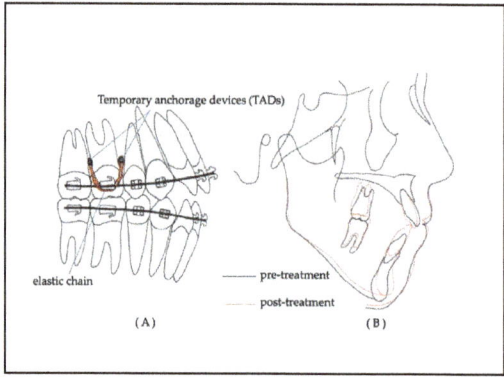

Figure 3. (**A**) A schema of orthodontic treatment of open bite with intruding molars using a multi-bracket appliance system and TADs. (**B**) Superimposition of cephalometric trace changes pre- and post-treatment.

In orthognathic surgery for skeletal open bite, only the mandible is positioned anteriorly and upward to the occlusal plane of the maxillary dentition, or the mandible is positioned anteriorly and upward with counterclockwise rotation by impacting the posterior region of the maxilla [15]. In other words, surgical orthodontic treatment reduces the lower facial height and surgically improves the vertical skeletal discrepancy. Therefore, this new treatment approach involving molar intrusion has been reported as a treatment method for skeletal open bite cases, mainly because it improves open bite by the same mechanism as surgical orthodontic treatment [16].

However, not all cases of skeletal open bite have been treated with molar intrusion, and there have been no reports on the criteria for the use of TADs in molar intrusion. Kamiyama et al. classified the structure of open bite into low position of anterior teeth, high position of molars, and vertical skeletal disharmony [17]. However, the main cephalometric assess points that determine the treatment strategy are unclear, and a comprehensive assessment is required to diagnose and make a decision on the treatment plan. In this study, we will report the treatment strategy for open bite cases by mainly examining the criteria for the indication of molar intrusion treatment as a retrospective study.

2. Materials and Methods

The subjects were 33 patients with open bite who visited the Tokyo Dental College Chiba Dental Center between 2012 and 2018. Criteria were defined to include cases that ended active treatment 1 year before, at which point the patients had overbite change within 1 mm and a positive overbite. The patients used a circumferential-type retainer after treatment. In addition, prior to treatment, ANB was more than $3.0°$, overbite was less than -2 mm, and deviation of menton from the mid-facial line was less than 2 mm as measured by the frontal cephalogram. Exclusion criteria were patients with severe tongue thrust, TMJ symptoms, especially progressive condylar resorption, and congenital abnormality such as craniofacial syndrome, cleft lip palate, and so on. Surgical orthodontic treatment was applied to 15 patients (Group S), and orthodontic treatment was applied to 18 patients, of which 8 cases underwent extrusion of anterior teeth (Group E) and 10 cases underwent intrusion of molars (Group I; Table 1). All cases were diagnosed, treated, and selected by six orthodontic specialists with more than 10 years of experience.

Table 1. Patients' characteristics.

	Surgical Orthodontic Treatment (Group S) $n = 15$	Intrusion of Molars (Group I) $n = 10$	Extrusion of Anterior Teeth (Group E) $n = 8$
sex	Male: 1 Female: 14	Male: 3 Female: 7	Male: 2 Female: 6
Age (average)	29.3 ± 13.8	20.6 ± 7.8	17.4 ± 10.4
Treatment plan			
Extraction case	4	7	5
Non-extraction case	11	3	3
Type of surgery			
SSRO	4		
SSRO + Le Fort 1	11		

SSRO: Sagittal split ramus osteotomy.

Measurements were made using a cephalometric radiograph and dental models of these subjects. Vertical and anterior–posterior measurements of skeletal and denture pattern in the cephalometric analysis were conducted, and overjet and overbite in the dental model analysis were measured. ANB and Wits appraisal were used for cephalometric anterior–posterior evaluation, while FMA, lower facial height, and palatal plane were used for vertical evaluation, which indicates the skeletal type (Figures 4 and 5).

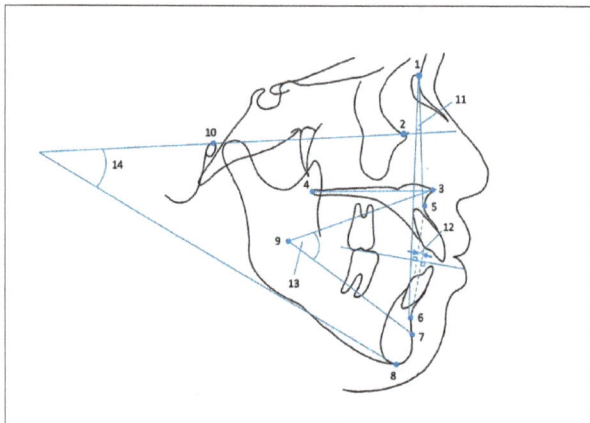

Figure 4. Cephalometric measurements (skeletal pattern). 1: nasion; 2: orbitale; 3: anterior nasal spine (ANS); 4: posterior nasal spine (PNS); 5: point A; 6: point B; 7: PM; 8: menton; 9: xi; 10: porion; 11: ANB angle; 12: Wits appraisal; 13: lower facial height; 14: mandibular plane angle (FMA). Palatal plane angle: the angle between the palatal plane connecting ANS and PNS and the Frankfort plane.

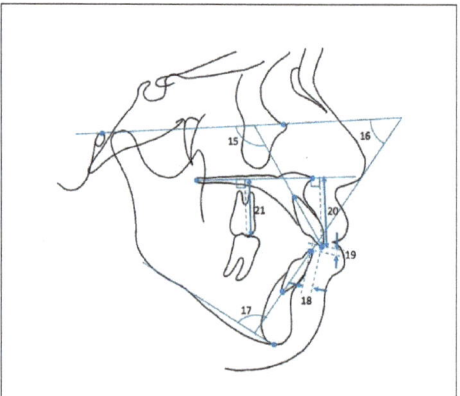

Figure 5. Cephalometric measurements (denture pattern). 15: U1 to FH plane angle (U1 to FH); 16: Frankfort mandibular incisor angle (FMIA); 17: incisor mandibular plane angle (IMPA); 18: overjet; 19: overbite; 20: upper incisor height; 21: upper molar height.

All measurements were taken manually by the same single researcher. Any measurement errors were re-measured by the researcher after a one-week interval. These measurements were compared between the three groups by one-way ANOVA and Tukey's analysis.

The measured items that showed significant difference ($p < 0.05$) among the three groups were selected to perform receiver operating characteristic (ROC) analysis, and the area under the curve (AUC) of the ROC curve was used to determine appropriate cephalometric parameters for the decision of treatment—specifically, deciding between extruding anterior teeth or intruding molars, or between intruding molars or adopting surgical orthodontic treatment. The treatment option criteria were also examined based on the cutoff point, which is the best combination of specificity and sensitivity.

The sample size was calculated using the mean and standard deviation of the pretreatment mandibular plane angle for each group from our preliminary study, which consisted of 20 subjects, with an alpha error of 80% and a beta error of 20%, requiring 7 patients in each group.

3. Results and Discussion

3.1. Comparison of the Mean Value of Pre-Treatment Measurements in the Three Groups

There was a significant difference in FMA between Group S and Group I and between Group S and Group E. Lower facial height also showed a significant difference between Group S and Group E (Table 2). Since the Japanese standard value for FMA is approximately 25° and that for lower facial height is roughly 49° [18], all of these items show extremely large values in Group E and Group I and values slightly larger than the standard in Group E. The larger the values, the longer the skeletal vertical length is, indicating a high-angle case. Furthermore, there were significant differences in upper molar height (UM height) and upper incisor height (UI height) between the groups.

Table 2. Comparison of pre-treatment mean values among the three groups.

	Group S	p-Value (S–I)	Group I	p-Value (I–E)	Group E	p-Value (E–S)
Overjet (mm)	4.5 ± 4.2	NS	3.9 ± 2.5	NS	3.8 ± 2.0	NS
Overbite (mm)	−4.2 ± 1.7	NS	−3.0 ± 1.0	NS	−3.5 ± 0.8	NS
ANB (°)	6.0 ± 1.8	NS	4.8 ± 2.1	NS	3.6 ± 1.4	NS
Wits appraisal (mm)	−1.4 ± 4.1	NS	−2.0 ± 4.7	NS	−4.0 ± 1.3	NS
FMA (°)	42.0 ± 5.0	0.002 **	33.6 ± 4.3	NS	28.5 ± 3.3	0.000 **
Lower facial height (°)	57.4 ± 4.4	NS	53.3 ± 6.7	NS	50.1 ± 2.2	0.023 *
Palatal plane (°)	4.9 ± 3.5	NS	2.9 ± 3.1	NS	3.2 ± 3.8	NS
U1 to FH (°)	114.8 ± 8.0	NS	117.7 ± 6.8	NS	120.2 ± 5.7	NS
FMIA (°)	45.0 ± 8.2	NS	50.1 ± 6.5	NS	46.8 ± 6.8	NS
IMPA (°)	92.7 ± 11.4	NS	92.0 ± 13.4	NS	102.0 ± 8.1	NS
UM height (mm)	28.8 ± 2.4	NS	26.8 ± 2.3	0.009 **	24.5 ± 3.4	0.009 **
UI height (mm)	34.0 ± 4.1	NS	30.8 ± 2.7	NS	29.5 ± 2.8	0.046 *

NS: not significantly different; * $p < 0.05$, ** $p < 0.01$: statistically significant difference.

It has been reported that skeletal open bites are characterized by a downward growth of the mandible with a steep mandibular plane angle and a dentoalveolar development of the maxilla [19,20]. The results of this study agree with this finding and show that those with skeletal vertical problems have a particularly high upper molar height [21]. The results suggest that in cases with severe vertical skeletal problems, surgery is used to reduce posterior elongation, as is molar intrusion. However, it has been reported that the amount of molar intrusion in cases with stable post-treatment is limited to about 2–3 mm [22,23]. Therefore, the treatment of molar intrusion would be applied to moderate skeletal problems.

ANB tended to be larger in Group S and Group I. This suggests that these cases displayed not only anterior–posterior problems but also vertical problems involving mandibular retrusion, i.e., clockwise rotation of the mandible with a steep mandibular plane [24,25]. In such cases, orthognathic surgery can be used to impact the posterior dentition, and molar intrusion can achieve counterclockwise rotation of the mandible [2]. This advances the mandible and improves the aesthetics of the lateral profile.

The overbite, which measures the vertical relationship of the anterior teeth, did not show significant difference among the three groups. This showed that it was not an indicator of whether the case was skeletal or dental and is not very relevant in treatment planning.

3.2. Discrimination of the Optimal Cephalometric Analysis Items to Be Used as Selection Criteria for the Three Treatment Plans

ROC analysis is known to be a useful analysis for comparing diagnostic capabilities. The diagnostic ability is mainly evaluated by the area under the ROC curve, and the further upward and left value on this curve is taken as the cutoff point and used as the diagnostic reference value. It has been widely used in the medical and dental fields and also in orthodontics [26,27].

Based on the results of Table 2, FMA, UM height, and UI height, which have *p*-values less than 0.05 and are appropriate as vertical indicators, were selected using ROC analysis. Table 3 shows that the AUC values of the ROC curves for Group S and Group I are the highest in FMA (Figure 6a). This indicates that FMA has better diagnostic accuracy in determining whether orthognathic surgery or molar intrusion is required. On the other hand, UM height and UI height have low AUC and are less reliable as criteria for open bite treatment (Figure 6b,c). The measurement of tooth height was considered to be biased because of the measurement errors that may occur on the cephalometric film where the left and right sides overlap and also because of individual differences in tooth size and length. In other words, these measurements are not suitable enough as a criterion for the diagnosis of open bite.

Table 3. Results of the ROC curve analysis for Group S and Group I.

Variable	AUC	Cutoff Point	*p*-Value	95% CI	Sensitivity	Specificity
FMA	0.91	37.5	0.00 **	0.78 1.00	0.88	0.80
UM height	0.73	26.5	0.04 *	0.47 0.98	0.50	0.9
UI height	0.72	31.0	0.05	0.48 0.96	0.50	0.80

NS: not significantly different; * $p < 0.05$, ** $p < 0.01$: statistically significant difference.

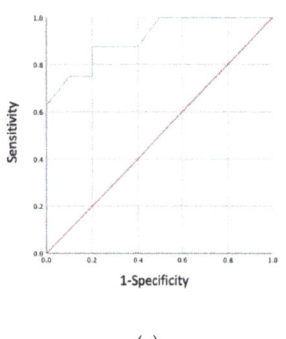
(a)

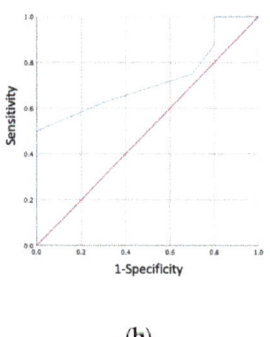
(b)

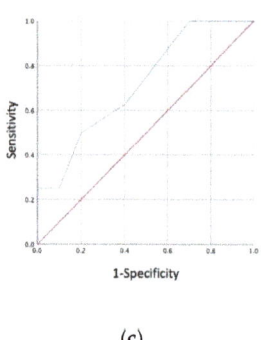
(c)

Figure 6. (a) The ROC curve of FMA measurement (between molar intrusion treatment and surgical orthodontic treatment); (b) the ROC curve of upper molar height measurement (between molar intrusion treatment and surgical orthodontic treatment); (c) the ROC curve of upper incisor height measurement (between molar intrusion treatment and surgical orthodontic treatment).

Table 4 also showed the highest AUC value for FMA (Figure 7a), but the value was lower than that of the results in Table 3. The AUC values for UM height and UI height were low (Figure 7b,c), as shown in Table 3. These results suggest that the borderline between orthognathic surgery and molar intrusion is clearer than the borderline between molar intrusion and anterior tooth extrusion.

Table 4. Results of the ROC curve analysis for Group I and Group E.

Variable	AUC	Cutoff Point	p-Value	95% Cl	Sensitivity	Specificity
FMA	0.87	30.0	0.03 *	0.52 0.92	0.67	0.70
UM height	0.75	25.3	0.04 *	0.47 0.88	0.67	0.75
UI height	0.60	32.0	0.46	0.45 0.90	0.67	0.50

NS: Not significantly different; * $p < 0.05$: statistically significant difference.

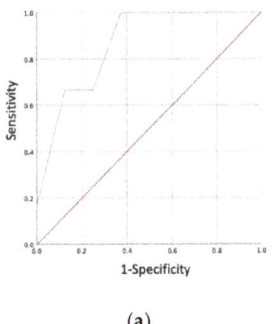
(a)

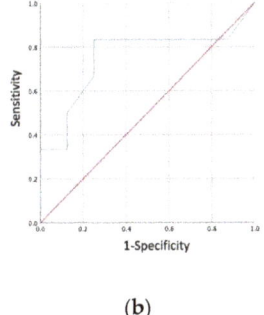
(b)

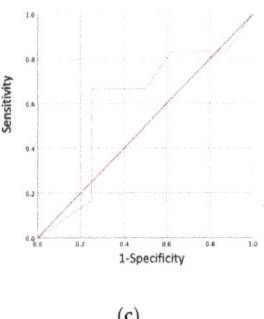
(c)

Figure 7. (a) The ROC curve of FMA measurement (between anterior teeth extrusion and molar intrusion); (b) the ROC curve of upper molar height measurement (between anterior teeth extrusion and molar intrusion); (c) the ROC curve of upper incisor height measurement (between anterior teeth extrusion and molar intrusion).

The cutoff point was determined as the value with the highest sensitivity and specificity. Table 3 shows that the borderline between the indications of orthognathic surgery and molar intrusion in FMA is 37.5°. This value seems to be extremely high, but this is due to the data consisting only of Japanese data. It is reported that the cephalometric norms of Japanese are characterized by mandibular retrusion, labial inclination of mandibular anterior teeth, steep mandibular plane, etc., compared to those of Caucasians, and generally tend to be high-angle facial type [28], explaining why the FMA in this study showed high values. This FMA value is regarded as reliable because it shows high sensitivity and specificity. On the other hand, the FMA showed a cutoff point of 30.0° as the borderline between molar intrusion and anterior tooth extrusion. This value has low sensitivity and specificity and is considered to be less reliable. This is due to molar intrusion being used for skeletal open bite cases as a method to avoid surgery [29], and the borderline between orthognathic surgery and molar intrusion becomes clearer, while the borderline between molar intrusion and anterior teeth extrusion remains unclear.

3.3. Study Limitations

The case selection for this study was from patients with ANB of more than 3°. In other words, we restricted the study to skeletal Class I or II and excluded Class III patients, on the grounds that molar intrusion is unsuitable for skeletal Class III treatment [30]. Patients with normal mandibular body length would present skeletal Class I and II malocclusions, while those with anterior–posterior disharmony display skeletal Class III malocclusion. Thus, the results of this study do not apply to skeletal Class III patients.

In addition, the sample size in this study satisfied the calculation, although it was less than that of similar studies. This may be due to the small sample size of the preliminary study used in the power analysis.

In our treatment, the method of molar intrusion using skeletal anchorage is not standardized—cases vary in having TADs implanted in the buccal alveolar region or palate.

In addition, even with molar intrusion, some percentage of the amount of improvement in overbite may also result in anterior tooth extrusion, which is considered a limitation of this study.

This study consisted of cases with stability one year after active treatment. Baek et al. reported a three-year follow-up in open bite molar intrusion cases. According to their study, 80% of the amount of molar relapse occurred in the first year [1]. Therefore, we set the follow-up period to one year, but a longer follow-up period is desirable as a future research prospect.

4. Conclusions

In this study, we suggested criteria for the treatment of open bite with molar intrusion. However, the diagnosis of open bite requires further careful consideration of treatment selection as there are many factors such as TMD and oral habits, and the diagnostic criteria need to be discussed with regard to long-term stability.

Author Contributions: Conceptualization, C.T. and Y.N.; methodology, Y.N.; validation, Y.N., M.Y.; formal analysis, C.T.; investigation, C.T.; data curation, C.T.; writing—original draft preparation, C.T.; writing—review and editing, Y.N., T.T., and M.Y.; visualization, C.T.; supervision, Y.N.; project administration, Y.N. All authors have read and agreed to the published version of the manuscript.

Funding: This research received no external funding.

Institutional Review Board Statement: This study protocol was approved by the Tokyo Dental College Ethics Committee (Approval No. 944).

Informed Consent Statement: Informed consent was obtained from all subjects involved in the study.

Data Availability Statement: The data presented in this study are available on request from the corresponding author.

Conflicts of Interest: The authors declare no conflict of interest.

References

1. Baek, M.S.; Choi, Y.J.; Yu, H.S.; Lee, K.J.; Kwak, J.; Park, Y.C. Long-Term Stability of Anterior Open-Bite Treatment by Intrusion of Maxillary Posterior Teeth. *Am. J. Orthod. Dentofac. Orthop.* **2010**, *138*, 396.e1–396.e9. [CrossRef]
2. Reichert, I.; Figel, P.; Winchester, L. Orthodontic Treatment of Anterior Open Bite: A Review Article—Is Surgery Always Necessary? *Oral Maxillofac. Surg.* **2014**, *18*, 271–277. [CrossRef]
3. Greenlee, G.M.; Huang, G.J.; Chen, S.S.H.; Chen, J.; Koepsell, T.; Hujoel, P. Stability of Treatment for Anterior Open-Bite Malocclusion: A Meta-Analysis. *Am. J. Orthod. Dentofac. Orthop.* **2011**, *139*, 154–169. [CrossRef]
4. De Freitas, M.R.; Beltrão, R.T.S.; Janson, G.; Henriques, J.F.C.; Cançado, R.H. Long-Term Stability of Anterior Open Bite Extraction Treatment in the Permanent Dentition. *Am. J. Orthod. Dentofac. Orthop.* **2004**, *125*, 78–87. [CrossRef]
5. Kim, Y.H.; Han, U.K.; Lim, D.D.; Serraon, M.L.P. Stability of Anterior Openbite Correction with Multiloop Edgewise Archwire Therapy: A Cephalometric Follow-up Study. *Am. J. Orthod. Dentofac. Orthop.* **2000**, *118*, 43–54. [CrossRef]
6. Jung, S.K.; Kim, T.W. The Relevance Analysis of Hyoid Bone Position to Skeletal or Dental Openbite and Dentofacial Characteristics. *Oral Surg. Oral Med. Oral Pathol. Oral Radiol.* **2015**, *120*, 528–533. [CrossRef]
7. Proffit, W.R.; Bailey, L.J.; Phillips, C.; Turvey, T.A. Long-Term Stability of Surgical Open-Bite Correction by Le Fort I Osteotomy. *Angle Orthod.* **2000**, *70*, 112–117. [CrossRef] [PubMed]
8. Lopez-Gavito, G.; Wallen, T.R.; Little, R.M.; Joondeph, D.R. Anterior Open-Bite Malocclusion: A Longitudinal 10-Year Postretention Evaluation of Orthodontically Treated Patients. *Am. J. Orthod.* **1985**, *87*, 175–186. [CrossRef]
9. Küçükkeleş, N.; Acar, A.; Demirkaya, A.A.; Evrenol, B.; Enacar, A. Cephalometric Evaluation of Open Bite Treatment with NiTi Arch Wires and Anterior Elastics. *Am. J. Orthod. Dentofac. Orthop.* **1999**, *116*, 555–562. [CrossRef]
10. Umemori, M.; Sugawara, J. Skeletal Anchorage System for Open-Bite Correction. *Am. J. Orthod. Dentofac. Orthop.* **1999**, *115*, 166–174.
11. Sherwood, K.H.; Burch, J.G.; Thompson, W.J. Closing Anterior Open Bites by Intruding Molars with Titanium Miniplate Anchorage. *Am. J. Orthod. Dentofac. Orthop.* **2002**, *122*, 593–600. [CrossRef]
12. Erverdi, N.; Keles, A.; Nanda, R. The Use of Skeletal Anchorage in Open Bite Treatment: A Cephalometric Evaluation. *Angle Orthod.* **2004**, *74*, 381–390. [CrossRef] [PubMed]
13. González Espinosa, D.; de Oliveira Moreira, P.E.; da Sousa, A.S.; Flores-Mir, C.; Normando, D. Stability of Anterior Open Bite Treatment with Molar Intrusion Using Skeletal Anchorage: A Systematic Review and Meta-Analysis. *Prog. Orthod.* **2020**, *21*. [CrossRef] [PubMed]

14. Sugawara, J.; Baik, U.B.; Umemori, M.; Takahashi, I.; Nagasaka, H.; Kawamura, H.; Mitani, H. Treatment and Posttreatment Dentoalveolar Changes Following Intrusion of Mandibular Molars with Application of a Skeletal Anchorage System (SAS) for Open Bite Correction. *Int. J. Adult Orthodon. Orthognath. Surg.* **2002**, *17*, 243–253.
15. Hoppenreijs, T.J.M.; Freihofer, H.P.M.; Stoelinga, P.J.W.; Tuinzing, D.B.; Van't Hof, M.A.; Van Der Linden, F.P.G.M.; Nottet, S.J.A.M. Skeletal and Dento-Alveolar Stability of Le Fort I Intrusion Osteotomies and Bimaxillary Osteotomies in Anterior Open Bite Deformities: A Retrospective Three-Centre Study. *Int. J. Oral Maxillofac. Surg.* **1997**, *26*, 161–175. [CrossRef]
16. Kuroda, S.; Sakai, Y.; Tamamura, N.; Deguchi, T.; Takano-Yamamoto, T. Treatment of Severe Anterior Open Bite with Skeletal Anchorage in Adults: Comparison with Orthognathic Surgery Outcomes. *Am. J. Orthod. Dentofac. Orthop.* **2007**, *132*, 599–605. [CrossRef] [PubMed]
17. Kamiyama, T.; Takiguti, H. Roentgeno-Cephalometric Analysis of Open Bite. *J. Jpn. Orthod. Soc.* **1958**, *17*, 31–40.
18. Alcalde, R.E.; Jinno, T.; Pogrel, M.A.; Matsumura, T. Cephalometric Norms in Japanese Adults. *J. Oral Maxillofac. Surg.* **1998**, *56*, 129–134. [CrossRef]
19. Subtelny, J.D.; Sakuda, M. Open-Bite: Diagnosis and Treatment. *Am. J. Orthod.* **1964**, *50*, 337–358. [CrossRef]
20. Nahoum, H.I. Vertical Proportions and the Palatal Plane in Anterior Open-Bite. *Am. J. Orthod.* **1971**, *59*, 273–282. [CrossRef]
21. Kucera, J.; Marek, I.; Tycova, H.; Baccetti, T. Molar Height and Dentoalveolar Compensation in Adult Subjects with Skeletal Open Bite. *Angle Orthod.* **2011**, *81*, 564–569. [CrossRef]
22. Alsafadi, A.S.; Alabdullah, M.M.; Saltaji, H.; Abdo, A.; Youssef, M. Effect of Molar Intrusion with Temporary Anchorage Devices in Patients with Anterior Open Bite: A Systematic Review. *Prog. Orthod.* **2016**, *17*. [CrossRef] [PubMed]
23. Scheffler, N.R.; Proffit, W.R.; Phillips, C. Outcomes and Stability in Patients with Anterior Open Bite and Long Anterior Face Height Treated with Temporary Anchorage Devices and a Maxillary Intrusion Splint. *Am. J. Orthod. Dentofac. Orthop.* **2014**, *146*, 594–602. [CrossRef]
24. Epker, B.N. Surgical-Orthodontic Collection of Openbite Deformity. *Angle Orthod.* **1977**, *71*, 278–299. [CrossRef]
25. Saltaji, H.; Flores-Mir, C.; Major, P.W.; Youssef, M. The Relationship between Vertical Facial Morphology and Overjet in Untreated Class II Subjects. *Angle Orthod.* **2012**, *82*, 432–440. [CrossRef]
26. Han, U.K.; Kim, Y.H. Determination of Class II and Class III Skeletal Patterns: Receiver Operating Characteristic (ROC) Analysis on Various Cephalometric Measurements. *Am. J. Orthod. Dentofac. Orthop.* **1998**, *113*, 538–545. [CrossRef]
27. Wardlaw, D.W.; Smith, R.J.; Hertweck, D.W.; Hildebolt, C.F. Cephalometrics of Anterior Open Bite: A Receiver Operating Characteristic (ROC) Analysis. *Am. J. Orthod. Dentofac. Orthop.* **1992**, *101*, 234–243. [CrossRef]
28. Ioi, H.; Nakata, S.; Nakasima, A.; Counts, A.L. Comparison of Cephalometric Norms between Japanese and Caucasian Adults in Antero-Posterior and Vertical Dimension. *Eur. J. Orthod.* **2007**, *29*, 493–499. [CrossRef]
29. Kuroda, S.; Katayama, A.; Takano-Yamamoto, T. Severe Anterior Open-Bite Case Treated Using Titanium Screw Anchorage. *Angle Orthod.* **2004**, *74*, 558–567. [CrossRef]
30. Akbaydogan, L.C.; Akin, M. Cephalometric Evaluation of Intrusion of Maxillary Posterior Teeth by Miniscrews in the Treatment of Open Bite. *Am. J. Orthod. Dentofac. Orthop.* **2021**, in press. [CrossRef] [PubMed]

Article

The Effects of Chewing Exercises on Masticatory Function after Surgical Orthodontic Treatment

Shinichi Negishi *, Kota Sato and Kazutaka Kasai

Department of Orthodontics, Nihon University School of Dentistry at Matsudo, Matsudo 102-8275, Japan; mako18008@g.nihon-u.ac.jp (K.S.); kasai.kazutaka@nihon-u.ac.jp (K.K.)
* Correspondence: negishi.shinichi@gmail.com; Tel.: +81-47-360-9410

Abstract: Recovery of oral function is one of the most important objectives of orthognathic surgery. This study investigated the effects of a chewing exercise on chewing patterns and other oral functions after sagittal split ramus osteotomy (SSRO). Ten subjects performed a chewing exercise. The control group comprised 19 patients. For masticatory function, the masticatory pattern, width, and height were assessed. For oral function, the occlusal, lip closure, and tongue pressure forces were measured. The chewing exercise was started 3 months after SSRO, and was performed for 5 min twice a day for 3 months. The masticatory pattern normalized in 60% of the patients and remained unchanged for the reversed and crossover types in 40% of the patients. In contrast, 21.0% of patients in the control group showed a change to the normal type. This may be a natural adaptation due to the changes in morphology. A more detailed study is needed to determine what does and does not improve with chewing exercise. The masticatory width significantly increased after performing the exercise. For oral function, a significant increase in the occlusal force was observed, with no significant difference in the control group. Chewing exercises immediately after SSRO improve masticatory patterns.

Keywords: chewing exercise; masticatory function; masticatory pattern

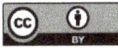

1. Introduction

One of the most important objectives of orthognathic surgery is the recovery of oral function. Numerous investigators have reported on oral function, including masticatory efficiency [1–6], muscle of mastication activity [5,7,8], occlusal force [2,3,9–12], masticatory movement [8,13,14], and occlusal contacts [3,4,10,11,15], following orthognathic surgery. After sagittal split ramus osteotomy (SSRO), the displacement of the proximal bone fragment often causes the condyle to move in the mandibular fossa, affecting the stability of the postoperative orthodontic treatment.

Okada et al. [16] reported that the displacement of bone fragments was compensated by resorption and the addition of the condyle. Furthermore, Kobayashi et al. [4] reported a significant change in masticatory efficiency after orthognathic surgery in patients with skeletal mandibular prognathism. Additionally, the normal chewing pattern showed a change in the condylar position compared with the abnormal chewing pattern. Kubota et al. [17] reported that the masticatory pattern normalizes after surgery for skeletal mandibular prognathism, but the preoperative masticatory movement pattern tends to be retained compared with the control group. This study investigated the effects of a chewing exercise on chewing patterns and other oral functions in patients with skeletal mandibular prognathism after SSRO.

2. Materials and Methods

2.1. Subjects

Eighty-nine patients with skeletal class III, who were not excluded based on the exclusion criteria, were selected from a total of 8625 patients in the clinic. Subsequently, 29 patients fulfilled the inclusion criteria, and 10 of these patients underwent mastication training. Ten subjects performed the chewing exercise after SSRO (4 men, 6 women; mean age, 27 years and 10 months, skeletal class III SSRO with mandibular setback) and were diagnosed with mandibular prognathism by the Department of Orthodontics, Nihon University, School of Dentistry at Matsudo. The control group comprised 19 patients (10 men, 9 women, with a mean age of 31 years and 9 months), who did not perform the masticatory exercise (skeletal class III SSRO with mandibular setback). The exclusion criteria were as follows: (1) dental caries and missing teeth; (2) syndrome, congenital deformity, or previous trauma; and (3) TMJ pain and dysfunction. The inclusion criteria were as follows: (1) asymmetry with a deviation of less than 4.0 mm from the facial midline; (2) fully erupted permanent dentition (without third molar); (3) needing mandibular setback by SSRO; (4) skeletal class III relationship determined by ANB angle; (5) absence of periodontal disease; and (6) no history of trauma (Figure 1).

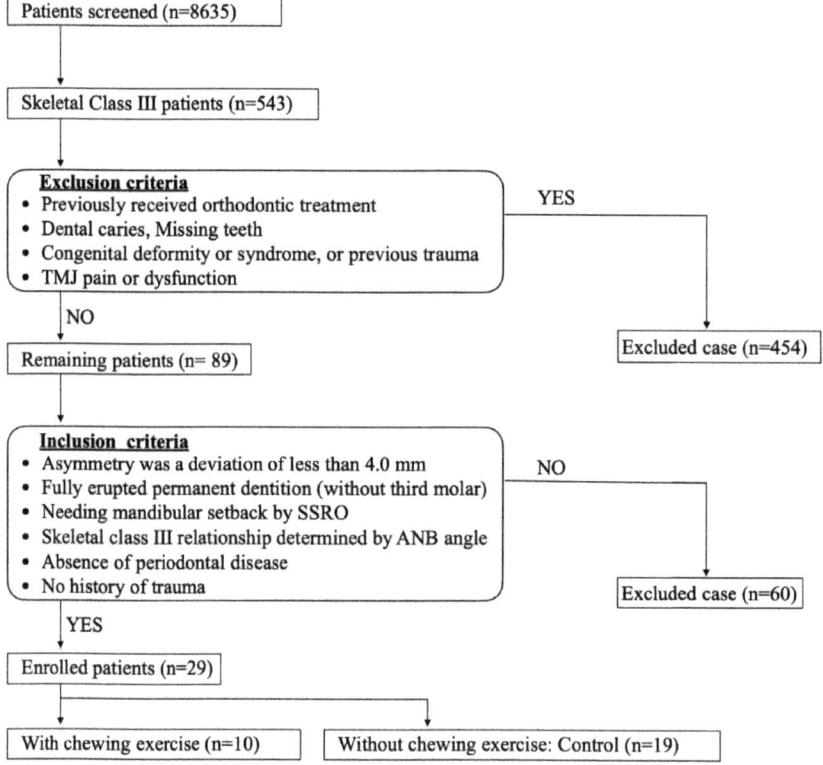

Figure 1. Flowchart of patient enrollment.

All data were taken before SSRO (T1) and 6 months after SSRO (T2). The chewing exercise was started at 3 months after SSRO, which coincides with the timing of bone fragment healing.

This study was approved by the Ethics Committee of Nihon University School of Dentistry at Matsudo (approval no. EC 17-003).

2.2. Methods of Measurement

2.2.1. Cephalometric Analysis

To investigate the maxillofacial morphology of the patients, lateral cephalograms were taken before SSRO (T1) and 6 months after SSRO (T2). Of the ten items measured through cephalometry, two were linear and eight were angular (Figure 2 and Table 1); the setback amount was also measured.

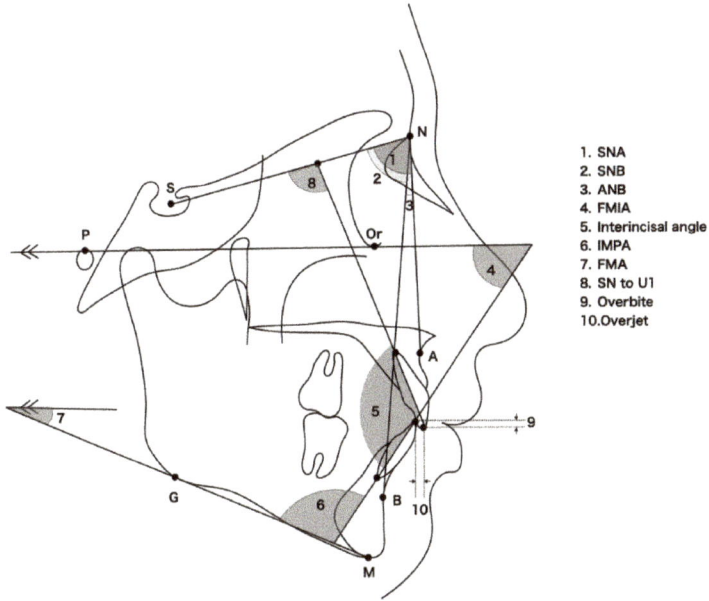

Figure 2. Cephalometric measurements: 1. SNA (degrees), 2. SNB (degrees), 3. ANB (degrees), 4. FMIA (degrees), 5. Interincisal angle (degrees), 6. IMPA (degrees), 7. FMA (degrees), 8. U1—SN (degrees), 9. Overbite (mm), 10. Overjet (mm).

Table 1. Cephalometric measurements.

	Exercise Group (n = 10)				Control Group (n = 19)				Statistical Significance			
	T1		T2		CT1		CT2			p-Value		
	Mean	SD	Mean	SD	Mean	SD	Mean	SD	T1-T2	CT1-CT2	T1-CT1	T2-CT2
Angle measurement												
SNA (°)	82.1	3.5	82.2	3.5	80.4	3.5	81.9	3.1	NS	NS	NS	NS
SNB (°)	83.5	4.3	81.1	4.3	80.7	4.1	78.6	3.0	**	**	NS	NS
ANB (°)	−1.5	3.1	1.1	2.4	−0.2	3.8	3.2	3.0	**	**	NS	NS
FMA (°)	30.1	4.8	30.4	4.8	29.8	4.3	30.2	3.9	NS	NS	NS	NS
FMIA (L1 to FH) (°)	65.8	8.5	67.4	7.4	59.3	9.9	60	6.4	NS	NS	NS	NS
IMPA (L1 to MP) (°)	84.2	5.3	82.3	4.7	90.9	9.1	89.7	7.8	NS	NS	NS	NS
U1 to SN (°)	114.9	8.0	112.7	8.9	111.3	8.6	110.3	8.4	NS	NS	NS	NS
Interincisal angle (°)	123.2	7.7	126.1	6.7	117.2	8.1	118.9	8.5	NS	NS	NS	NS
Liner measurement												
Overjet (mm)	−0.1	4.9	3.1	1.9	−3.2	3.6	2.6	2.6	**	**	NS	NS
Overbite (mm)	0.4	1.5	2.0	1.7	0.8	1.0	2.4	1.3	*	**	NS	NS

NS, non-significant. * $p < 0.05$, ** $p < 0.01$.

2.2.2. Three-Dimensional Computed Tomography (3D CT) Analysis

Three-dimensional CT image reconstruction.

The 3D CT scanning method was performed as reported by Imamura [18], and 3DCT images were used at T1 and T2. The images were produced using an Aquilion 64 CT scanner (Toshiba Medical Systems Tokyo, Japan). The image parameters were tube current, 100 mA; tube voltage, 120 kV; slice thickness, 1 mm; field of view, 240 mm × 240 mm. The patient was scanned from the chin to the glabella. A laser was used to stabilize the position of the patient's head. The vertical axis of the laser was the front view and the transverse axis of the laser was the plane between the tragia and the left side orbit. The occlusion was captured in a centric occlusion position with the lips lightly closed. The CT data were then taken and converted into Digital Imaging and Communications in Medicine (DICOM) format and then into Standard Triangulated Language (STL) format using DICOM software (OsiriX, Newton Graphics, Hokkaido Japan). The data were generated using 3D volume rendering software (Artec Studio 9, Artec 3D, Luxembourg City, Luxembourg). 3DCT image reconstruction was performed after rendering of the cranial and mandibular bones.

Defining the spatial coordinate system (3D CT images).

The standard coordinates of the STL were set using 3D image analysis software (Body-Rugle, Medic Engineering, Kyoto, Japan). On the CT images, the coordinates were determined with reference to the superior border of the right and left external auditory canal poles (Po) and the right inferior orbital border (Or). The Frankfurt horizontal (FH) plane (axial plane) connected the Po and Or on both sides. The Coronal plane was drawn perpendicular to the axial direction through Po on both sides. The sagittal plane was defined as the plane passing through the center of Po from left to right and perpendicular to the axial direction. The X axis was the line defined through the left and right Po. The Y axis was a straight line through the center of the left and right Po and perpendicular to the FH plane. The Z axis (Figure 3) was the line through the origin and perpendicular to the X axis. The left side of the X axis was [+], the top side of the Y axis was [+], and the front side of the Z axis was [+].

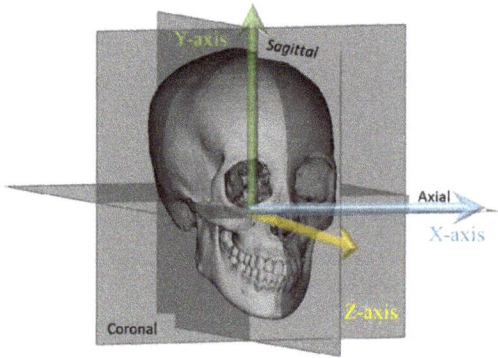

Figure 3. Definition of the coordinate system for the CT image. The X axis was set by the right and left center of porions and orbitales. The Y axis was perpendicular to the X axis and through the right and left porions. The Z axis was perpendicular to the X and Y axes and through the center of the right and left orbitals.

Changes in the position of the proximal bone fragment and condyle.

The method described by Imamura [19] was used. In addition, 3D CT images at T1 and T2 were superimposed to measure changes in the position of the proximal bone fragments and condyle.

To measure changes in the proximal fragment, 3D CT images of the mandible were superimposed by 3D image analysis software (Body-Rugle, Medic Engineering, Kyoto, Japan), using the least squares method. The software calculated the optimal position using an algorithm based on mutual information of each data set, and superimposed T1 and T2. The landmarks of the proximal fragment were the outermost points of the condyle (Lp), the coronoid process (Cp), and the vestibular incision (An), which were set on a coordinate axis. The amount of change in the position was then calculated (Figure 4).

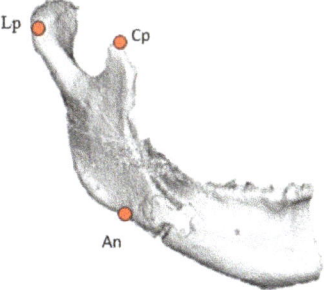

Figure 4. Setting landmarks of proximal bone fragment. Lp: lateral point, Cp: coronoid process, An: antegonial notch.

From the coronal view of the CT image, the midsagittal line (line B) was defined as the line joining the base of the vomer and the midpoint of the clivus of the sphenoid. The axial condylar angle was measured as the angle between Line B and the line crossing Lp-Mp (the most medial point) of the condyle (Figure 5).

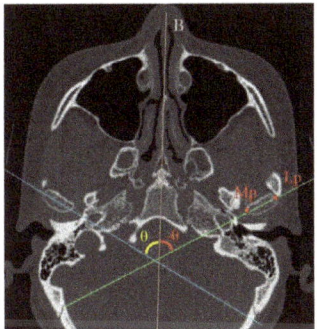

Figure 5. Landmarks, reference line, and angular measurement of condyle on an axial plane.

The median sagittal line (line B) was defined as a line connecting the base of the vomer to the midpoint of the clivus of the sphenoid. The angle crossing the lateral point-medial point of the condyle was measured as the axial condylar angle.

2.2.3. Analysis of Chewing Pattern

The masticatory movements were measured by Gnatho-Hexagraph III (GC Corporation, Tokyo, Japan). The method of measurement was based on the method reported by Suzuki et al. [19]. A mandibular clutch was set on the patient's mandibular anterior incisors. Then, the patient's head was allowed to relax in a sitting position without being fixed. The FH plane was horizontal to the floor of the treatment room, and the headframe and facebow were placed. The reference plane was the bilateral upper edge of the external acoustic meatus. The FH plane was defined as the upper edge of the external auditory meatus and the inferior edge of the left orbit. The measurement points were the mandibular condyle, the mesial buccal cusp of the mandibular first molar, and the contact point of the mandibular central incisor. The patient was instructed to masticate freely with chewing gum. After the gum had softened, the patient was instructed to masticate the gum alternately on one side for 30 s. Masticatory movement was recorded. One piece (1.5 g) of regular chewing gum (100% xylitol chewing gum; Oral Care, Tokyo, Japan) was used for the test. A total of 10 masticatory strokes (strokes 5–14) on the dominant-hand side were analyzed in the masticatory cycle of the mandibular incisor region. The masticatory patterns were analyzed using software attached to a device measuring jaw movements. The masticatory width and height were calculated based on the average of 10 masticatory cycles. The chewing patterns were classified as follows: a normal pattern (from centric occlusion, the mandible moves downward and then laterally toward the chewing side or the non-chewing side, before returning to centric occlusion along a concave, convex, or linear path); a reversed pattern (R pattern; the reverse of normal chewing; the mandible moves laterally first before moving downward and then returning to centric occlusion); or a crossover pattern (C pattern; the mandible moves slightly laterally, downward, and slightly laterally again and then returns to centric occlusion), as shown in Figures 6 and 7.

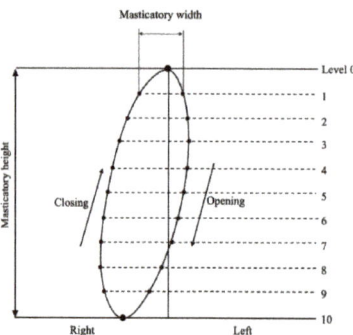

Figure 6. Measurement of the masticatory width and height. With an intercuspal position of 0 and a mean maximum mouth opening position of 10, the opening and closing path distances of the mouth were measured at levels from 1 to 9. The mean value was calculated and used as the masticatory width.

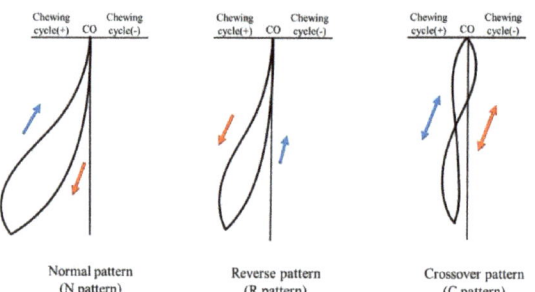

Figure 7. Schematic drawing of a chewing cycle from the frontal view.

A chewing exercise using chewing gum (NOTIME, LOTTE Co. Ltd., Tokyo, Japan) was started 3 months after surgery and was performed for 5 min twice a day for 3 months. The patients recorded the exercise conditions on the check sheets.

2.2.4. Analysis of Oral Function

Occlusal force (OF): An OF meter (GM10, Nagano Keiki Co. Ltd., Tokyo, Japan), as shown in Figure 8, was used to measure the OF. The maximum OFs applied by the left and right first molars were measured twice, and the highest values were recorded for each subject.

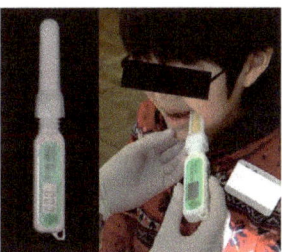

Figure 8. Occlusal force measurement. The occlusal force was measured using GM10 (Nagano Keiki Co. Ltd., Tokyo, Japan). The subjects were seated in the Frankfurt horizontal plane parallel to the floor. The sensor was placed in the maxillary first molar, and the occlusal force was measured.

Lip closure force (LCF) was measured using Lip De Cum LDC-110R® (Cosmo Instruments Co. Ltd., Tokyo, Japan), shown in Figure 9. The analyzer consists of a sensor with a lip adapter and a digital display [20]. The lip closure force analyzer (Lip De Cum®) was set up with a lip holder (Ducklings®) placed on the sensor. The lip closure force was measured while the patient was seated (with the FH plane parallel to the floor plane) and was instructed to close the upper and lower lips with maximum force. The LCF was measured three times, and the highest value was recorded for each subject.

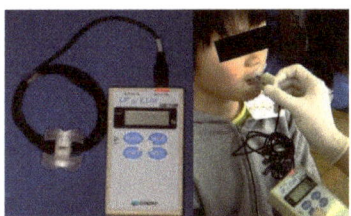

Figure 9. Lip closure force measurement. The lip closure force was measured using a Lip de Cum® LDC-110R (Cosmo Instruments Co. Ltd., Tokyo, Japan). The subjects were seated with the Frankfurt horizontal plane parallel to the floor. Duckling lip holders were placed between the lips and the maximum lip closure force was measured in the intercuspal position.

Tongue pressure force (TPF): The TPF was measured using a TPM-01 (JMS Co. Ltd., Hiroshima, Japan), as shown in Figure 10. For the measurement of TPF, the patient was instructed to hold the cylinder so that the balloon was placed between the tongue and the anterior region of the palate with the lips closed. Then, three times in one-minute intervals, the patient pressed the balloon against the palate for seven seconds. The measurements were made based on previous reports [21]. The reproducibility of these measurements between sessions was checked before this study. The greatest of the three measurements was taken as the TPF for each patient.

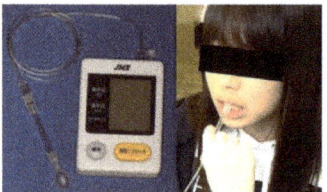

Figure 10. Tongue pressure force measurement. The tongue pressure force was measured using a TPM01 (JMS Co. Ltd., Hiroshima, Japan). The patient sat with the Frankfurt plane parallel to the clinic floor. The balloon was inserted into the mouth, and the patient was instructed to lightly bite down on the hard ring with the upper and lower central incisors, to secure the balloon to the anterior part of the palate.

2.2.5. Statistical Analyses

We performed a sample size calculation using data derived from a preliminary study [22]. On the basis of these results, we calculated the sample size and determined that 10 subjects and 19 controls were required.

To test the intra-inspector reliability, 10 cephalometric films were randomly selected by one person and traced and measured by the inspector twice, two weeks apart [23,24]. The selected cephalometric films were blinded to the patient's name. Each film was then taken and randomized by assigning it to an inspector. Intra-class correlation coefficients (r) were calculated from cephalometric films of T1 and T2 to assess reliability. Confidence intervals of 95% were considered statistically reliable, and the R values calculated for each variable ranged between 0.95 and 1.00. Furthermore, the random error was assessed using the Dahlberg equation, and the measurement error ranged from 0.10 to 0.19. Statistical analyses were performed using the JMP 14 software, SAS for Universities Edition (SAS Institute Inc., Cary, NC, USA). Means and standard deviations were calculated for each cephalometric and oral function value, and are presented in Tables 1 and 2. The Shapiro–Wilk normality test confirmed the normality of the sample distribution in each group (both $p > 0.05$). The Wilcoxon rank-sum test was used to examine the values of T1, T2, and each control group value.

Table 2. Oral function measurements.

	Exercise Group (n = 10)				Control Group (n = 19)				Statistical Significance			
	T1		T2		CT1		CT2		*p*-Value			
	Mean	SD	Mean	SD	Mean	SD	Mean	SD	T1-T2	CT1-C2	T1-C1	T2-C2
Oral function measurements												
Masticatory width (mm)	1.7	0.9	3.0	1.3	1.4	1.0	1.2	0.8	*	NS	NS	**
Masticatory height (mm)	15.2	3.6	15.2	5.1	12	4.9	12.4	4.6	NS	NS	NS	NS
Occlusal force (N)	209.4	98.9	261.5	91.3	204.6	124	222.5	144.8	*	NS	NS	*
Lip closure force (N)	11.4	9.4	8.2	3.0	7.6	3.0	8.5	2.8	NS	NS	NS	NS
Tongue pressure force (Kpa)	27.0	6.2	29.0	5.9	22	13.2	29.6	9.3	NS	NS	NS	NS

NS, non-significant. * $p < 0.05$, ** $p < 0.01$.

3. Results

3.1. Cephalometric Analysis

Analysis of the molar relationship showed bilateral angle class III findings in all patients. The mean preoperative orthodontic treatment period was 2 years and 10 months (control group: 3 years and 3 months), the mean postoperative orthodontic treatment period was 9 months (control group: 8 months), and the mean total orthodontic treatment period was 3 years and 7 months (control group: 3 years and 11 months). Due to the extraction of the maxillary first premolar in the preoperative orthodontic treatment, the patient's molar relationship changed to angle class II after SSRO. The mean amount of mandibular setback by SSRO was 5.8 ± 4.2 (control: 6.2 ± 5.2) mm, with a difference of less than 2 mm between the left and right sides. The mean ANB angle (derived from the maxilla, nasion, and mandible) in the patient group at T2 did not differ significantly from that of the controls at T2 (Table 1).

3.2. Chewing Cycle and Oral Function Analysis

Chewing cycles were assessed for chewing pattern, masticatory width, and masticatory height. The chewing pattern changed to normal in 60.0% of the patients and did not change in 40.0% of the patients. In the control group, 21.0% changed to normal, and 79.0% did not change from reversed or crossover type (Figure 11). Masticatory width significantly increased, with no significant difference in the control group. Although oral function showed a significant increase in OF, there was no significant difference in LCF and TPF, with no significant difference observed in the control group (Table 2).

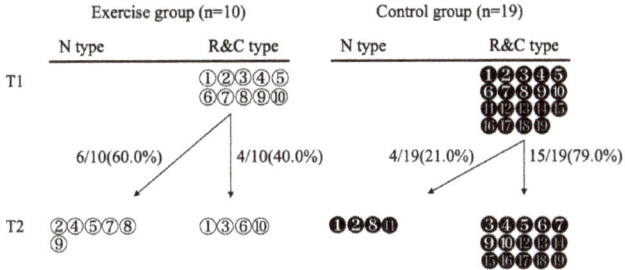

Figure 11. Changes in chewing patterns between T1 and T2.

3.3. Measurement of Changes in Position in the Proximal Bone Fragment and Condyle

The displacement of the proximal bone fragment from T1 to T2 after SSRO is shown in Table 3. The Lp changed by 0.1 externally, superiorly, and anteriorly; Cp changed externally, superiorly by 0.1 mm, and anteriorly by 0.2 mm; and An changed externally by 0.1 mm, superiorly by 0.6 mm, and posteriorly by 0.5 mm. There was no significant difference between the value of each measurement and the control group (Table 3).

Table 3. Comparison between exercise group and control group of proximal bone fragment and axial condylar angle between T1 and T2.

	Exercise Group (n = 10)								Control Group (n = 19)							
	X		Y		Z		θ		X		Y		Z		θ	
	Mean	SD	Mean	SD	Mean	SD	Mean	SD	Mean	SD	Mean	SD	Mean	SD	Mean	SD
Lp (mm)	−0.1	0.4	0.1	0.1	0.1	0.5			−0.2	1.3	0.2	1.0	0.4	0.7		
Cp (mm)	−0.1	0.4	0.1	0.5	0.2	0.6			−0.7	2.3	0.1	2.5	−0.2	0.9		
An (mm)	0.1	0.8	−0.6	3.4	−0.5	2.3			−0.9	2.8	2.4	2.2	−1.9	4.0		
Condylar angle (°)							3.0	1.1							3.0	3.9

Lp: Lateral point Cp: Coronoid process An: Antegonial notch.

4. Discussion

This study evaluated chewing patterns, oral function, and condylar position before and after orthognathic surgery with a chewing exercise in patients with skeletal class III SSRO. SSRO is widely performed for surgical orthodontic treatment of patients with jaw deformities. Imamura [18] reported that changes in the mandible after SSRO included external and superior displacement of the proximal bone fragment within a short timeframe, which induced the external, superior, and internal rotation of the condyle, resulting in bone remodeling from the external to the anterosuperior condyle. Thus, after SSRO, changes in the proximal bone fragments may cause unpredictable reactions in the mandibular position and occlusion.

Several studies have reported that there were no significant differences between the preoperative chewing cycle duration or peak velocity and the corresponding postoperative values [25,26]. However, Okada et al. [16] reported that after and before orthognathic surgery, the chewing pattern changed in approximately 50% of patients from the narrow type (chopping) to the broader (grinding) type, and the condylar position also changed due to condylar resorption. Furthermore, Kubota et al. [17] reported that the chewing pattern changed from chopping to grinding after SSRO. The results of our study's control group are consistent with those reported previously [16,17]. A previous study suggested that chewing exercises after orthognathic surgery improve masticatory efficiency and bite force [27]. Harzer et al. [28] stated that the setback of the mandible by SSRO improves the activity of the masticatory muscles. It was also reported that improved occlusal contact increases bite force [29]. Our previous study in Japan suggested that a chewing exercise for grown-up children facilitates an increase in oral function and changes in chewing patterns [30]. The results of the present study are similar to those of the previous studies of chewing exercises. The masticatory pattern changed to the normal type in 60% of the patients and remained unchanged from the reversed and crossover type in 40% of the patients. Three of the four patients with no change had a crossbite molar occlusion on their first visit. The results suggest that longer or more demanding chewing exercises are needed to change masticatory movements. In contrast, 21.0% of the patients in the control group showed a change to the normal type. This may be a natural adaptation due to the changes in morphology. A more detailed study is needed to determine what does and what does not improve with chewing exercises.

Okada et al. [16] suggested that patients with a broader chewing pattern after SSRO undergo condylar remodeling. This may be a compensation mechanism for the change in the proximal fragment's position caused by SSRO. Based on the present study's results of the chewing exercise compared with the control group, the chewing exercise group showed a change in chewing pattern to the normal type (broader). In this study, the amount of change in the proximal fragment was less than that reported by Okada et al. because the asymmetry case was excluded, but the proximal fragment moved in a distal rotation around the condyle. The amount of movement of the proximal fragment was less than that of the control group without training, suggesting that the chewing exercise may have affected the adaptation of the proximal fragment to the postoperative position. This result suggests that the purpose of chewing exercise is to adapt the chewing pattern to occlusion and jaw position after SSRO. In clinical practice, it is important to provide chewing exercises to patients who do not adapt chewing patterns to occlusion after SSRO. However, our investigation has a limitation: it did not include long-term follow-ups with sufficient subjects. The control group, which did not conduct the chewing exercise, may have been able to adapt their form and function with a longer follow-up period. In the future, longer-term observations will be made to investigate the remodeling of the condyle after improvement with a chewing exercise.

5. Conclusions

- Chewing patterns change to the normal type in 60% of the patients by performing a chewing exercise after SSRO.
- In the control group with no chewing exercise, 21% of the subjects spontaneously changed to the normal type of mastication.
- Chewing exercises can be useful to normalize masticatory movements after SSRO.

Author Contributions: Conceptualization, S.N. and K.K.; methodology, S.N.; software, K.S.; validation, S.N. and K.K.; formal analysis, S.N.; investigation, S.N.; resources, K.S.; data curation, K.S.; writing—original draft preparation, S.N.; writing—review and editing, S.N.; visualization, S.N.; supervision, K.K.; project administration, K.K. All authors have read and agreed to the published version of the manuscript.

Funding: This research received no external funding.

Institutional Review Board Statement: The study was conducted according to the guidelines of the Declaration of Helsinki, and approved by the Ethics Committee of Nihon University School of Dentistry at Matsudo (approval no. EC 17-003).

Informed Consent Statement: Informed consent was obtained from all subjects involved in the study.

Conflicts of Interest: The authors declare no conflict of interest.

References

1. Hidaka, O.; Iwasaki, M.; Saito, M.; Morimoto, T. Influence of Clenching Intensity on Bite Force Balance, Occlusal Contact Area, and Average Bite Pressure. *J. Dent. Res.* **1999**, *78*, 1336–1344. [CrossRef]
2. Braber, W.; Glas, H.; Bilt, A.; Bosman, F. Masticatory function in retrognathic patients, before and after mandibular advancement surgery. *J. Oral Maxillofac. Surg.* **2004**, *62*, 549–554. [CrossRef] [PubMed]
3. Hoon, J.Y.; Kwon, I.J.; Akram, A.A.; Yoojung, S.; Bongju, K.; Soung, M.K. Effects of chewing exerciser on the recovery of masticatory function recovery after orthognathic surgery: A single-center randomized clinical trial, a preliminary study. *Medicina* **2020**, *56*, 483.
4. Kobayashi, T.; Honma, K.; Shingaki, S.; Nakajima, T. Changes in Masticatory Function after Orthognathic Treatment in Patients with Mandibular Prognathism. *Br. J. Oral Maxillofac. Surg.* **2001**, *39*, 260–265. [CrossRef]
5. Raustia, A.M.; Oikarinen, K.S. Changes in Electric Activity of Masseter and Temporal Muscles after Mandibular Sagittal Split Osteotomy. *Int. J. Oral Maxillofac. Surg.* **1994**, *23*, 180–184. [CrossRef]
6. Shinogaya, T.; Bakke, M.; Thomsen, C.E.; Vilmann, A.; Matsumoto, M. Bite Force and Occlusal Load in Healthy Young Subjects—A Methodological Study. *Eur. J. Prosthodont. Restor. Dent.* **2000**, *8*, 11–15.
7. Ingervall, B.; Ridell, A.; Thilander, B. Changes in Activity of the Temporal, Masseter and Lip Muscles after Surgical Correction of Mandibular Prognathism. *Int. J. Oral Surg.* **1979**, *8*, 290–300. [CrossRef]
8. Ueki, K.; Marukawa, K.; Hashiba, Y.; Nakagawa, K.; Degerliyurt, K.; Yamamoto, E. Changes in the duration of the chewing cycle in patients with skeletal class III with and without asymmetry before and after orthognathic surgery. *J. Oral Maxillofac. Surg.* **2009**, *67*, 67–72. [CrossRef]
9. Choi, Y.J.; Lim, H.; Chung, C.J.; Park, K.H.; Kim, K.H. Two-year follow-up of changes in bite force and occlusal contact area after intraoral vertical ramus osteotomy with and without Le Fort I osteotomy. *J. Oral Maxillofac. Surg.* **2014**, *43*, 742–747. [CrossRef]
10. Iwase, M.; Ohashi, M.; Tachibana, H.; Toyoshima, T.; Nagumo, M. Bite Force, Occlusal Contact Area and Masticatory Efficiency before and after Orthognathic Surgical Correction of Mandibular Prognathism. *Int. J. Oral Maxillofac. Surg.* **2006**, *35*, 1102–1107. [CrossRef]
11. Ohkura, K.; Harada, K.; Morishima, S.; Enomoto, S. Changes in Bite Force and Occlusal Contact Area after Orthognathic Surgery for Correction of Mandibular Prognathism. *Oral Surg. Oral Med. Oral Pathol. Oral Radiol. Endod.* **2001**, *91*, 141–145. [CrossRef] [PubMed]
12. Nakata, Y.; Ueda, H.M.; Kato, M.; Tabe, H.; Shikata-Wakisaka, N.; Matsumoto, E. Changes in stomatognathic function induced by orthognathic surgery in patients with mandibular prognathism. *J. Oral Maxillofac. Surg.* **2007**, *65*, 444–451. [CrossRef] [PubMed]
13. Ueki, K.; Marukawa, K.; Hashiba, Y.; Nakagawa, K.; Degerliyurt, K.; Yamamoto, E. Assessment of the relationship between the recovery of maximum mandibular opening and the maxillomandibular fixation period after orthognathic surgery. *J. Oral Maxillofac. Surg.* **2008**, *66*, 486–491. [CrossRef]
14. Farella, M.; Michelotti, A.; Bocchino, T.; Cimino, R.; Laino, A.; Steenks, M.H. Effects of orthognathic surgery for class III malocclusion on signs and symptoms of temporomandibular disorders and on pressure pain thresholds of the jaw muscles. *J. Oral Maxillofac. Surg.* **2007**, *36*, 583–587. [CrossRef]
15. Harada, K.; Watanabe, M.; Ohkura, K.; Enomoto, S. Measure of bite force and occlusal contact area before and after bilateral sagittal split ramus osteotomy of the mandible using a new pressure-sensitive device: A preliminary report. *J. Oral Maxillofac. Surg.* **2000**, *58*, 370–373. [CrossRef]
16. Okada, H.; Suzuki, Y.; Imamura, R.; Ishii, K.; Negishi, S.; Kasai, K. The Relationship between Chewing Patterns and Displacement of the Proximal Bone Fragment and Morphological Changes in Condyle after Sagittal Split Ramus Osteotomy. *J. Oral Sci.* **2020**, *18*, 332–343. [CrossRef]
17. Kubota, T.; Yagi, T.; Tomonari, H.; Ikemori, T.; Miyawaki, S. Influence of Surgical Orthodontic Treatment on Masticatory Function in Skeletal Class III Patients. *J. Oral Rehabil.* **2015**, *42*, 733–741. [CrossRef]
18. Imamura, R. Assessment of the Position and Morphology of the Condylar Head of Mandible after Sagittal Split Rmaus Osteotomy: Apostoperative Comparative Study from 1 to 6 Months. *J. Oral Sci.* **2017**, *14*, 139–151.

19. Suzuki, Y.; Saitoh, K.; Imamura, R.; Ishii, K.; Negishi, S.; Imamura, R.; Yamaguchi, M.; Kasai, K. Relationship between Molar Occlusion and Masticatory Movement in Lateral Deviation of the Mandible. *Am. J. Orthod. Dentofacial Orthop.* **2017**, *151*, 1139–1147. [CrossRef]
20. Ibrahim, F.; Arifin, N.; Rahim, Z.H.A. Effect of Orofacial Myofunctional Exercise Using an Oral Rehabilitation Tool on Labial Closure Strength, Tongue Elevation Strength and Skin and Skin Elasticity. *J. Phys. Ther. Sci.* **2013**, *25*, 11–14. [CrossRef]
21. Hayashi, R.; Tsuga, K.; Hosokawa, R.; Yoshida, M.; Sato, Y.; Akagawa, Y. A Novel Handy Probe for Tongue Pressure Measurement. *Int. J. Prosthodont.* **2002**, *15*, 385–388.
22. Faul, F.; Erdfelder, E.; Buchner, A.; Lang, A.G. Statistical power analyses using G*Power 3.1: Tests for correlation and regression analyses. *Behav. Res. Methods* **2009**, *41*, 1149–1160. [CrossRef]
23. Ko, W.-C.E.; Huang, C.S.; Lo, L.J.; Chen, Y.R. Longitudinal observation of mandibular motion pattern in patients with skeletal Class III malocclusion subsequent to orthognathic surgery. *J. Oral Maxillofac. Surg.* **2012**, *70*, 158–168.
24. Gjørup, H.; Kjaer, I.; Sonnesen, L.; Beck-Nielsen, S.S.; Haubek, D. Morphological Characteristics of Frontal Sinus and Nasal Bone Focusing on Bone Resorption and Apposition in Hypophosphatemic Rickets. *Orthod. Craniofac. Res.* **2013**, *16*, 246–255. [CrossRef] [PubMed]
25. Takeda, H.; Nakamura, Y.; Handa, H.; Ishii, H.; Hamada, Y.; Seto, K. Examination of Masticatory Movement and Rhythm before and after Surgical Orthodontics in Skeletal Class III Patients with Unilateral Posterior Cross-Bite. *J. Oral Maxillofac. Surg.* **2009**, *67*, 1844–1849. [CrossRef]
26. Yashiro, K.; Takada, K. Improvements in Smoothness of Chewing Cycles in Adults with Mandibular Prognathism after Surgery: A Longitudinal Study. *J. Oral Rehabil.* **2013**, *40*, 418–428. [CrossRef] [PubMed]
27. Kato, K.; Kobayashi, T.; Kato, Y.; Takata, Y.; Yoshizawa, M.; Saito, C. Changes in Masticatory Functions after Surgical Orthognathic Treatment in Patients with Jaw Deformities: Efficacy of Masticatory Exercise Using Chewing Gum. *J. Oral Maxillofac. Surg.* **2012**, *24*, 147–151. [CrossRef]
28. Harzer, W.; Worm, M.; Gedrange, T.; Schneider, M.; Wolf, P. Myosin Heavy Chain mRNA Isoforms in Masseter Muscle before and after Orthognathic Surgery. *Oral Surg. Oral Med. Oral Pathol. Oral Radiol. Endod.* **2007**, *104*, 486–490. [CrossRef]
29. Ferrario, V.F.; Serrao, G.; Dellavia, C.; Caruso, E.; Sforza, C. Relationship between the Number of Occlusal Contacts and Masticatory Muscle Activity in Healthy Young Adults. *Cranio* **2002**, *20*, 91–98. [CrossRef]
30. Negishi, S.; Hayashi, R.; Saitoh, K.; Kasai, K. Influence of Masticatory Exercises Using Hard Chewing Gum on Chewing Pattern and First Molar of Mixed Dentition. *Orthod Waves Jpn* **2010**, *69*, 156–162. [CrossRef]

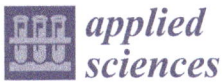

Article

Influence of Pre-Etched Area and Functional Monomers on the Enamel Bond Strength of Orthodontic Adhesive Pastes

Yuriko Tezuka [1], Yasuhiro Namura [1,2,*], Akihisa Utsu [3], Kiyotaka Wake [3], Yasuki Uchida [1,2], Mizuki Inaba [1,2], Toshiki Takamizawa [4,5] and Mitsuru Motoyoshi [1,2]

[1] Department of Orthodontics, Nihon University School of Dentistry, Tokyo 101 8310, Japan; deyu20250@g.nihon-u.ac.jp (Y.T.); uchida.yasuki@nihon-u.ac.jp (Y.U.); inaba.mizuki@nihon-u.ac.jp (M.I.); motoyoshi.mitsuru@nihon-u.ac.jp (M.M.)
[2] Division of Clinical Research, Dental Research Center, Nihon University School of Dentistry, Tokyo 101 8310, Japan
[3] Department of Oral Structural and Functional Biology, Nihon University Graduate School of Dentistry, Tokyo 101 8310, Japan; deak20007@g.nihon-u.ac.jp (A.U.); deki20024@g.nihon-u.ac.jp (K.W.)
[4] Department of Operative Dentistry, Nihon University School of Dentistry, Tokyo 101 8310, Japan; takamizawa.toshiki@nihon-u.ac.jp
[5] Division of Biomaterials Science, Dental Research Center, Nihon University School of Dentistry, Tokyo 101 8310, Japan
* Correspondence: namura.yasuhiro@nihon-u.ac.jp; Tel.: +81-33219-8000

Abstract: This study was performed to investigate the influence of pre-etching area and functional monomers in orthodontic adhesive pastes on enamel bond strength. Bovine enamel was partially pre-etched with phosphoric acid for 30 s over areas with a diameter of 1.0, 2.0 or 3.0 mm, and metal brackets were then bonded with or without functional monomers in the orthodontic adhesive paste. For the baseline groups, the whole adherent area was pre-etched. The shear bond strength (SBS) and adhesive remnant index (ARI) were determined. The adhesive paste/enamel interfaces were observed by scanning electron microscopy (SEM). Although the adhesive paste with functional monomers showed higher SBS than the functional monomer-free adhesive paste in all groups, there were no significant differences in SBS between them regardless of the pre-etched area. The SBS increased with increasing pre-etched area in both orthodontic adhesive pastes. In SEM images of adhesive paste/enamel interfaces, although adhesive with functional monomers showed excellent adaptation, the functional monomer-free adhesive paste showed gap formation at the interface. These findings suggested that the pre-etching area greatly influenced bond strength, regardless of the presence or absence of the functional monomer in the orthodontic adhesive paste.

Keywords: orthodontic adhesive paste; functional monomer; pre-etched area

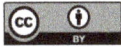

1. Introduction

In recent years, the number of bonding steps has decreased not only for direct resin composite restorations, but also for direct bonding techniques in orthodontic treatment. Simplified bonding procedures are very user-friendly and reduce technique sensitivity [1]. Single-step self-etching adhesive systems combine the functions of etching, priming and bonding into a single bottle [2], which contains acidic functional monomers that simultaneously decalcify and prime the tooth substrate. Functional monomers based on phosphoric or carboxylic acid ester exhibit strong bond strength with enamel and dentin [3]. The chemical bond between hydroxyapatite (HAp) and functional monomers plays an important role in long-lasting bond performance, in conjunction with micromechanical interlocking.

Functional monomers have been utilised in other resin-based materials, such as self-adhesive resin cements, self-adhesive flowable restorative materials and orthodontic adhesive pastes. These materials do not require etching, priming and bonding procedures, as the self-adherent materials can simply be applied to the tooth substrate. However, there are adhesion concerns, due to low elastic modulus and gap formation at marginal regions, about using these materials on enamel without any pre-treatment, because they have weaker etching capabilities than previous adhesive systems [4,5]. Therefore, selective etching is recommended for retention of restorations. In orthodontic treatment using bonding brackets, phosphoric acid pre-etching is the standard bonding procedure. On the other hand, when the pre-etched area extends beyond the area covered with resin bonding agents, there are concerns about the risk of caries, progression of enamel deficiency and staining during and after orthodontic treatment [6].

Bonding orthodontic brackets does not necessarily require extremely strong adhesive, because the brackets are physically removed after treatment. A previous study reported that moderate bond strength (6–8 MPa) may be necessary to maintain orthodontic brackets [7], but a bond strength of 13.7 MPa or more may lead to cracking of the enamel when debonding the brackets [8]. Therefore, pre-etching a limited area of enamel, in combination with the use of an adhesive containing functional monomers, may be helpful to reduce the risk of over-etching while ensuring sufficient retention of brackets. However, little information is available about the enamel bonding effectiveness of such techniques.

This study was performed to investigate the influence of the pre-etched area and functional monomers in orthodontic adhesive pastes on enamel bond strength and the ultrastructure at the adhesive paste/enamel interface. The null hypotheses were as follows: the enamel bond strength of different orthodontic adhesive pastes would not differ according to the presence or absence of functional monomers, and the enamel bond strength would not differ according to the pre-etched area. Therefore, in order to compare their adhesive effects, adhesion strength was examined by shear bond strength test and adhesive state at the enamel–adhesive interface was evaluated by adhesive remnant index, Knoop hardness test and scanning electron microscopy observation.

2. Materials and Methods

2.1. Shear Bond Strength

The samples, consisting of 72 bovine mandibular incisors, were divided into eight groups of nine specimens each. Bovine enamel was employed due to being an acceptable substrate for bonding testing [9]. The enamel was flattened and polished up to #2000-grit with silicon carbide paper. The pre-etching (Transbond XT Etching Gel; 3M Unitek, Monrovia, CA, USA https://www.3m.com/3M/en_US/p/c/dental-orthodontics/ accessed on 16 August 2021; and GC Ortho Etching Gel; GC Ortholy, Tokyo, Japan, https://www.gcortholy.com/ accessed on 16 August 2021, application time; 30 s) was performed in circles of different areas (diameter: 1.0, 2.0 or 3.0 mm). The area was standardised with a hole in a 0.2 mm-thick polypropylene sheet (Figure 1). The pre-etched surface was rinsed and dried for 20 s. A paste (Transbond XT [TB]; 3M Unitek (functional monomer-free), or Universal Bond [UB]; GC Ortholy (containing functional monomer)) was smeared on the bracket and pressed against the pre-etched enamel surface. After removing the excess paste, the mesio-distal portion of the bracket was irradiated with an LED curing unit (Valo; Ultradent Products, South Jordan, UT, USA, https://www.ultradent.com/ accessed on 16 August 2021) for 20 s. After being stored in distilled water (37 °C for 24 h), each specimen was tested in shear mode using a universal testing machine (5567; Instron, Norwood, MA, USA, https://www.instron.com/ accessed on 16 August 2021, experimental environment; 23 ± 1 °C and 50 ± 5% relative humidity) at a crosshead speed of 1 mm/min. Shear bond strength (SBS) was calculated as the peak load at failure divided by the bonded area (12.8 mm^2) of the bracket base. For the baseline groups, the bracket was bonded to a pre-etched enamel surface that was the same size as the bracket base. The SBSs of the baseline groups were measured under the same conditions described above.

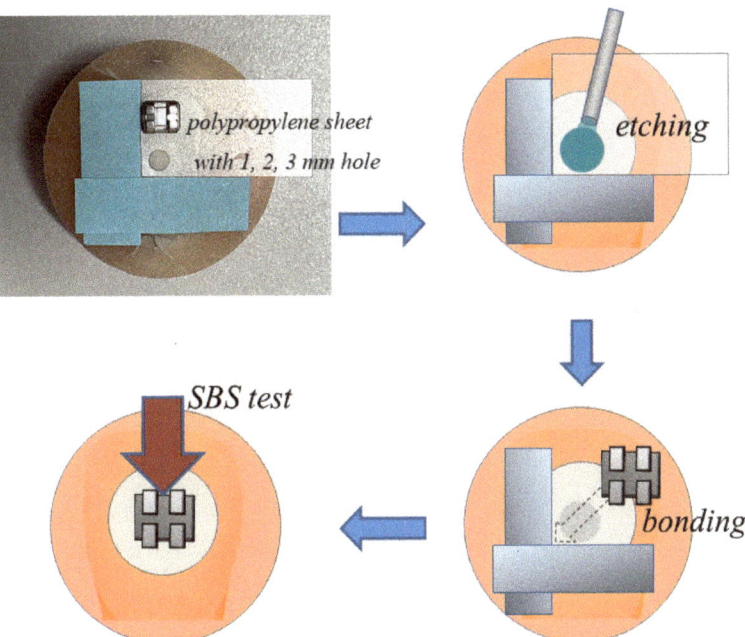

Figure 1. Bonding procedures.

2.2. Adhesive Remnant Index

After the SBS test, the tooth and bracket sides of each debonded specimen were examined under an optical microscope (SZ-3003; As One, Osaka, Japan) at 15× magnification. The residual adhesive on each tooth was assessed based on the adhesive remnant index (ARI) [10].

2.3. Knoop Hardness Numbers of Orthodontic Adhesive Pastes

To define orthodontic adhesive paste thickness, an adhesive tape with a hole (internal diameter, 2 mm; thickness, 100 μm) was attached to transparent matrix tape (Matrix Tape and Dispenser; 3M Oral Care), which was then put on a flat enamel surface. The paste was condensed into the hole of the adhesive tape and a metal bracket was then pressed on the paste. Light irradiation was performed from two different sides for 20 s. The bonded specimens were stored under conditions of 100% humidity at 37 °C for 24 h, prior to measurement of the Knoop hardness number (KHN) at the centre of the adhesive paste bonded to the bracket (from the indentation), following application of a load (98.7 mN) with a microhardness tester (HMV-2; Shimadzu, Kyoto, Japan, https://www.shimadzu.com/ accessed on 16 August 2021, application time; 15 s). Ten specimens were prepared for each adhesive paste and the mean values were calculated.

2.4. Scanning Electron Microscopy

The cross section of the bonded brackets was observed using scanning electron microscopy (SEM) (ERA-8800FE; Elionix Ltd., Tokyo, Japan, https://www.elionix.co.jp/ accessed on 16 August 2021) to determine the ultrastructure of the adhesive paste/enamel interfaces. Bonded specimens were fabricated as described for the SBS test and stored in distilled water at 37 °C for 24 h, before being embedded in epoxy resin (Epon 812; Nisshin EM, Tokyo, Japan) and sectioned longitudinally. All specimens were examined under the operating condition of a voltage of 10 kV.

2.5. Statistical Analysis

Statistical power analysis indicated the need for seven specimens for SBS tests. Descriptive statistics were calculated using a statistical analysis software (SPSS Inc., Chicago, IL, USA). Kolmogorov–Smirnov and Leven tests were performed to assess normality and homogeneity of variance. Analysis of variance followed by the Games–Howell post hoc test was used for statistical comparison of SBS values [11]. For comparison of ARI between the pre-etching areas and the adhesives, the Chi-squared test with Yates' correction was performed [12]. Student's t test was conducted for comparison of KHN.

3. Results

3.1. SBS

The SBSs of TB and UB are presented in Table 1. For the baseline groups, the mean SBS of TB was 12.3 MPa and that of UB was 13.3 MPa. For the 1 mm- and 2 mm-diameter pre-etched groups, the mean SBSs of TB were 2.7 and 3.5 MPa, and those of UB were 2.9 and 5.2 MPa, respectively. For the 3 mm-diameter pre-etched groups, the mean SBS of TB was 6.7 MPa, whereas that of UB was 10.0 MPa. The 1 and 2 mm groups with both adhesives, and the 3 mm group with TB, indicated significantly lower SBS values than the baseline groups. On the other hand, there was no significant difference in SBS between the 3 mm group and baseline group with UB. When comparing different materials with the same pre-etched area, UB showed higher SBS values than TB.

Table 1. Shear bond strength by pre-etched area.

	Pre-Etching Area (mm^2)	Proportion of Bonding Area Pre-etched	TB		UB	
			Mean ± SD (MPa)	Group *	Mean ± SD (MPa)	Group *
1 mm	0.8	0.06	2.7 ± 1.3	a	2.9 ± 1.1	a
2 mm	3.1	0.24	3.5 ± 1.3	a	5.2 ± 2.3	a, b
3 mm	7.1	0.55	6.7 ± 1.5	b, c	10.0 ± 2.6	c, d
Baseline (bracket base dimension: 3.2 mm × 4.0 mm)	12.8	1.00	12.3 ± 3.0	d	13.3 ± 4.3	d

* Different letters indicate a significant difference ($p < 0.05$). Abbreviation: SD, standard deviation.

3.2. Adhesive Remnant Index

The ARI results are presented in Table 2. For TB, no significant differences in failure mode were observed among groups with different pre-etched areas. For UB, significant differences in failure mode were observed among the groups and the ARI tended to increase with increasing pre-etched area.

Table 2. ARI scores by pre-etched area.

	TB				UB			
Score	0	1	2	3	0	1	2	3
1 mm	7	2	0	0	9	0	0	0
2 mm	5	4	0	0	6	0	3	0
3 mm	4	3	2	0	0	3	6	0
Baseline	6	2	1	0	2	0	2	5
Chi-square value	1.6364				27.4168			
(p value)	($p = 0.996$)				($p = 0.0012$)			

ARI scores: 0, no adhesive left on tooth surface; 1, less than 50% of adhesive left on tooth surface; 2, more than 50% of adhesive left on tooth surface; and 3, all adhesive left on the tooth surface [8].

3.3. KHN of Orthodontic Adhesive Pastes

The KHNs of the tested orthodontic adhesive pastes are presented in Table 3. The mean KHN of UB was 6.2 ± 1.0 and that of TB was 16.5 ± 1.6.

Table 3. KHN for different orthodontic adhesive pastes.

TB		UB	
Mean ± SD	Group *	Mean ± SD	Group *
16.5 ± 1.6	a	6.2 ± 1.0	b

* Different letters indicate a significant difference ($p < 0.05$). Abbreviation: SD, standard deviation.

3.4. SEM Observations

SEM images of adhesive paste/enamel interfaces in the 2 mm groups are shown in Figures 2 and 3. For TB (Figure 2), although the pre-etched region (white arrow in Figure 2a) indicated excellent adaptation between demineralised enamel substrate and the adhesive paste, the non-etched region showed a gap between the enamel and adhesive paste. For UB (Figure 3), excellent adaptation between enamel substrate and the adhesive paste was observed in both the pre-etched and non-etched regions (Figure 3c,e). Adhesive paste interpenetration with enamel as resin tags was clearly observed in the pre-etched region with both adhesive pastes (Figures 2c and 3c).

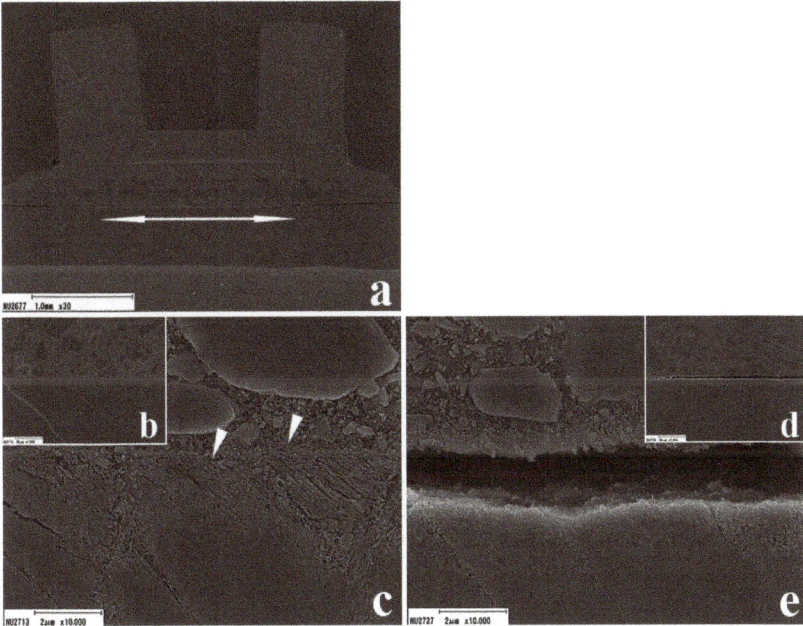

Figure 2. Representative SEM images of the orthodontic adhesive paste/enamel interface in TB. In the pre-etched area, excellent adaptation was observed (arrow), but gap formation was observed at both edges of the bracket base ((**a**): magnification 30×). In the pre-etched region ((**b**): magnification 1000×, (**c**): magnification 10,000×), compression of the enamel surface was observed (arrowheads). In the non-etched region, detachment between adhesive paste and enamel was observed ((**d**): magnification 1000×, (**e**): magnification 10,000×).

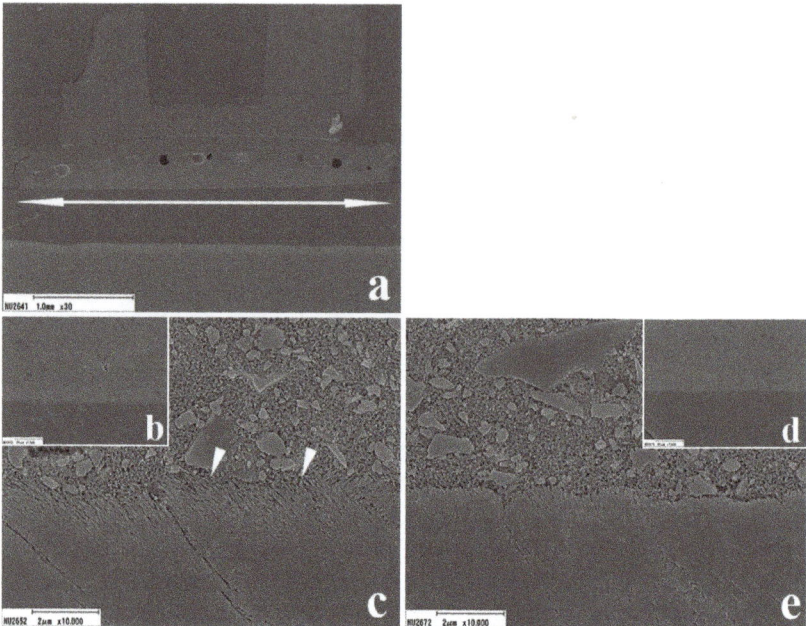

Figure 3. Representative SEM images of the orthodontic adhesive paste/enamel interface in UB. The whole interface (arrow range) region showed excellent adaptation ((**a**): magnification 30×). In the pre-etched region ((**b**): magnification 1000 ×, (**c**): magnification 10,000×), a typical etching pattern and resin enamel tags were clearly observed (arrowheads). The non-etched region ((**d**): magnification 1000×, (**e**): magnification 10,000×) showed neither the typical etching pattern nor resin enamel tags.

4. Discussion

In this study, bovine enamel was employed as a substitute for human enamel because of the difficulty of collecting the latter in the same condition [13]. To maximise the similarity to clinical orthodontic treatment with direct bonding of brackets, it would have been best to use intact enamel in the experiment. However, the undulations of bovine enamel are deeper and broader than those of human enamel. Therefore, the adherent enamel surfaces were ground flat to standardise the methodology and ensure both an appropriate adherent area for the bonded assembly and a uniform stress distribution [14,15].

Various types of functional monomer have been employed in different types of adhesive systems, such as phosphoric acid ester, carboxylic acid and alcohol functional monomers [16]. The functional monomers 10-methacryloyloxydecyl dihydrogen phosphate (MDP) and 4-methacryloxyethyl trimellitate anhydride (4-META) have often been employed in orthodontic adhesive systems [17,18]. In this study, UB contained MDP as a functional monomer, but there were no significant differences in SBS between UB and the functional monomer-free orthodontic adhesive paste TB, regardless of the pre-etched area. Therefore, the first null hypothesis, that the enamel SBS in different orthodontic adhesive pastes would not differ according to the presence or absence of functional monomers in the adhesive paste, was not rejected. An optimal orthodontic adhesive system would not fail during treatment, and would allow easy debonding of the brackets on completion of treatment [19]. Previous studies have reported that the ideal enamel bond strength of orthodontic brackets ranges from 6 to 13.7 MPa [5,6]. Excessive enamel bond strength may cause damage to the intact enamel surface when debonding brackets [20]. In this study, the baseline and 3 mm groups were within the range of ideal bond strength for both materials. Although UB showed higher SBS values than TB, the difference was not significant in any pre-etched group. This can be explained by the lower mechanical properties of

UB due to the presence of functional monomers. The incompatibility between residual acidic monomer and the other resin monomers, and the low pH of functional monomers, may inhibit polymerization, resulting in lower mechanical properties [21,22]. This was supported by the results of the KHN and ARI evaluation. UB showed a significantly lower KHN and marked increases in the rates of ARI scores 2 and 3 than TB.

However, on SEM images, although UB in the 2 mm group showed excellent adaptation in both pre-etched and non-etched regions, TB in the 2 mm group showed gap formation between the enamel and adhesive paste in the non-etched region. This gap formation between the adhesive paste and enamel substrate may be a cause of caries, staining and bracket failure during orthodontic treatment. Therefore, orthodontic adhesive paste containing functional monomers may improve the integrity of the interface even in non-etched regions due to its chemical bonding ability.

On investigation of the influence of the pre-etched area on the enamel SBS, no significant differences were observed in SBS with UB between the 3 mm and baseline groups. On the other hand, the functional monomer-free adhesive paste TB showed significantly lower SBSs in the partially pre-etched groups than the baseline group, regardless of the pre-etched area. Therefore, the second null hypothesis, that the enamel bond strength would not differ by pre-etched area, was rejected. Although enamel HAp is considered less amenable to chemical reaction with functional monomers than dentin HAp [23,24], the functional monomer in the orthodontic adhesive may enhance enamel bond effectiveness. However, it may be difficult to reach the minimum enamel bond strength requirement without phosphoric acid pre-etching, even when orthodontic adhesive pastes contain functional monomers. Takamiya et al. investigated the bond effectiveness of five self-adhesive flowable resin composites without any pre-treatment, and recommended selective enamel etching for these materials [25]. Based on previous investigations of self-adhesive materials and the outcomes of this study, it may be necessary to pre-etch at least half of the bracket base area in the case of UB.

It is difficult to compare the outcomes of in vitro experiments and clinical situations directly. In addition, the bond strength value is influenced by many factors, such as the type of bond strength test, adherent substrate, material selection, adherent conditions, caries prophylaxis treatment, etc. [26–28]. In this study, the adherent enamel surface was ground flat to standardise conditions, but this introduces an important difference from the clinical situation. The outer surface of intact enamel, i.e., the prismless layer, has stronger resistance to acid than a prismatic one. In a previous investigation of self-etching adhesive systems for intact enamel using different etching strategies, unground enamel without pre-etching showed significantly lower bond performance than ground enamel, but no significant difference was observed between ground and unground enamel with pre-etching [29]. It was suggested that mechanical interlocking is more important for intact enamel adhesion than chemical bonding. Hence, phosphoric acid pre-etching is necessary for securing brackets during treatment, even when using orthodontic adhesive pastes marketed as self-adhesive.

Although there has been a study showing the enamel bonding effectiveness of UB, little information is available on this material [30]. On the other hand, TB has been used in many studies, often as a control material [31–33]. In this study, to standardise the bonding protocol between TB and UB, we omitted the priming step of TB. The primer composition of TB is similar to typical bonding agents and does not contain any functional monomers. In a previous study, SEM revealed no ultrastructure differences in the etched enamel region according to primer application [34]. In addition, previous laboratory studies demonstrated comparable tensile bond strength with and without primer application [35–37]. These findings suggest that primer application may not influence enamel bond effectiveness or morphological features in the vicinity of the interface of TB, and that the bonding procedures used in the baseline and partially pre-etched groups did not cause problems.

Regarding the ARI, a significant difference was detected in UB, but not TB, according to the pre-etched area. UB tended to show an increase in the rate of ARI scores of 2 and 3 with increasing pre-etched area. Remnant adhesive paste on the enamel surface should be removed with rotary rather than hand instruments [38]. Although grinding and polishing the adhesive remnant on the tooth surface may be time-consuming, this method is safe and gentle [39]. Therefore, adhesive paste containing functional monomers with partial pre-etching may be preferable to functional monomer-free adhesive paste because of adaptation and improved treatment of the debonded enamel surface.

5. Conclusions

Within the limitations of this study, we concluded that:

1. Enamel bond strengths of orthodontic adhesive pastes increased with increasing pre-etched area.
2. SEM revealed no gap formation in the vicinity of the interface with UB, in contrast to TB.
3. For UB, adhesive failure at the adhesive paste/bracket interface increased as a higher proportion of the bonding area was pre-etched.

These findings suggest that the pre-etching area markedly influences enamel bond effectiveness regardless of the presence or absence of functional monomers in orthodontic adhesive paste.

Author Contributions: Conceptualization, Y.N. and T.T.; methodology, Y.N., Y.T. and Y.U.; validation, Y.U. and M.I.; formal analysis, Y.N.; investigation, Y.T., A.U. and K.W.; resources, Y.T.; data curation, K.W.; writing—original draft preparation, Y.N.; writing—review and editing, T.T. and M.M.; visualization, Y.N.; supervision, M.M.; project administration, Y.N.; funding acquisition, Y.N. and T.T. All authors have read and agreed to the published version of the manuscript.

Funding: This work was supported in part by a Grant-in-Aid for Scientific Research (no. 19K10158) from the Japan Society for the Promotion of Science. This project was also supported by the Sato Fund in 2021.

Institutional Review Board Statement: Not applicable.

Data Availability Statement: The data are contained within the article and/or available from the corresponding author upon reasonable request.

Acknowledgments: Not applicable.

Conflicts of Interest: The authors declare no conflict of interest.

References

1. de Assis, C.; Lemos, C.; Gomes, J.; Vasconcelos, B.; Moraes, S.; Braz, R.; Pellizzer, E.P. Clinical efficiency of self-etching one-step and two-step adhesives in NCCL: A systematic review and meta-analysis. *Oper. Dent.* **2020**, *45*, 598–607. [CrossRef] [PubMed]
2. Patcas, R.; Eliades, T. Structure/property relationships in orthodontic ceramics. In *Orthodontic Applications of Biomaterials*; Eliades, T., Brantley, W.A., Eds.; Woodhead Publishing: Cambridge, UK, 2017; p. 225.
3. Van Landuyt, K.L.; Yoshida, Y.; Hirata, I.; Snauwaert, J.; De Munck, J.; Okazaki, M.; Suzuki, K.; Lambrechts, P.; Van Meerbeek, B. Influence of the chemical structure of functional monomers on their adhesive performance. *J. Dent. Res.* **2008**, *87*, 757–761. [CrossRef] [PubMed]
4. Takamizawa, T.; Barkmeier, W.W.; Latta, M.A.; Berry, T.P.; Tsujimoto, A.; Miyazaki, M. Simulated Wear of Self-Adhesive Resin Cements. *Oper. Dent.* **2016**, *41*, 327–338. [CrossRef] [PubMed]
5. Imai, A.; Takamizawa, T.; Sugimura, R.; Tsujimoto, A.; Ishii, R.; Kawazu, M.; Saito, T.; Miyazaki, M. Interrelation among the handling, mechanical, and wear properties of the newly developed flowable resin composites. *J. Mech. Behav. Biomed. Mater.* **2019**, *89*, 72–80. [CrossRef]
6. Hess, E.; Campbell, P.M.; Honeyman, A.L.; Buschang, P.H. Determinants of enamel decalcification during simulated orthodontic treatment. *Angle Orthod.* **2011**, *81*, 836–842. [CrossRef] [PubMed]
7. Reynolds, I.R. A review of direct orthodontic bonding. *Br. J. Orthod.* **1975**, *2*, 171–179. [CrossRef]
8. Retief, D.H. Failure at the dental adhesive-etched enamel interface. *J. Oral Rehabil.* **1974**, *1*, 265–294. [CrossRef]
9. Soares, F.Z.; Follak, A.; da Rosa, L.S.; Montagner, A.F.; Lenzi, T.L.; Rocha, R.O. Bovine tooth is a substitute for human tooth on bond strength studies: A systematic review and meta-analysis of in vitro studies. *Dent. Mater.* **2016**, *32*, 1385–1393. [CrossRef]
10. Årtun, K.; Bergland, S. Clinical trials with crystal growth conditioning as an alternative to acid-etch enamel pretreatment. *Am. J. Orthod.* **1984**, *85*, 333–340. [CrossRef]

11. Namura, Y.; Takamizawa, T.; Uchida, Y.; Inaba, M.; Noma, D.; Takemoto, T.; Miyazaki, M.; Motoyoshi, M. Effects of composition on the hardness of orthodontic adhesives. *J. Oral Sci.* **2020**, *62*, 48–51. [CrossRef]
12. Masucci, C.; Cipriani, L.; Defraia, E.; Franchi, L. Transverse relationship of permanent molars after crossbite correction in deciduous dentition. *Eur. J. Orthod.* **2017**, *39*, 560–566. [CrossRef] [PubMed]
13. Yassen, G.H.; Platt, J.A.; Hara, A.T. Bovine teeth as substitute for human teeth in dental research: A review of literature. *J. Oral Sci.* **2011**, *53*, 273–282. [CrossRef] [PubMed]
14. Braga, R.R.; Meira, J.B.; Boaro, L.C.; Xavier, T.A. Adhesion to tooth structure: A critical review of "macro" test methods. *Dent. Mater.* **2010**, *26*, e38–e49. [CrossRef] [PubMed]
15. Sirisha, K.; Rambabu, T.; Shankar, Y.R.; Ravikumar, P. Validity of bond strength tests: A critical review: Part I. *J. Conserv. Dent.* **2014**, *17*, 305–311. [CrossRef] [PubMed]
16. Yoshida, Y.; Nagakane, K.; Fukuda, R.; Nakayama, Y.; Okazaki, M.; Shintani, H.; Inoue, S.; Tagawa, Y.; Suzuki, K.; De Munck, J.; et al. Comparative study on adhesive performance of functional monomers. *J. Dent. Res.* **2004**, *83*, 454–458. [CrossRef]
17. Costa, A.C.; Sabóia, V.; Marçal, F.; Sena, N.; De Paula, D.; Ribeiro, T.; Feitosa, V. In vitro evaluation of experimental self-adhesive orthodontic composites used to bond ceramic brackets. *Materials* **2019**, *12*, 419. [CrossRef]
18. Saito, K.; Sirirungrojying, S.; Meguro, D.; Hayakawa, T.; Kasai, K. Bonding durability of using self-etching primer with 4-META/ MMA-TBB resin cement to bond orthodontic brackets. *Angle Orthod.* **2005**, *75*, 260–265. [CrossRef]
19. Theodorakopoulou, L.P.; Sadowsky, P.L.; Jacobson, A.; Lacefield, W., Jr. Evaluation of the debonding characteristics of 2 ceramic brackets: An in vitro study. *Am. J. Orthod. Dentofac. Orthop.* **2004**, *125*, 329–336. [CrossRef]
20. Azzeh, E.; Feldon, P.J. Laser debonding of ceramic brackets: A comprehensive review. *Am. J. Orthod. Dentofac. Orthop.* **2003**, *123*, 79–83. [CrossRef]
21. Sanares, A.M.; Itthagarun, A.; King, N.M.; Tay, F.R.; Pashley, D.H. Adverse surface interactions between one-bottle light-cured adhesives and chemical-cured composites. *Dent. Mater.* **2001**, *17*, 542–556. [CrossRef]
22. Zorzin, J.; Petschelt, A.; Ebert, J.; Lohbauer, U. pH neutralization and influence on mechanical strength in self-adhesive resin luting agents. *Dent. Mater.* **2012**, *28*, 672–679. [CrossRef] [PubMed]
23. Yoshihara, K.; Yoshida, Y.; Hayakawa, S.; Nagaoka, N.; Irie, M.; Ogawa, T.; Van Landuyt, K.L.; Osaka, A.; Suzuki, K.; Minagi, S.; et al. Nanolayering of phosphoric acid ester monomer on enamel and dentin. *Acta Biomater.* **2011**, *7*, 3187–3195. [CrossRef]
24. Yaguchi, T. Layering mechanism of MDP-Ca salt produced in demineralization of enamel and dentin apatite. *Dent. Mater.* **2017**, *33*, 23–32. [CrossRef] [PubMed]
25. Takamiya, H.; Tsujimoto, A.; Teixeira, E.C.; Jurado, C.A.; Takamizawa, T.; Barkmeier, W.W.; Latta, M.A.; Miyazaki, M.; Garcia-Godoy, F. Bonding and wear properties of self-adhesive flowable restorative materials. *Eur. J. Oral Sci.* **2021**, *31*, e12799. [CrossRef]
26. Finnema, K.J.; Ozcan, M.; Post, W.J.; Ren, Y.; Dijkstra, P.U. In-vitro orthodontic bond strength testing: A systematic review and meta-analysis. *Am. J. Orthod. Dentofac. Orthop.* **2010**, *137*, 615–622.e3. [CrossRef]
27. Salz, U.; Bock, T. Testing adhesion of direct restoratives to dental hard tissue—A review. *J. Adhes. Dent.* **2010**, *12*, 343–371. [CrossRef] [PubMed]
28. Lanteri, V.; Segù, M.; Doldi, J.D.H.; Butera, A.D.H. Pre-bonding prophylaxis and brackets detachment: An experimental comparison of different methods. *Int. J. Clin. Dent.* **2014**, *7*, 191–197.
29. Takeda, M.; Takamizawa, T.; Imai, A.; Suzuki, T.; Tsujimoto, A.; Barkmeier, W.W.; Latta, M.A.; Miyazaki, M. Immediate enamel bond strength of universal adhesives to unground and ground surfaces in different etching modes. *Eur. J. Oral Sci.* **2019**, *127*, 351–360. [CrossRef] [PubMed]
30. Ok, U.; Aksakalli, S.; Eren, E.; Kechagia, N. Single-component orthodontic adhesives: Comparison of the clinical and in vitro performance. *Clin. Oral Investig.* **2021**, *25*, 3987–3999. [CrossRef] [PubMed]
31. Romano, F.L.; Tavares, S.W.; Nouer, D.F.; Consani, S.; Magnani, M.B.B.A. Shear bond strength of metallic orthodontic brackets bonded to enamel prepared with Self-Etching Primer. *Angle Orthod.* **2005**, *75*, 849–853. [CrossRef]
32. Cunha, T.M.A.; Behrens, B.A.; Nascimento, D.; Retamoso, L.B.; Lon, L.F.S.; Tanaka, O.; Guariza Filho, O. Blood contamination effect on shear bond strength of an orthodontic hydrophilic resin. *J. Appl. Oral Sci.* **2012**, *20*, 89–93. [CrossRef] [PubMed]
33. Wan, A.; Razak, W.S.; Sherriff, M.; Bister, D.; Seehra, J. Bond strength of stainless steel orthodontic brackets bonded to prefabricated acrylic teeth. *J. Orthod.* **2017**, *44*, 105–109. [CrossRef]
34. Jörgensen, K.D.; Shimokobe, H. Adaptation of resinous restorative materials to acid etched enamel surfaces. *Scand. J. Dent. Res.* **1975**, *83*, 31–36. [CrossRef]
35. O'Brien, K.D.; Watts, D.C.; Read, M.J. Light cured direct bonding—Is it necessary to use a primer? *Eur. J. Orthod.* **1991**, *13*, 22–26. [CrossRef]
36. Tang, A.T.; Björkman, L.; Adamczak, E.; Andlin-Sobocki, A.; Ekstrand, J. In vitro shear bond strength of orthodontic bondings without liquid resin. *Acta Odontol. Scand.* **2000**, *58*, 44–48. [CrossRef] [PubMed]
37. Bazargani, F.; Magnuson, A.; Löthgren, H.; Kowalczyk, A. Orthodontic bonding with and without primer: A randomized controlled trial. *Eur. J. Orthod.* **2016**, *38*, 503–507. [CrossRef] [PubMed]

38. Janiszewska-Olszowska, J.; Szatkiewicz, T.; Tomkowski, R.; Tandecka, K.; Grocholewicz, K. Effect of orthodontic debonding and adhesive removal on the enamel - current knowledge and future perspectives—Asystematic review. *Med. Sci. Monit.* **2014**, *20*, 1991–2001. [CrossRef]
39. Proffit, W.R. The third stage of comprehensive treatment: Finishing. In *Contemporary Orthodontics*, 5th ed.; Proffit, W.R., Fields, H.W., Sarver, D.M., Eds.; Mosby Elsevier: St Louis, MI, USA, 2013; pp. 582–605.

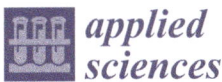

Article

Heat Generation and Temperature Control during Bone Drilling for Orthodontic Mini-Implants: An In Vitro Study

Ibrahim Barrak [1,*], Gábor Braunitzer [2], József Piffkó [1] and Emil Segatto [1]

[1] Craniofacial Unit, Department of Oral and Maxillofacial Surgery, Faculty of Medicine, University of Szeged, 6725 Szeged, Hungary; piffkojozsef@gmail.com (J.P.); dr@segatto.hu (E.S.)
[2] Dicomlab Dental Ltd., 6725 Szeged, Hungary; gabor.braunitzer@dicomlab.com
* Correspondence: barrakibrahim@gmail.com; Tel.: +36-70-611-5247

Abstract: Background: The purpose of our in vitro study was to evaluate the impact of different irrigation fluid temperatures in combination with different drilling speeds on intraosseous temperature changes during mini-implant site preparation. Methods: Porcine ribs were used as bone specimens. Grouping determinants were as follows: irrigation fluid temperature (10 and 20 °C) and drilling speed (200, 600, 900, and 1200 RPM). The axial load was controlled at 2.0 kg. Temperature measurements were conducted using K-type thermocouples. Results: Extreme increments were observed only in the unirrigated groups. Irrigation invariably made a significant difference within groups defined by the same drilling speed. The comparison of the different temperature irrigation fluids (10 and 20 °C) in combination with the same drilling speed (200, 600, 900, or 1200 rpm) resulted in a statistically significant difference between the two different temperatures, whereas the use of irrigation fluid at a controlled room temperature of 20 °C showed significantly higher temperature changes. Conclusions: Based on the results of the study, we conclude that irrigation while preparing a pilot hole for a self-tapping orthodontic miniscrew is of utmost importance, even at low drilling speeds. The temperature of the cooling fluid does influence local temperature elevation to a significant extent.

Keywords: orthodontic screw; mini-implant; pre-drilling; heat production; temperature; irrigation; cooled irrigation; safety; bone drilling

Citation: Barrak, I.; Braunitzer, G.; Piffkó, J.; Segatto, E. Heat Generation and Temperature Control during Bone Drilling for Orthodontic Mini-Implants: An In Vitro Study. *Appl. Sci.* **2021**, *11*, 7689. https://doi.org/10.3390/app11167689

Academic Editor: Mitsuru Motoyoshi

Received: 29 June 2021
Accepted: 14 August 2021
Published: 21 August 2021

Publisher's Note: MDPI stays neutral with regard to jurisdictional claims in published maps and institutional affiliations.

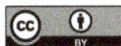

Copyright: © 2021 by the authors. Licensee MDPI, Basel, Switzerland. This article is an open access article distributed under the terms and conditions of the Creative Commons Attribution (CC BY) license (https://creativecommons.org/licenses/by/4.0/).

1. Introduction

Anchorage in the orthodontic field can be defined as a resistance to unwanted tooth movement [1]. To achieve such resistance, anchorage units are utilized. A stable anchorage unit is a crucial element of successful orthodontic treatment. To achieve the required anchorage, dental implants, palatal implants, mini-plates, or mini-implants have been used [2–4]. These devices are attached to the basal bone or the alveolar process of the maxilla or the mandible; therefore, they provide skeletal anchorage. Given that they are in place only for the duration of the orthodontic treatment, they are usually referred to as temporary anchorage devices (TADs). In 1997, Kanomi introduced mini-implants that were specifically developed to provide stable anchorage during orthodontic treatment [5]. Because of their many advantages (versatility, independence of patient adherence, minimal surgical invasiveness, low morbidity, relative affordability, and good patient acceptance), mini-implants have become especially popular among orthodontists [6–8]. Despite their short length and small diameter, mini-implants offer stable anchorage for different types of tooth movement, including retraction, distalization, mesialization, and intrusion [9,10]. In terms of insertion, two main kinds of mini-implants may be distinguished: self-drilling, which does not require a pilot hole, and non-self-drilling (i.e., self-tapping), which requires the drilling of a pilot hole before the implant placement. Complications of this approach to anchorage include injury of the roots of the neighboring teeth, implant loosening, and even implant fracture [11]. Uemura and his colleagues concluded that mini-implant stability could be influenced by implant diameter, inflammation of the peri-implant tissues, cortical bone thickness, and high mandibular plane angle [12]. It was also found that temperature elevation at the level of the cortical bone and higher torque during insertion may result in an early implant loss [9,13,14]. Some studies reported lower success rates with mandibular mini-implants [11,13,15–17] due to microcracks caused by over-torquing in thick and hard bone [9] and the consequent excessive heat production. Tachibana and co-workers achieved optimal insertion torque by pre-drilling, and this way they managed to avoid osteonecrosis [9]. In contrast, Gurdán et al. reported that pre-drilling for 1.6 mm self-drilling mini-implants with a 1 mm diameter pilot drill did not decrease intraosseous temperatures when the mini-implant was placed into a model mandible [18]. Matsuoka et al. measured the heat production during the placement of self-drilling mini-implants without the preparation of the pilot hole, and they found that self-drilling at speeds higher than 150 rpm causes thermal damage [14]. Uemura and co-workers concluded that the ratio of the diameter of the pilot hole and the mini-implant is an important factor in implant stability [12]. Despite the beneficial advantages of adequate predrilling on implant stability, the drilling procedure itself can have effects on intraosseous temperature during mini-implant placement. During the rotary cutting of the drills, the generated heat may accumulate locally, especially at the level of the denser cortical bone, which can eventually lead to necrosis [19]. The characteristics of the bone (whether the cortex of the mandible or the cortical bone of the anterior palate) can also lead to an increased risk of overheating during drilling. It is amply documented in the literature that osteonecrosis occurs when the intraosseous temperature rises to 47 °C [16,20]. To our knowledge, intraosseous heat generation during pre-drilling of a pilot hole at different drilling speeds in combination with irrigation fluids of different temperature has not been previously investigated in the literature. The purpose of our in vitro study was to evaluate the impact of different irrigation fluid temperatures in combination with different drilling speeds on intraosseous temperature changes during mini-implant site preparation.

2. Materials and Methods

2.1. Bone Model

Porcine ribs were used for the experiments because of their favorable anatomical and thermophysical characteristics [18,21,22]. The study conducted by Kim and his colleagues [23] concluded that cortical bone thickness falls in a range of approximately 1.14–1.49 mm for the human maxilla at the sites of orthodontic implant placement. The specimens selected were in the above-mentioned range between 1.2 and 1.5 mm (as can be seen in Figure 1), which is also a widely used value in the literature [9].

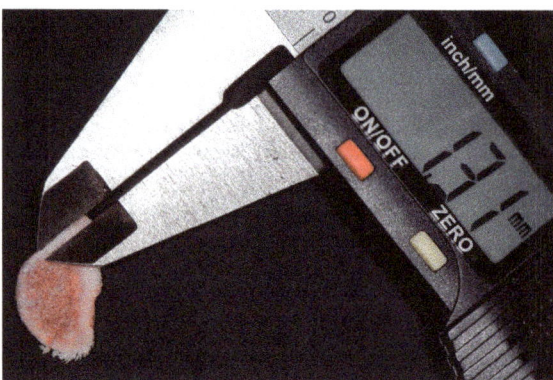

Figure 1. Porcine rib model used for the in vitro experiment with a cortical bone thickness of 1.31 mm.

Sener et al. [24] proved in their study that the increase in intraosseous temperature elevation was greater in the cortical layer of the bone in comparison to the deeper parts of the drilled cavity. This finding has also been confirmed by other studies [25,26]. Bones were taken from the same animal, and the animals were not killed for the sake of the experiments. The specimens were all stored at a temperature of −10 °C in normal saline when not used as it is suggested by Sedlin and Hirsch [27].

2.2. Setup

Drillings were performed in accordance with the manual of the Benefit orthodontic implant system (PSM Medical Solutions, Tuttlingen, Germany) with a diameter of 1.4 mm as can be seen in Figure 2.

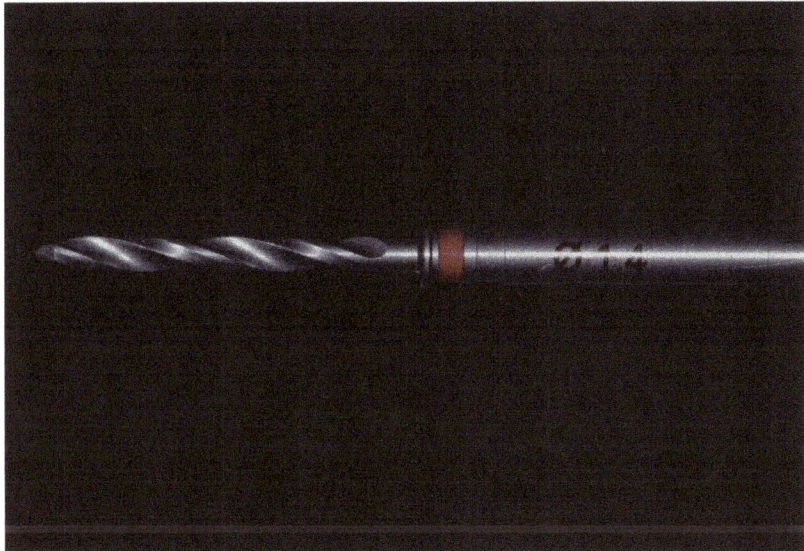

Figure 2. 1.4 mm diameter drill used for the investigation.

Osteotomies were carried out at the drilling speeds of 200, 600, 900, and 1200 rpm; all of these mentioned were used in the literature [18,28,29]. We also compared the use of irrigation fluids at different temperatures (20 and 10 °C) with no irrigation. A total of 40 drillings were performed in each of the 12 groups. Entry points for the freehand groups were marked on the surface of the bone specimens.

Studies suggest that the maximum temperature increment can be observed in the cortical layer of the bone [24–26]. Therefore, we performed temperature measurements in the cortical layer of the bone. K-type thermocouples were used for temperature measurements with a connected measurement device (HoldPeak 885A, HoldPeak; Zhuhai, Guangdong, China). The thermocouples were consistently placed into a cavity prepared with a 1.5 mm diameter implant drill and a depth control of 1.2 mm; therefore, we could ensure that the depth of the cavity never exceeded the cortical layer. Measurement cavities were positioned at a 1.00 mm horizontal distance from the 1.4 mm drilling canal. The thermocouple was placed touching the lateral bony wall of the cavity being closer to the implant bed to be drilled, followed by tight filling with bone chips derived from rib specimens of the same animal, and the hole was thoroughly sealed with plasticine to maintain adequate insulation (Figure 3).

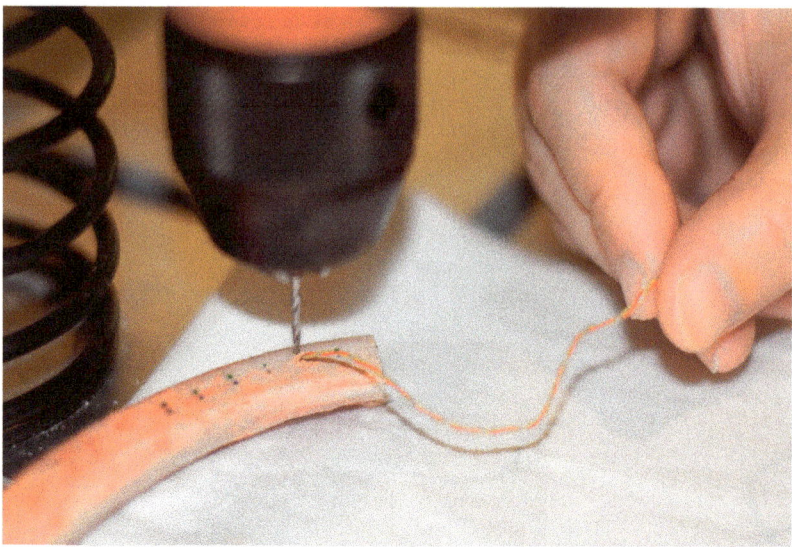

Figure 3. A close-up of the experimental setting.

A constant axial load of 2.0 kg was used, as it can be considered as a low hand pressure, and it is extensively used in the literature, as it can be seen in reviews also concerning the topic [21,30–32]. The constant load was achieved by placing a weight on top of the drilling apparatus and then manipulating the resistance in a way that the load exerted by the tip of the drill was 2.0 kg. A bench drill with an adjustable drilling speed was used for the experiments (Bosch PBD 40; Bosch, Stuttgart, Germany). The specimens were heated up to a temperature of 37 °C. Drillings with temperature measurement were only executed if the baseline temperature of the bone was between 35 and 37 °C. A single drilling lasted 5–10 s.

A constantly controlled external irrigation was provided by a widely known, accepted, and used surgical unit (INTRAsurg 300, KaVo Dental GmbH, Biberach/Riß, Germany), and the standard cannula of another system was used (W&H). The cannula was safely and precisely attached to the drilling machine, and it was directed toward the drill bit. The flow rate was 100 mL/min as recommended in the literature [33–36]. The temperature of the irrigation fluid was either 20 ± 1 °C or 10 ± 1 °C. The temperature of the irrigation fluid was always checked with an infrared thermometer before every measurement.

The full setup can be seen in Figure 4. All the drilling procedures were conducted in the same air-conditioned room, where the temperature was controlled within the range of 20 ± 1 °C.

2.3. Collection of Data and Statistical Analysis

Baseline and peak temperatures were collected to one decimal point in a spreadsheet file in Microsoft Excel 2013 15.0 (Microsoft Corporation, Redmond, WA, USA). Temperature elevations were calculated as peak temperature minus baseline temperature to one decimal point using the spreadsheet. The data were analyzed in SPSS 23.0 (Armonk, NY, USA, IBM). The normality of distributions was tested with the Shapiro–Wilk test. As non-normal distributions were observed, Kruskal–Wallis ANOVA was used.

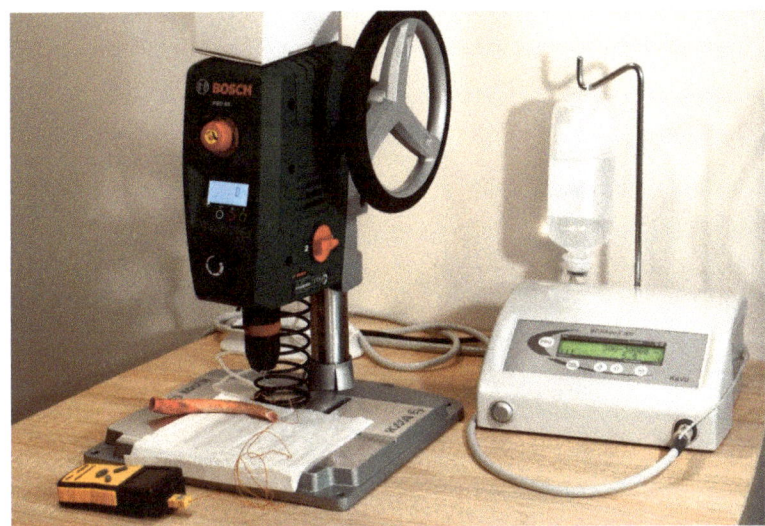

Figure 4. The study setting, including the bench drill, and the irrigation system (provided by the surgical unit).

3. Results

The descriptive statistics of the measured thermal changes are given in Table 1.

Table 1. Mean temperature rises, maximum and minimum of temperature rises, groups divided by different drilling speeds, and temperature of the irrigation fluid.

Grouping Number	Drilling Speed (rpm)	Temperature of Irrigation Fluid (°C)	Number of Drillings	Mean (SD) Temperature Rise (°C)	Maximum Temperature Rise (°C)	Minimum Temperature Rise (°C)	Median Temperature Value (°C)
1	200	10	40	−2.45 (0.57)	−1.30	−3.50	−2.50
2	200	20	40	0.05 (0.07)	0.20	0.00	0.00
3	200	no irrigation	40	2.22 (0.71)	3.80	1.20	2.10
4	600	10	40	−1.76 (0.35)	−1.00	−2.80	−1.80
5	600	20	40	1.02 (0.33)	1.30	0.00	1.20
6	600	no irrigation	40	3.75 (0.97)	6.10	2.00	3.75
7	900	10	40	−1.02 (0.38)	0.20	−1.30	−1.15
8	900	20	40	1.48 (0.56)	2.60	0.50	1.30
9	900	no irrigation	40	5.92 (1.14)	9.50	4.40	5.90
10	1200	10	40	−0.18 (0.23)	1.30	0.00	0.10
11	1200	20	40	1.86 (0.65)	3.40	1.20	1.70
12	1200	no irrigation	40	7.76 (1.59)	11.50	4.70	7.45

SD: Standard deviation.

Almost all pairwise comparisons indicated significant difference at $p < 0.05$; the exceptions are given in Table 2.

In three groups, the measured temperature increment was >5 °C (no irrigation at 600, 900, and 1200 rpm). In one group, the temperature increment was ≥10 °C (no irrigation at 900 and 1200 rpm). Thus, extreme increments were observed only in the unirrigated groups. Irrigation invariably made a significant difference within groups defined by the same drilling speed. The use of a 20 °C irrigation fluid resulted in a lower temperature increment, which remained in the safe zone throughout the use of every drilling speed (200, 600, 900, and 1200 rpm). In all of the groups with 10 °C external irrigation, the measured temperature changes were negative in comparison to the baseline cortical intraosseous temperature, despite the drilling procedure. This might be the result of the cooling effect of the irrigation fluid being more pronounced than the heat-producing effect of the drilling. The comparison of the different temperature irrigation fluids (10 and 20 °C) in combination with the same drilling speed (200, 600, 900, or 1200 rpm) resulted in a statistically significant difference between the two different temperatures, whereas the use of irrigation fluid at a controlled room temperature of 20 °C showed significantly higher temperature changes.

A graphical summary of the results is given in Figure 5.

Table 2. The non-significant differences can be seen after the pairwise comparison.

Grouping Number	Drilling Speed (rpm)	Temperature of Irrigation Fluid (°C)	No significant Difference Could Be Observed $p < 0.05$
1	200	10	4
2	200	20	7, 10
3	200	no irrigation	6, 8, 11
4	600	10	1, 7
5	600	20	8, 10
6	600	no irrigation	3, 9
7	900	10	2, 4
8	900	20	3, 5, 11, 12
9	900	no irrigation	6, 12
10	1200	10	2, 5
11	1200	20	3, 8
12	1200	no irrigation	8, 9

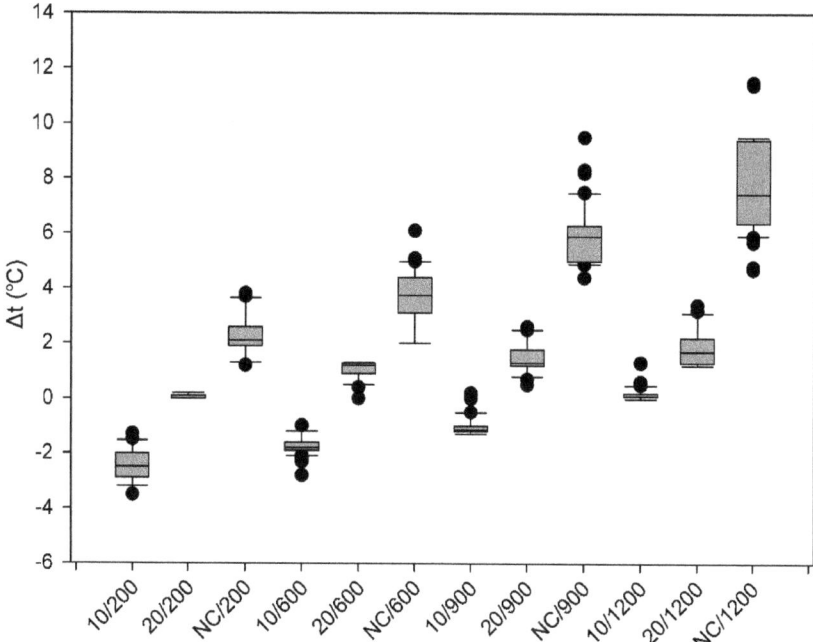

Figure 5. Temperature changes across the study groups. The lower margin of the boxes shows the 25th percentile, the line within the boxes marks the median, and the upper margin of the boxes indicates the 75th percentile. The error bars (whiskers) above and below the boxes indicate the 90th and 10th percentiles. The black dots represent the outliers. Labels of the X-axis: temperature of cooling fluid (°C)/rpm; NC: no cooling.

4. Discussion

Anchorage control is a key factor of success in clinical orthodontics [11]. According to the literature, miniscrew failure can be traced back to multiple factors, including bone density, the thickness of the cortical bone, screw length, diameter and design (shape of the screw thread), insertion angle and torque, the type of the miniscrew (self-drilling or self-tapping), the amount and direction of loading, the length of the treatment period, microfracture of the alveolar bone, and overheating [1,16,37,38].

Intraosseous heat generation can seriously interfere with the local homeostatic conditions of the bone. A temperature increase to 40 °C initiates hyperemia; however, if the thermal elevation continues and reaches 53 °C, blood flow stops entirely [20,39]. Eriksson and colleagues reported that the threshold for thermal damage to osseous structures fell between 44 and 47 °C [39,40]. This means that for the measurements of our study, where the baseline temperature was a mean of 36 °C, safe temperature elevation fell between Δt = 8–11 °C, depending on the exact baseline temperature of any given specimen. The results are interpreted accordingly. Drilling at 1200 rpm without any irrigation resulted in a mean temperature elevation of Δt = 7.76 °C, with elevations reaching Δt = 11.5 °C, which is unacceptable in terms of safety. The apparently moderate mean temperature elevation of Δt = 5.92 °C for the 900 rpm/no irrigation group might suggest that drilling at this speed without irrigation could be safe, but note that the maximum elevation in this group was still in the unsafe range (Δt = 9.5 °C). The mean temperature elevations without irrigation at 200 rpm (Δt = 2.22 °C) and 600 rpm (Δt = 3.74 °C) remained in the safe range. Elevation maxima did not exceed the safety threshold either. This might give the impression that bone drilling without irrigation at low speeds is completely safe. Reality appears to be a bit more complicated. Iyer and co-workers concluded that a temperature elevation of only 4.3 °C caused a significant difference in the quality of the newly formed bone around an implant [41]. In other words, it seems that thermal harm is not necessarily linked to extreme heat elevations: lower temperatures can do harm too but not immediately and not necessarily in the form of some necrotic process. This corroborates the repeated conclusion that intraosseous heat elevation is best kept as low as possible, which means that no bone drilling should happen without irrigation. While this conclusion is commonplace in implant dentistry done with implants of regular dimensions, less is known about the situation with mini-implants, which is exactly what motivated our study. From our data, it seems that this smaller system (i.e., drills of a smaller diameter and a shallower/narrower bony socket) is even more sensitive to heat generation (and the presence or absence of cooling), even at low speeds.

The effects of the use of cooled irrigation fluids in bone drilling are also relatively under investigated. The results of Isler et al. [42] suggest that the use of 4 °C saline might have a positive effect on bone healing. Sener and his colleagues [24] concluded that 10 °C saline can be more effective at keeping temperatures under control in an implant preparation setting than 25 °C saline, whereas Kondo et al. [43] demonstrated the superiority of cold irrigation fluid in minimizing temperature elevation in a neurosurgical setting, where strict temperature control is crucial to protect the nervous tissue. Our research group found that a 10 °C saline solution provides sufficient external cooling during normal implant site preparation with lower temperature increments as compared to room temperature (20 °C) irrigation [33,35,36]. As for the results of the present study, the use of both 10 and 20 °C significantly reduced heat generation at all speeds. At any speed, there was a statistically significant difference in temperature elevation, depending on the temperature of the irrigation fluid (and compared to the no-irrigation condition), which corroborates our above conclusion about the sensitivity of the system.

The most important limitation of this study is its in vitro nature. Care was taken, though, that the key elements and parameters of the model (such as the cortical thickness of the bone and the axial load) are accepted in the literature. Furthermore, to our knowledge, this is the first study to examine multiple aspects of heat generation and control within the same model in connection with orthodontic anchorage and with a clinically relevant drill bit diameter (Ø = 1.4 mm).

Another relative limitation is that the exact drilling time was not considered, while it obviously appears in the literature as a factor [21,44–47]. However, the results suggest that within the short timeframe we used (no drilling lasted more than 10 s), time was not a clinically significant factor (there was only one instance in only one group when the temperature increment exceeded the generally accepted safety limit).

5. Conclusions

Based on the results and the relevant literature, and within the limitations of this study, we conclude that irrigation while preparing a pilot hole for a self-tapping orthodontic miniscrew is of utmost importance, even at low drilling speeds. In such cases, the working area is small, which, without proper irrigation, probably makes the system more susceptible to heat concentration than what can be observed during regular (i.e., prosthetic) implant surgery. As a general conclusion, it is recommendable that, when preparing the site for these miniscrews, the clinician should observe the "lowest possible speed with constant irrigation" principle known from implant dentistry. As for the temperature of the cooling fluid, this does influence local temperature elevation to a significant extent, but the difference does not seem to be relevant from a clinical point of view. However, it does not necessarily mean that it does not influence healing. This should be clarified in histological studies.

Author Contributions: Conceptualization, J.P., I.B., and E.S.; methodology J.P., I.B. and E.S.; software, G.B. and I.B.; validation, G.B. and I.B.; formal analysis, G.B. and I.B.; investigation, I.B.; resources I.B.; data curation, G.B. and I.B.; writing—original draft preparation, G.B., I.B. and E.S.; writing—review and editing, G.B., I.B., J.P. and E.S.; visualization, G.B. and I.B.; supervision, G.B., J.P. and E.S. All authors have read and agreed to the published version of the manuscript.

Funding: This research received no external funding.

Institutional Review Board Statement: Not applicable.

Informed Consent Statement: Not applicable.

Data Availability Statement: Not applicable.

Acknowledgments: The authors would like to thank PSM Medical Solutions Ltd. for their support of the drill bits. The authors would like to thank Nikolett Langó for her help during visualization of the article.

Conflicts of Interest: The authors declare no conflict of interest.

References

1. Papadopoulos, M.A.; Tarawneh, F. The use of miniscrew implants for temporary skeletal anchorage in orthodontics: A comprehensive review. *Oral Surg. Oral Med. Oral Pathol. Oral Radiol. Endod.* **2007**, *103*, e6–e15. [CrossRef]
2. Tsui, W.K.; Chua, H.D.; Cheung, L.K. Bone anchor systems for orthodontic application: A systematic review. *Int. J. Oral Maxillofac. Surg.* **2012**, *41*, 1427–1438. [CrossRef]
3. Afrashtehfar, K.I.; Del Fabbro, M. Clinical performance of zirconia implants: A meta-review. *J. Prosthet. Dent.* **2020**, *123*, 419–426. [CrossRef]
4. Lyu, X.; Guo, J.; Chen, L.; Gao, Y.; Liu, L.; Pu, L.; Lai, W.; Long, H. Assessment of available sites for palatal orthodontic mini-implants through cone-beam computed tomography. *Angle Orthod.* **2020**, *90*, 516–523. [CrossRef] [PubMed]
5. Kanomi, R. Mini-implant for orthodontic anchorage. *J. Clin. Orthod.* **1997**, *31*, 763–767.
6. Reichow, A.M.; Melo, A.C.; de Souza, C.M.; Castilhos, B.B.; Olandoski, M.; Alvim-Pereira, C.C.; Alvim-Pereira, F.; Trevilatto, P.C. Outcome of orthodontic mini-implant loss in relation to interleukin 6 polymorphisms. *Int. J. Oral Maxillofac. Surg.* **2016**, *45*, 649–657. [CrossRef] [PubMed]
7. Wilmes, B.; Drescher, D. Impact of bone quality, implant type, and implantation site preparation on insertion torques of mini-implants used for orthodontic anchorage. *Int. J. Oral Maxillofac. Surg.* **2011**, *40*, 697–703. [CrossRef] [PubMed]
8. Afrashtehfar, K.I. Patient and miniscrew implant factors influence the success of orthodontic miniscrew implants. *Evid. Based Dent.* **2016**, *17*, 109–110. [CrossRef]

9. Tachibana, R.; Motoyoshi, M.; Shinohara, A.; Shigeeda, T.; Shimizu, N. Safe placement techniques for self-drilling orthodontic mini-implants. *Int. J. Oral Maxillofac. Surg.* **2012**, *41*, 1439–1444. [CrossRef]
10. Wilmes, B.; Rademacher, C.; Olthoff, G.; Drescher, D. Parameters affecting primary stability of orthodontic mini-implants. *J. Orofac. Orthop. Fortschr. Kieferorthopadie* **2006**, *67*, 162–174. [CrossRef]
11. Kuroda, S.; Sugawara, Y.; Deguchi, T.; Kyung, H.M.; Takano-Yamamoto, T. Clinical use of miniscrew implants as orthodontic anchorage: Success rates and postoperative discomfort. *Am. J. Orthod. Dentofac. Orthop.* **2007**, *131*, 9–15. [CrossRef]
12. Uemura, M.; Motoyoshi, M.; Yano, S.; Sakaguchi, M.; Igarashi, Y.; Shimizu, N. Orthodontic mini-implant stability and the ratio of pilot hole implant diameter. *Eur. J. Orthod.* **2012**, *34*, 52–56. [CrossRef]
13. Motoyoshi, M.; Hirabayashi, M.; Uemura, M.; Shimizu, N. Recommended placement torque when tightening an orthodontic mini-implant. *Clin. Oral Implant. Res.* **2006**, *17*, 109–114. [CrossRef]
14. Matsuoka, M.; Motoyoshi, M.; Sakaguchi, M.; Shinohara, A.; Shigeede, T.; Saito, Y.; Matsuda, M.; Shimizu, N. Friction heat during self-drilling of an orthodontic miniscrew. *Int. J. Oral Maxillofac. Surg.* **2011**, *40*, 191–194. [CrossRef] [PubMed]
15. Cheng, S.J.; Tseng, I.Y.; Lee, J.J.; Kok, S.H. A prospective study of the risk factors associated with failure of mini-implants used for orthodontic anchorage. *Int. J. Oral Maxillofac. Implant.* **2004**, *19*, 100–106.
16. Park, H.S.; Jeong, S.H.; Kwon, O.W. Factors affecting the clinical success of screw implants used as orthodontic anchorage. *Am. J. Orthod. Dentofac. Orthop.* **2006**, *130*, 18–25. [CrossRef] [PubMed]
17. Wu, T.Y.; Kuang, S.H.; Wu, C.H. Factors associated with the stability of mini-implants for orthodontic anchorage: A study of 414 samples in Taiwan. *J. Oral Maxillofac. Surg.* **2009**, *67*, 1595–1599. [CrossRef]
18. Gurdan, Z.; Vajta, L.; Toth, A.; Lempel, E.; Joob-Fancsaly, A.; Szalma, J. Effect of pre-drilling on intraosseous temperature during self-drilling mini-implant placement in a porcine mandible model. *J. Oral Sci.* **2017**, *59*, 47–53. [CrossRef] [PubMed]
19. Abouzgia, M.B.; James, D.F. Temperature rise during drilling through bone. *Int. J. Oral Maxillofac. Implant.* **1997**, *12*, 342–353.
20. Eriksson, R.A.; Albrektsson, T. The effect of heat on bone regeneration: An experimental study in the rabbit using the bone growth chamber. *J. Oral Maxillofac. Surg.* **1984**, *42*, 705–711. [CrossRef]
21. Mohlhenrich, S.C.; Modabber, A.; Steiner, T.; Mitchell, D.A.; Holzle, F. Heat generation and drill wear during dental implant site preparation: Systematic review. *Br. J. Oral Maxillofac. Surg.* **2015**, *53*, 679–689. [CrossRef]
22. Quaranta, A.; Andreana, S.; Spazzafumo, L.; Piemontese, M. An in vitro evaluation of heat production during osteotomy preparation for dental implants with compressive osteotomes. *Implant Dent.* **2013**, *22*, 161–164. [CrossRef] [PubMed]
23. Kim, H.J.; Yun, H.S.; Park, H.D.; Kim, D.H.; Park, Y.C. Soft-tissue and cortical-bone thickness at orthodontic implant sites. *Am. J. Orthod. Dentofac. Orthop.* **2006**, *130*, 177–182. [CrossRef] [PubMed]
24. Sener, B.C.; Dergin, G.; Gursoy, B.; Kelesoglu, E.; Slih, I. Effects of irrigation temperature on heat control in vitro at different drilling depths. *Clin. Oral Implant. Res.* **2009**, *20*, 294–298. [CrossRef]
25. Stelzle, F.; Frenkel, C.; Riemann, M.; Knipfer, C.; Stockmann, P.; Nkenke, E. The effect of load on heat production, thermal effects and expenditure of time during implant site preparation—An experimental ex vivo comparison between piezosurgery and conventional drilling. *Clin. Oral Implant. Res.* **2014**, *25*, e140–e148. [CrossRef] [PubMed]
26. Augustin, G.; Davila, S.; Udiljak, T.; Vedrina, D.S.; Bagatin, D. Determination of spatial distribution of increase in bone temperature during drilling by infrared thermography: Preliminary report. *Arch. Orthop. Trauma Surg.* **2009**, *129*, 703–709. [CrossRef] [PubMed]
27. Sedlin, E.D.; Hirsch, C. Factors affecting the determination of the physical properties of femoral cortical bone. *Acta Orthop. Scand.* **1966**, *37*, 29–48. [CrossRef] [PubMed]
28. Nam, O.; Yu, W.; Choi, M.Y.; Kyung, H.M. Monitoring of Bone Temperature During Osseous Preparation for Orthodontic Micro-Screw Implants: Effect of Motor Speed and Ressure. *Key Eng. Mater.* **2006**, *321–323*, 1044–1047. [CrossRef]
29. Wilmes, B.; Ottenstreuer, S.; Su, Y.Y.; Drescher, D. Impact of implant design on primary stability of orthodontic mini-implants. *J. Orofac. Orthop. Fortschr. Kieferorthopadie* **2008**, *69*, 42–50. [CrossRef] [PubMed]
30. Mishra, S.K.; Chowdhary, R. Heat generated by dental implant drills during osteotomy-a review: Heat generated by dental implant drills. *J. Indian Prosthodont. Soc.* **2014**, *14*, 131–143. [CrossRef] [PubMed]
31. Tehemar, S.H. Factors affecting heat generation during implant site preparation: A review of biologic observations and future considerations. *Int. J. Oral Maxillofac. Implant.* **1999**, *14*, 127–136.
32. Pandey, R.K.; Panda, S.S. Drilling of bone: A comprehensive review. *J. Clin. Orthop. Trauma* **2013**, *4*, 15–30. [CrossRef]
33. Barrak, I.; Boa, K.; Joob-Fancsaly, A.; Varga, E.; Sculean, A.; Piffko, J. Heat Generation During Guided and Freehand Implant Site Preparation at Drilling Speeds of 1500 and 2000 RPM at Different Irrigation Temperatures: An In Vitro Study. *Oral Health Prev. Dent.* **2019**, *17*, 309–316. [CrossRef] [PubMed]
34. Barrak, I.; Joob-Fancsaly, A.; Braunitzer, G.; Varga, E., Jr.; Boa, K.; Piffko, J. Intraosseous Heat Generation During Osteotomy Performed Freehand and Through Template With an Integrated Metal Guide Sleeve: An In Vitro Study. *Implant Dent.* **2018**, *27*, 342–350. [CrossRef] [PubMed]
35. Barrak, I.; Joob-Fancsaly, A.; Varga, E.; Boa, K.; Piffko, J. Effect of the Combination of Low-Speed Drilling and Cooled Irrigation Fluid on Intraosseous Heat Generation During Guided Surgical Implant Site Preparation: An In Vitro Study. *Implant Dent.* **2017**, *26*, 541–546. [CrossRef]

36. Boa, K.; Barrak, I.; Varga, E., Jr.; Joob-Fancsaly, A.; Varga, E.; Piffko, J. Intraosseous generation of heat during guided surgical drilling: An ex vivo study of the effect of the temperature of the irrigating fluid. *Br. J. Oral Maxillofac. Surg.* **2016**, *54*, 904–908. [CrossRef]
37. Papageorgiou, S.N.; Zogakis, I.P.; Papadopoulos, M.A. Failure rates and associated risk factors of orthodontic miniscrew implants: A meta-analysis. *Am. J. Orthod. Dentofac. Orthop.* **2012**, *142*, 577–595 e577. [CrossRef]
38. Inoue, M.; Kuroda, S.; Yasue, A.; Horiuchi, S.; Kyung, H.M.; Tanaka, E. Torque ratio as a predictable factor on primary stability of orthodontic miniscrew implants. *Implant Dent.* **2014**, *23*, 576–581. [CrossRef]
39. Eriksson, A.R.; Albrektsson, T. Temperature threshold levels for heat-induced bone tissue injury: A vital-microscopic study in the rabbit. *J. Prosthet. Dent.* **1983**, *50*, 101–107. [CrossRef]
40. Eriksson, A.R.; Albrektsson, T.; Albrektsson, B. Heat caused by drilling cortical bone. Temperature measured in vivo in patients and animals. *Acta Orthop. Scand.* **1984**, *55*, 629–631. [CrossRef]
41. Iyer, S.; Weiss, C.; Mehta, A. Effects of drill speed on heat production and the rate and quality of bone formation in dental implant osteotomies. Part II: Relationship between drill speed and healing. *Int. J. Prosthodont.* **1997**, *10*, 536–540. [PubMed]
42. Isler, S.C.; Cansiz, E.; Tanyel, C.; Soluk, M.; Selvi, F.; Cebi, Z. The effect of irrigation temperature on bone healing. *Int. J. Med. Sci.* **2011**, *8*, 704–708. [CrossRef] [PubMed]
43. Kondo, S.; Okada, Y.; Iseki, H.; Hori, T.; Takakura, K.; Kobayashi, A.; Nagata, H. Thermological study of drilling bone tissue with a high-speed drill. *Neurosurgery* **2000**, *46*, 1162–1168. [CrossRef] [PubMed]
44. Ginta, T.; Ariwahjoedi, B. Cutting Force and Temperature Variation in Bone Drilling—A Review. *Adv. Mater. Res.* **2014**, *845*, 934–938. [CrossRef]
45. Ben Achour, A.; Petto, C.; Meissner, H.; Hipp, D.; Nestler, A.; Lauer, G.; Teicher, U. The Influence of Thrust Force on the Vitality of Bone Chips Harvested for Autologous Augmentation during Dental Implantation. *Materials* **2019**, *12*, 3695. [CrossRef]
46. Teicher, U.; Ben Achour, A.; Nestler, A.; Brosius, A.; Lauer, G. Process based analysis of manually controlled drilling processes for bone. *AIP Conf. Proc.* **2018**, *1960*, 070025. [CrossRef]
47. Pellicer-Chover, H.; Penarrocha-Oltra, D.; Aloy-Prosper, A.; Sanchis-Gonzalez, J.C.; Penarrocha-Diago, M.A.; Penarrocha-Diago, M. Comparison of peri-implant bone loss between conventional drilling with irrigation versus low-speed drilling without irrigation. *Med. Oral Patol. Oral Cir. Bucal* **2017**, *22*, e730–e736. [CrossRef]

Article

Effect of Adhesive Application Method on the Enamel Bond Durability of a Two-Step Adhesive System Utilizing a Universal Adhesive-Derived Primer

Toshiki Takamizawa [1,*], Munenori Yokoyama [1], Keiichi Sai [1], Sho Shibasaki [1], Wayne W. Barkmeier [2], Mark A. Latta [2], Akimasa Tsujimoto [3] and Masashi Miyazaki [1]

1 Department of Operative Dentistry, Nihon University School of Dentistry, Tokyo 101-8310, Japan; demu20022@g.nihon-u.ac.jp (M.Y.); sai.keiichi@nihon-u.ac.jp (K.S.); shibasaki.shou@nihon-u.ac.jp (S.S.); miyazaki.masashi@nihon-u.ac.jp (M.M.)
2 Department of General Dentistry, Creighton University School of Dentistry, Omaha, NE 68102, USA; waynebarkmeier@creighton.edu (W.W.B.); mlatta@creighton.edu (M.A.L.)
3 Department of Operative Dentistry, University of Iowa College of Dentistry, Iowa City, IA 52242, USA; akimasa-tsujimoto@uiowa.edu
* Correspondence: takamizawa.toshiki@nihon-u.ac.jp

Abstract: This study aimed to evaluate the effect of the adhesive application method on the durability of the enamel bond and the thickness of the adhesive layer. A new-generation two-step universal adhesive system, G2-Bond Universal, and two conventional two-step adhesive systems were utilized. The shear bond strength to bovine enamel was measured after thermal cycling in both etch-and-rinse and self-etch modes. Fifteen specimens were divided into three groups as follows: Group I, wherein a strong air stream was applied over the bonding agent for 5 s; Group II, wherein a gentle air stream was applied over the bonding agent for 5 s; and Group III, which was prepared as in Group II, followed by the application of a second layer of the bonding agent and a gentle air stream for 5 s. The durability of the enamel bond and thickness of the tested adhesives were influenced by the application method in both etching modes. The application method used in Group II appeared to be most suitable in terms of the bonding of the adhesives to the enamel. The new-generation two-step self-etch adhesive, comprising a universal adhesive-derived primer and a hydrophobic bonding agent, showed superior bond performance to the conventional two-step adhesive systems.

Keywords: two-step adhesive system; universal adhesive-derived primer; adhesive layer thickness; enamel bond durability

1. Introduction

The methods used to apply adhesives can considerably influence the clinical outcomes, regardless of the adhesive system utilized [1,2]. Previous studies investigated the bond effectiveness of various adhesive systems using different adhesive application methods and concluded that bond performance and morphological features in the vicinity of the resin–tooth interface were strongly influenced by the adhesive application method [3–6]. For instance, a warm air blow technique [1], the etching mode [4], an active application technique [5,6], and double-layer application [7–9] have been reported to improve the bonding performance of universal adhesives. Some of these techniques also influence the morphological features at the interface between the adhesive layer and the tooth substrate and the thickness of the adhesive layer [7–9].

The configuration of the tooth cavity is highly variable—depending on the location, depth, and size of the lesion, and the defects of the tooth substrate—and can influence not only the contraction stress of the resin composite but also the methods of adhesive application, air blowing, and filling [10,11]. The thickness of the adhesive layer might vary within the cavity. Furthermore, the thickness of the adhesive layer depends on the viscosity of the adhesive, the method used to apply the adhesive, and the strength of the air blow stream [7–9]. When comparing the thickness of the adhesive layer between multiple-step adhesive systems and single-step self-etch adhesive systems, including universal adhesive systems, the adhesive layers in the three-step etch-and-rinse and two-step self-etch adhesive systems were approximately five times thicker than those in the single-step self-etch adhesives [12]. A thicker adhesive layer is thought to improve the bond performance because it reduces the concentration of local stress, suppresses crack propagation, and decreases the relative thickness of the oxygen inhibited layer [7–9]. Hashimoto et al. [13] investigated the effect of consecutive coatings of the three-step adhesive system on the dentin microtensile bond strength and concluded that the bond strengths increased with each coating, up to four coats; no increase in bond strength was observed after more than four coats. However, the optimal thickness of the adhesive layer remains controversial and may vary among the different adhesive systems and tooth substrates. Phosphoric acid pre-etching has profound effects on the immediate and long-term bond durability because of the creation of a strong mechanical interlocking between the adhesive layer and the enamel substrate [14].

A recently introduced two-step adhesive system comprises a 2-hydroxyethyl methacrylate (HEMA)-free universal adhesive-derived primer and a hydrophobic bonding agent without any solvents or functional monomers. This adhesive system showed superior bond durability under thermal stress and long-term water storage when compared with conventional two-step self-etch adhesives, regardless of the tooth substrate or etching mode used [15]. Moreover, Tamura et al. [16] showed that the enamel and dentin bond durability achieved under fatigue stress by the new two-step adhesive system was equivalent to that attained by a gold standard two-step self-etch adhesive, Clearfil SE Bond. Thus, this new adhesive system might be able to achieve a durable bond performance and can be used in the clinical setting owing to the presence of a universal adhesive-derived primer. However, there is little information regarding the bond performance of this two-step adhesive system when applied using different methods.

This study aimed to investigate the effect of the adhesive application method on the durability of the enamel bond and the thickness of the adhesive layer using the new two-step adhesive system and compare it with those of the conventional two-step self-etch adhesive systems. The null hypotheses were as follows: (i) the enamel bond durability of the universal adhesive-derived two-step adhesive system (under thermal stress) would vary with the different application methods used, and (ii) the trend of enamel bond durability based on the different application methods used would not differ from those observed using the tested conventional two-step adhesive systems.

2. Materials and Methods

2.1. Study Materials

Table 1 lists the two-step adhesive systems used in this study. An adhesive system utilizing a universal adhesive-derived primer, G2-Bond Universal (GU, GC, Tokyo, Japan), was used. Additionally, two conventional two-step adhesive systems, Clearfil SE Bond 2 (CS, Kuraray Noritake Dental, Tokyo, Japan) and OptiBond eXTRa (OX, Kerr, Brea, CA, USA), were used for comparison. The phosphoric acid etching agent Ultra-Etch was obtained from Ultradent Products (South Jordan, UT, USA), and the resin composite Clearfil AP-X was obtained from Kuraray Noritake Dental. A light-emitting diode curing unit with an internal tip diameter of 10 mm (Valo; Ultradent Products) was used, and a light irradiance of 1000 mW/cm^2 (standard mode) was maintained during the course of the experiment.

Table 1. Materials used in this study.

Code	Adhesive System (Lot. No.)	Main Components	pH (Primer)	Manufacturer
CS	Clearfil SE Bond 2 (Primer: 5852494) (Adhesive: 5847004)	Primer: MDP, HEMA, water, initiators Adhesive: MDP, HEMA, bis-GMA, initiators, microfiller	2.0	Kuraray Noritake Dental, Tokyo, Japan
GU	G2-Bond Universal (Primer: 190711) (Adhesive: 190711)	Primer: 4-MET, MDP, MDTP, dimethacrylate monomer, acetone, water, photoinitiator, filler Adhesive: dimethacrylate monomer, bis-GMA, filler, photoinitiator	1.5	GC, Tokyo, Japan
OX	OptiBond eXTRa Universal (Primer: 58470004) (Adhesive: 5852494)	Primer: GPDM, HEMA, acetone, ethyl alcohol Adhesive: GPDM, HEMA, glycerol dimethacrylate, ethyl alcohol, sodium hexafluorosilicate	1.6	Kerr, Brea, CA, USA
	Resin Composite	Main Components		Manufacturer
	Clearfil AP-X (N416213)	bis-GMA, TEGDMA, silane barium glass filler, silane silica filler, silanated colloidal silica, CQ, pigments, others		Kuraray Noritake Dental

MDP: 10-methacryloyloxydecyl dihydrogen phosphate, HEMA: 2-hydroxyethyl methacrylate, bis-GMA: 2,2-bis[4-(2-hydroxy-3-methacryloyloxypropoxy) phenyl] propane, 4-MET: 4-methacryloyloxyethyl trimellitate, MDTP:10-methacryloyloxydecyl dihydrogen thiophosphate, GPDM: glycerol dimethacrylate dihydrogen phosphate, TEGDMA: triethyleneglycol dimethacrylate, CQ: dl-camphorquinone.

2.2. Specimen Preparation

Bovine teeth were used as a substitute for human teeth. Approximately two-thirds of the apical root of each tooth was removed using a diamond-impregnated disk in a precision sectioning saw (IsoMet 1000 Precision Sectioning Saw; Buehler, Lake Bluff, IL, USA). The labial surfaces were subjected to mechanical grinding/polishing (Ecomet 4; Buehler) with a wet #180-grit silicon carbide (SiC) paper (Fuji Star Type DDC; Sankyo Rikagaku, Saitama, Japan) to create a flat enamel surface, approximately 8 mm in diameter. The prepared tooth was then inserted in self-curing acrylic resin (Tray Resin II; Shofu, Kyoto, Japan) to expose the flattened enamel surface. The adherent enamel bonding surfaces were wet polished using #240-grit SiC paper followed by #320-grit SiC paper (Fuji Star Type DDC). We used 810 bovine teeth for SBS tests and 180 teeth for adhesive layer thickness measurements (Figure 1).

2.3. Adhesive Application Protocol and Thermal Cycling

As part of the design process for this study, we assumed that variations in clinical bonding procedures might result in the creation of different adhesive layer thicknesses. Such variation may occur in clinical situations due to misunderstanding of bonding procedures, cavity configuration, or errors in handling. We therefore designed protocols to generate adhesive layers of different thicknesses. Table 2 shows the adhesive application protocols for the adhesives. Fifteen specimens were prepared to determine the shear bond strength (SBS) to enamel in the self-etch mode (SE mode, without phosphoric acid pre-etching) and etch-and-rinse mode (ER mode, phosphoric acid pre-etching for 15 s). The bonded area was standardized as the center of the labial surface. For the ER mode, 35% phosphoric acid was applied to the enamel surface for 15 s, before applying the primer, and rinsed with water spray from a dental syringe for 15 s. For both etching modes, the primers were applied to the adherent surface following the manufacturers' instructions. The 15 specimens were divided into three groups on the basis of the application method as follows:

Group I: a strong stream of air was applied over the bonding agent for 5 s;

Group II: a gentle stream of air was applied over the bonding agent for 5 s (the strength of the air blow was similar to that recommended by each manufacturers' instructions);

Group III: prepared as in Group II followed by the application of a second layer of the bonding agent and a gentle air blow for 5 s.

The bonding agent-treated enamel surfaces were light irradiated for 10 s. The bonded specimens were created by clamping the plastic molds (height, 2.0 mm; internal diameter, 2.38 mm; Ultradent Products) in a fixture against the adherent surfaces. The resin composite was condensed into the mold and light irradiated for 20 s. All steps in the bonding procedures were conducted by a single operator over the course of the whole experiment. After removing the excessive bonding agent with a sharp scalpel, we subjected the bonded specimens to thermal cycling (TC) after storage in 37 °C distilled water for 24 h. The specimens were subjected to either 10,000 or 30,000 TCs between 5 °C and 55 °C, with a dwell time of 30 s, before the SBS test [6]. Baseline specimens were stored in distilled water at 37 °C for 24 h before the SBS test (24 h groups).

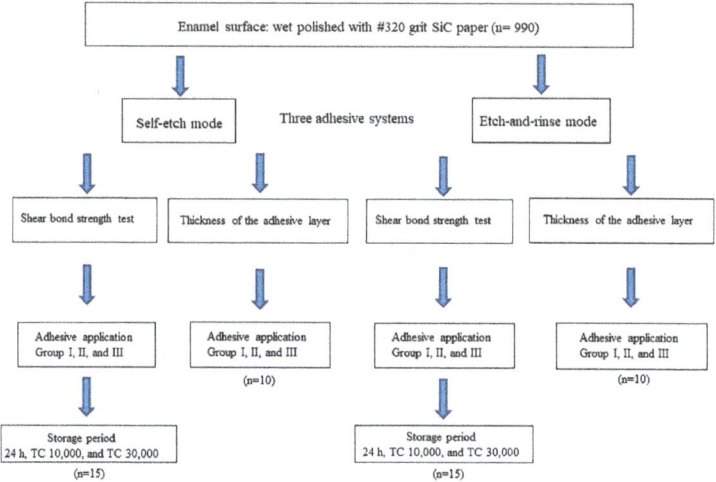

Figure 1. Flow diagram of this study.

2.4. SBS Tests

Notched-edge SBS tests were conducted in accordance with ISO 29022 [17]. The bonded specimens were fixed with an Ultradent shearing fixture and loaded to failure at a crosshead speed of 1.0 mm per min using a universal testing machine (Type 5500R; Instron, Norwood, MA, USA). The SBS values (MPa) were calculated by dividing the peak load at failure by the area of the bonded enamel. The debonded sites on the enamel surfaces and the debonded resin composite rods were observed using an optical microscope (SZH-131; Olympus, Tokyo, Japan) to evaluate the failure mode. When more than 80% of the adherent area was occupied by the adhesive, resin composite, or enamel substrate, the failure mode was classified as an adhesive failure, cohesive failure in resin, or cohesive failure in enamel, respectively. Other failure patterns, such as partially adhesive and partially cohesive, were classified as mixed failures [8].

2.5. Thickness of the Adhesive Layer

To determine the thickness of the adhesive layer in each group, we observed the resin/enamel interfaces using a confocal laser scanning microscope (CLSM, VK-8700; Keyence, Osaka, Japan). Ten bonded specimens per group were made, as described earlier, and embedded in epoxy resin (Epon 812; Nisshin EM, Tokyo, Japan). The embedded specimens were longitudinally sectioned with a precision sectioning saw (IsoMet 1000 Precision Sectioning Saw). The sectioned surfaces were wet polished using #4000-grit SiC paper and a sequence of carbide polishing papers (Struers, Cleveland, OH, USA). The resin/enamel interfaces of all the specimens were observed under the CLSM, and the thickness of the adhesive layer was measured using the software supplied with the CLSM. Profilometric measurements were conducted in three regions, at the center and two further points located one-quarter of the interface length from the center of the specimen, and the mean values were calculated for each group.

Table 2. Application protocols for pre-etching and two-step adhesive systems.

Etching-Mode		Pre-Etching Protocol
SE (self-etch)		Phosphoric acid pre-etching was not performed.
ER (etch-and-rinse)		Enamel surfaces were phosphoric acid etched for 15 s. Etched surface was rinsed with water for 15 s and air-dried.
Adhesive	Group	Adhesive Application Protocol
CS	I	Primer was applied to air-dried enamel surface for 20 s followed by medium air pressure for 5 s. Bonding agent was then applied to the primed surface and a strong stream of air was applied over the bonding agent for 5 s. Light irradiated for 10 s.
	II	Primer was applied to air-dried enamel surface for 20 s followed by medium air pressure for 5 s. Bonding agent was then applied to the primed surface and was gently air thinned for 5 s. Light irradiated for 10 s.
	III	After bonding procedure of Group II without light irradiation, another layer of bonding agent was applied and was gently air thinned for 5 s. Bonding agent was light irradiated for 10 s.
GU	I	Primer was applied to air-dried enamel surface for 10 s and then a strong stream of air was applied over the liquid primer for 5 s. Bonding agent was then applied to the primed surface and a strong stream of air was applied over the bonding agent for 5 s. Light irradiated for 10 s.
	II	Primer was applied to air-dried enamel surface for 10 s and then a strong stream of air was applied over the primer for 5 s. Bonding agent was then applied to the primed surface and was gently air thinned for 5 s. Light irradiated for 10 s.
	III	After bonding procedure of Group II without light irradiation, another layer of bonding agent was applied and was gently air thinned for 5 s. Light irradiated for 10 s.
OX	I	Primer was applied to air-dried enamel surface with rubbing action for 20 s. Medium air pressure was applied to the surface for 5 s. Bonding agent was applied to the primed surface with rubbing action for 15 s, and then a strong stream of air was applied over the bonding agent for 5 s. Light irradiated for 10 s.
	II	Primer was applied to air-dried enamel surface with rubbing action for 20 s. Medium air pressure was applied to the surface for 5 s. Bonding agent was applied to the primed surface with rubbing action for 15 s and then gently air thinned for 5 s. Light irradiated for 10 s.
	III	After bonding procedure of Group II without light irradiation another layer of bonding agent was applied and was gently air thinned for 5 s. Light irradiated for 10 s.

Strength of air-blow for each protocol; Group I: strong air stream; Group II: gentle air stream (similar to each manufacturer's instructions); Group III: gentle air stream was applied to each adhesive layer.

2.6. Scanning Electron Microscopy Observations

Representative adhesive treated enamel surfaces and resin/enamel interfaces were observed using scanning electron microscopy (SEM; ERA-8800FE; Elionix, Tokyo, Japan). The enamel surfaces were treated, following the manufacturers' instructions, and rinsed with acetone and water. Additionally, the prepared specimen with #320-grit SiC paper, with and without 35% phosphoric acid pre-etching for 15 s, but not rinsed with acetone, were evaluated (baseline) to compare the morphological changes after adhesive treatment.

Bonded specimens stored in 37 °C distilled water for 24 h were embedded in the epoxy resin (Epon 812) and longitudinally sectioned with a precision sectioning saw. The sectioned surfaces of the resin/enamel interfaces were polished to a high gloss using abrasive disks (Fuji Star Type DDC) followed by diamond pastes (DP-Paste; Struers,

Ballerup, Denmark) down to a particle size of 0.25 μm, followed by ultrasonic cleaning for 20 min. The specimens were dehydrated in a graded series of tert-butyl alcohol (50% for 20 min, 75% for 20 min, 95% for 20 min, and 100% for 2 h) and transferred from the final 100% bath to a freeze dryer (Model ID-3; Elionix) for 30 min. The specimens with the resin/enamel interfaces were then subjected to argon–ion beam etching (EIS-200ER; Elionix) for 45 s with the ion beam (accelerating voltage, 1.0 kV; ion current density, 0.4 mA/cm^2) directed perpendicular to the polished surface [12]. Finally, all the specimens were coated with a thin film of gold using a sputter coater (Quick Coater Type SC-701; Sanyu Electron, Tokyo, Japan). Further observations were performed under a field emission SEM at an operating voltage of 10 kV.

2.7. Statistical Analysis

A statistical power analysis (G Power calculator) indicated that at least 13 specimens were required to effectively measure the SBS in each group and 9.4 measurements of the thickness of the adhesive layer were required per group. The parameters used were as follows: f = 0.25, α = 0.05, β = 0.2, and power = 0.8. Hence, the experiments were performed using 15 specimens for the SBS test and 10 specimens for the thickness measurements. Post hoc power tests were performed on the gathered data, and the sample size was found to be adequate.

The homogeneity of variance (Bartlett's test) and distribution of normality (Shapiro–Wilk test) were confirmed before analysis of variance (ANOVA) was performed. In the case of the SBS data, the groups that underwent the SE and ER modes were analyzed separately, and three-way ANOVA followed by Tukey's honest significant difference (HSD) test (α = 0.05) was used to analyze each data set. The following factors were used: adhesive application method, TC period, and adhesive system. One-way ANOVA, followed by Tukey's HSD test (α = 0.05), was used for comparisons within subsets.

In the case of the thickness measurements, three-way ANOVA, followed by Tukey's HSD test (α = 0.05), was used to analyze the full data set using the following factors: etching mode, adhesive application method, and adhesive system. The statistical analyses were performed using a statistical analysis software system (Sigma Plot 13; SPSS, Chicago, IL, USA).

3. Results

3.1. SBS in SE Mode

The SBS values of the enamel under TC in the SE mode are presented in Table 3 and Figure 2. Three-way ANOVA showed that all the factors significantly influenced the values and that all interactions were significant ($p < 0.001$).

The mean SBS values in the SE mode ranged from 29.9 to 43.8 MPa in CS, 35.5 to 47.7 MPa in GU, and 29.0 to 39.7 MPa in OX. Considering the trends of SBS in the different application groups, we found that all the adhesives showed higher SBS values in Group II than in Groups I and III, regardless of the storage period. All adhesives in Group II showed significantly higher SBS values than those at 24 h in Group I and at TC 30,000 in Group III. In Group I, although no significant differences in SBS values were observed among the storage periods in the CS subgroup, GU and OX presented with significantly higher SBS values at TC 10,000 and TC 30,000 than at 24 h (Table 3). In Group II, no significant differences were observed among the storage periods for all three adhesives, whereas in Group III, although no significant differences in the SBS values were observed among the various storage periods for CS and GU, OX presented with a significantly higher value at TC 10,000 in comparison with those at the other storage periods. Furthermore, GU showed higher SBS values than the other adhesives, regardless of the storage period or application group. In particular, GU presented with significantly higher SBS values than the other adhesives at all storage periods in Group I and at 24 h and TC 10,000 in Group II.

Table 3. Influence of application method on enamel bond strength (SE mode).

	Group I			Group II			Group III		
	24 h	TC 10,000	TC 30,000	24 h	TC 10,000	TC 30,000	24 h	TC 10,000	TC 30,000
CS	32.8 (3.2) [bCD]	33.9 (4.5) [bCD]	29.9 (1.8) [cD]	41.2 (2.5) [bA]	43.7 (3.2) [bA]	43.8 (1.7) [aA]	39.6 (3.9) [aAB]	35.9 (4.9) [bBC]	36.0 (4.5) [abBC]
GU	35.5 (1.6) [aB]	47.4 (3.1) [aA]	44.2 (2.1) [aA]	46.9 (4.4) [aA]	47.7 (1.8) [aA]	45.9 (2.7) [aA]	36.3 (4.5) [aB]	39.4 (3.0) [aB]	37.8 (3.5) [aB]
OX	29.9 (1.5) [cD]	35.1 (1.8) [bBC]	34.0 (2.2) [bC]	37.9 (2.0) [cAB]	39.4 (3.1) [cA]	38.3 (4.4) [bAB]	29.0 (2.4) [bD]	39.7 (2.6) [aA]	32.9 (3.4) [bCD]

n = 15, mean (SD) in MPa. Same lower-case letters in vertical columns indicate no difference at 5% significance level. Same capital letters in horizontal rows indicate no difference at 5% significance level. Values in parentheses indicate standard deviation.

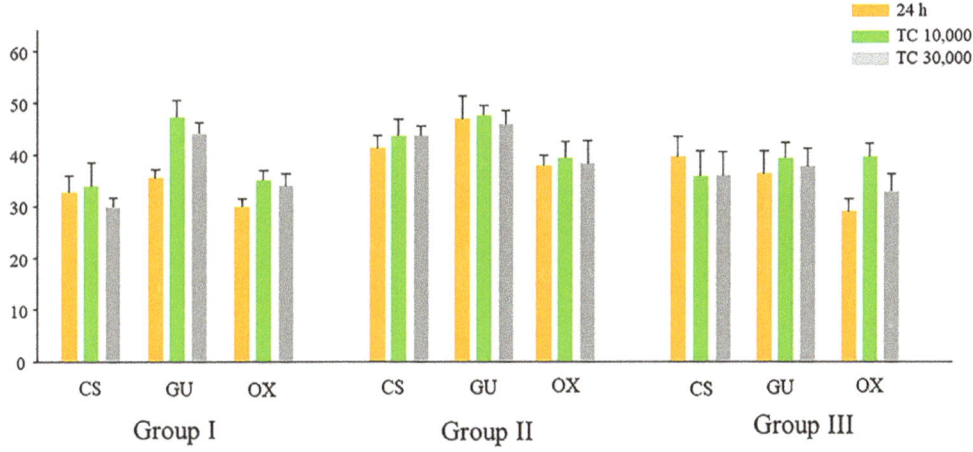

Figure 2. Influence of application method on enamel SBS (SE mode).

3.2. SBS in ER Mode

Table 4 and Figure 3 present the enamel SBS values in the ER mode under TC. Three-way ANOVA showed that all the factors significantly influenced the values and that all interactions were significant ($p < 0.001$).

The mean SBS values in the SE mode ranged from 38.4 to 48.3 MPa in CS, 38.0 to 51.6 MPa in GU, and 30.9 to 44.9 MPa in OX. All the adhesives showed higher SBS values in Group II than in Groups I and III, regardless of the storage period (Table 4). In particular, the SBS values of all three adhesives at TC 10,000 in Group II were significantly higher than at the other storage periods in Groups I and III, except for GU at TC 10,000 and TC 30,000 in Group I. In Group I, although no significant differences in SBS values were observed among the storage periods in the case of CS, GU and OX presented with significantly higher values after TC than at 24 h (Table 4). In Group II, no significant differences among the storage periods were observed in the cases of CS and GU. Similarly, no significant differences among the storage periods were observed in the case of CS in Group III; however, GU and OX presented with significantly lower SBS values at TC 30,000 than at the other storage periods. The SBS values in OX were significantly lower than in the other adhesives during most of the storage periods, regardless of the application group (Table 4). Furthermore, GU and OX showed significantly higher SBS values in the ER mode at 24 h than in the SE mode. However, no significant differences in the SBS values of the three adhesives were observed between the SE and ER modes at TC 30,000 in Group III.

Table 4. Influence of application method on enamel bond strength (ER mode).

	Group I			Group II			Group III		
	24 h	TC 10,000	TC 30,000	24 h	TC 10,000	TC 30,000	24 h	TC 10,000	TC 30,000
CS	* 42.0 (2.5) ^{aBC}	* 41.3 (3.9) ^{bBC}	* 43.6 (3.2) ^{bB}	* 44.3 (4.0) ^{bAB}	* 48.3 (3.7) ^{aA}	43.9 (2.6) ^{bAB}	42.6 (3.1) ^{aBC}	38.4 (4.6) ^{bCD}	38.0 (2.5) ^{aD}
GU	* 41.9 (3.2) ^{aBC}	49.1 (4.5) ^{aA}	* 50.0 (2.5) ^{aA}	* 50.1 (3.7) ^{aA}	* 50.8 (2.8) ^{aA}	* 51.6 (2.7) ^{aA}	* 42.7 (2.5) ^{aB}	* 43.9 (2.3) ^{aB}	38.0 (2.3) ^{aC}
OX	* 36.2 (4.1) ^{bCD}	* 40.3 (2.5) ^{bB}	* 40.5 (2.5) ^{cB}	* 41.6 (3.1) ^{bAB}	* 44.9 (1.9) ^{bA}	39.9 (2.3) ^{cB}	* 33.9 (2.5) ^{bDE}	39.0 (1.4) ^{bBC}	30.9 (2.9) ^{bE}

n = 15, mean (SD) in MPa. Same lower-case letters in vertical columns indicate no difference at 5% significance level. Same capital letters in horizontal rows indicate no difference at 5% significance level. Values in parentheses indicate standard deviation. Asterisk indicates significant differences between SE mode and ER mode at 5% significance level.

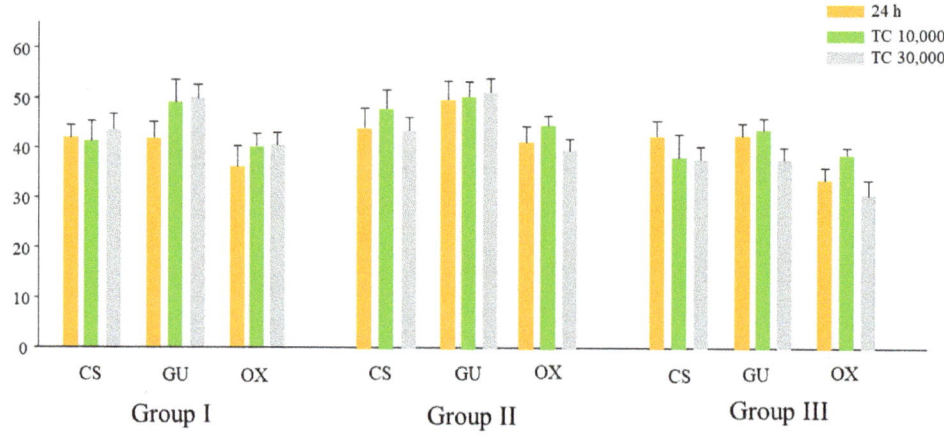

Figure 3. Influence of application method on enamel SBS (ER mode).

3.3. Failure Mode Analysis of Debonded Specimens after SBS

Figure 4 shows the frequencies of the failure modes in the tested adhesive systems. In the SE mode, all the adhesive systems in the 24 h and TC 30,000 groups predominantly presented with adhesive failure, regardless of the application method. The proportion of mixed or cohesive failure in the enamel was markedly higher in Group II at TC 10,000 than the other groups. In the ER mode, the frequencies of mixed and cohesive failure in enamel were higher than those in the SE mode. In particular, CS and GU showed higher frequencies of these failure modes in Group II at 24 h and TC 10,000 than in the other groups.

3.4. Thickness of the Adhesive Layer

Table 5 and Figure 5 present the thicknesses of the adhesive layer in the different adhesive systems under different application methods. Three-way ANOVA revealed that although the application method and adhesive systems used significantly influenced the thickness of the adhesive layer ($p < 0.001$), the etching mode did not have any influence ($p = 0.974$). The three-way interaction between the etching mode, application method, and type of adhesive system was not significant ($p = 0.987$). Although the two-way interaction between the application method and type of adhesive system used was significant ($p < 0.05$), other interactions, such as those between the etching mode and application method and etching mode and type of adhesive system used, were not significant ($p = 0.697$ and $p = 0.873$, respectively).

The mean adhesive thickness ranged from 8.2 to 20.2 μm in Group I, 34.4 to 56.9 μm in Group II, and 105.9 to 158.7 μm in Group III (Table 5). In Group I, GU showed a significantly thicker adhesive layer than the other adhesive systems in both etching modes. In Group II, although no significant differences were observed between GU and CS, OX showed a significantly thinner adhesive layer than the other adhesive systems in both etching modes.

In Group III, GU showed a significantly thicker adhesive layer than OX in both etching modes. The coefficient of variation (CV) was obtained from the mean adhesive thickness and standard deviation. The CV ranged from 7.6% to 15.9% in Group I, 13.5% to 26.8% in Group II, and 22.5% to 35.8% in Group III. The CV tended to increase with the increase in thickness of the adhesive thickness (Group I < Group II < Group III), regardless of the adhesive system.

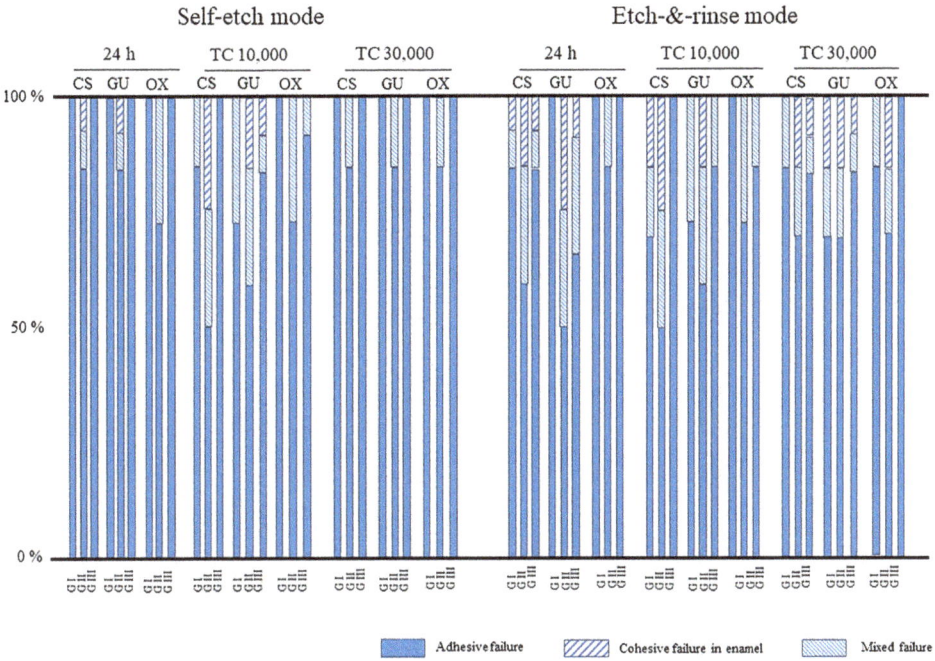

Figure 4. Failure mode analysis of the debonded enamel specimens. CS: Clearfil SE Bond 2, GU: G2-Bond Universal, OX: OptiBond eXTRa, TC: thermal cycle, G I/II/III: Group I/II/III.

Table 5. Thickness of adhesive layer in different application methods in different adhesive systems.

	Group I		Group II		Group III	
	SE	ER	SE	ER	SE	ER
CS	8.9 (0.7) [bC] [7.9%]	9.2 (0.7) [bC] [7.6%]	49.6 (7.1) [aB] [14.3%]	52.5 (7.5) [aB] [14.3%]	134.4 (48.1) [abA] [35.8%]	134.6 (47.7) [abA] [35.4%]
GU	19.2 (3.1) [aC] [15.6%]	20.2 (2.7) [aC] [13.4%]	52.9 (10.9) [aB] [20.6%]	56.9 (7.7) [aB] [13.5%]	158.7 (39.4) [aA] [24.8%]	157.8 (38.5) [aA] [24.4%]
OX	8.2 (1.3) [bC] [15.9%]	8.2 (1.2) [bC] [14.6%]	34.4 (8.2) [bB] [23.8%]	37.0 (9.9) [bB] [26.8%]	115.1 (25.9) [bA] [22.5%]	105.9 (25.0) [bA] [23.6%]

n = 12, mean (SD) in μm. Same lower-case letters in vertical columns indicate no difference at 5% significance level. Same capital letters in horizontal rows indicate no difference at 5% significance level. Values in parentheses indicate standard deviation. Percentage values in brackets indicate coefficient of variation.

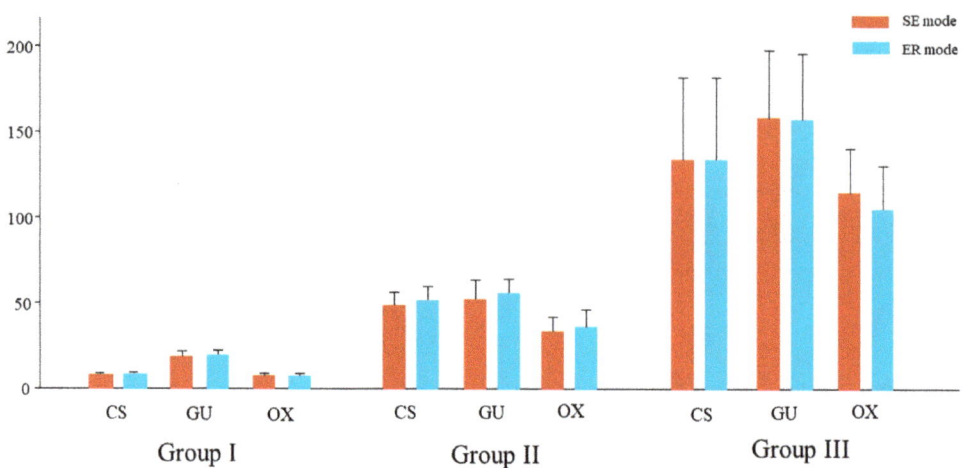

Figure 5. Thickness of adhesive layer in different application methods in different adhesive systems.

3.5. SEM Observations

Representative SEM images of treated and baseline enamel surfaces are shown in Figure 6. The baseline specimen ground with SiC papers exhibited scratch marks from the carbide polishing paper; additionally, the smear layer along with some enamel fragments was observed (Figure 6A). In the baseline specimen treated with phosphoric acid, the smear layer was completely removed, and a typical etching pattern was observed (Figure 6B). All the adhesive systems had a similar morphological appearance in the SE mode; most of the smear layer was dissolved, and a shallow etching pattern was observed. Particularly, the enamel rods were more clearly observed in OX than in the other adhesive systems (Figure 6G). Conversely, in the ER mode, although the adhesive systems showed similar morphological appearances to those of the baseline specimen treated with phosphoric acid, the spicular etching pattern appeared to be collapsed in OX (Figure 6H).

Figures 7–9 show representative resin/enamel interfaces. All the adhesive systems showed excellent adaptation between the adhesive layer and the decalcified enamel substrate in both etching modes. No clear differences were observed in the thickness of the adhesive layer in the different etching modes, regardless of the adhesive system or application method used. In Group I (Figure 7), the thickness of the adhesive layers in CS and OX were similar (approximately 10 μm), but GU presented with twice the thickness of the other adhesive systems. In Groups II and III (Figures 8 and 9), the thickness of the adhesive layers in CS and GU were similar and higher than that in OX. In the ER mode, the smear layer was completely dissolved, and adhesive interpenetration with enamel as resin tags was clearly observed, regardless of the adhesive system or application method used. On the contrary, enamel resin tags were not clearly seen in the SE mode, regardless of the adhesive system or application used. Part of the smear layer remained on the treated surface and created a hybrid layer (Figures 7C, 8C and 9A,C,E), which was infiltrated by the resin monomers in some instances. The ultrastructure of the adhesive layer was dependent on the adhesive system used. Unlike CS and GU, somewhat larger irregular fillers (approximately 0.1–0.5 μm in size) and nano-sized fillers were observed in OX. The thickness of the adhesive layer differed with the different adhesive systems and application methods used.

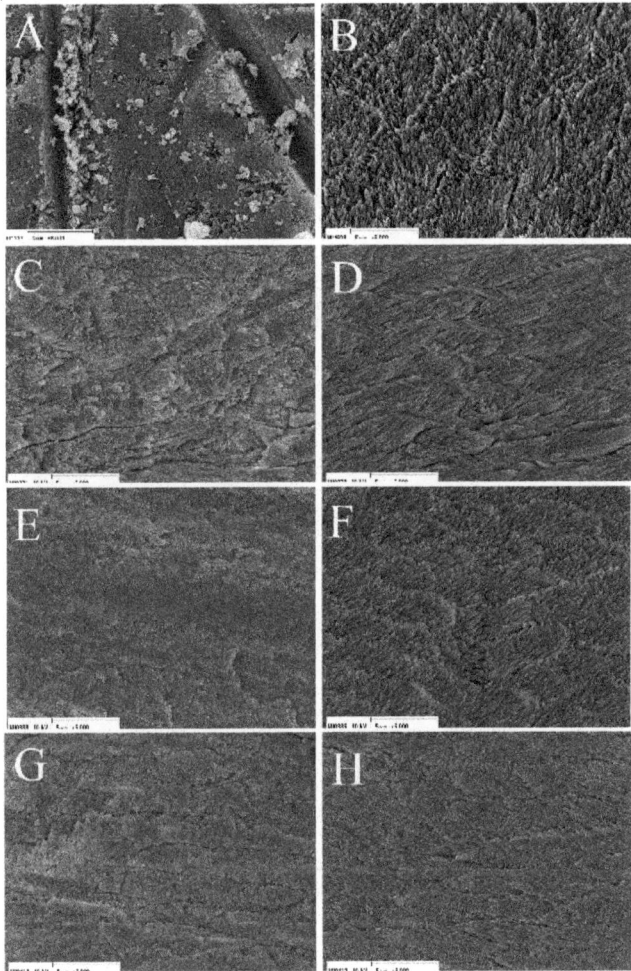

Figure 6. Representative SEM images of the treated enamel surface. (**A**) Ground with SiC paper #320 (×5000). (**B**) Phosphoric acid etching for 15 s (×5000). (**C**) CS in SE mode (×5000). (**D**) CS in ER mode (×5000). (**E**) GU in SE mode (×5000). (**F**) GU in ER mode (×5000). (**G**) OX in SE mode (×5000). (**H**) OX in ER mode (×5000).

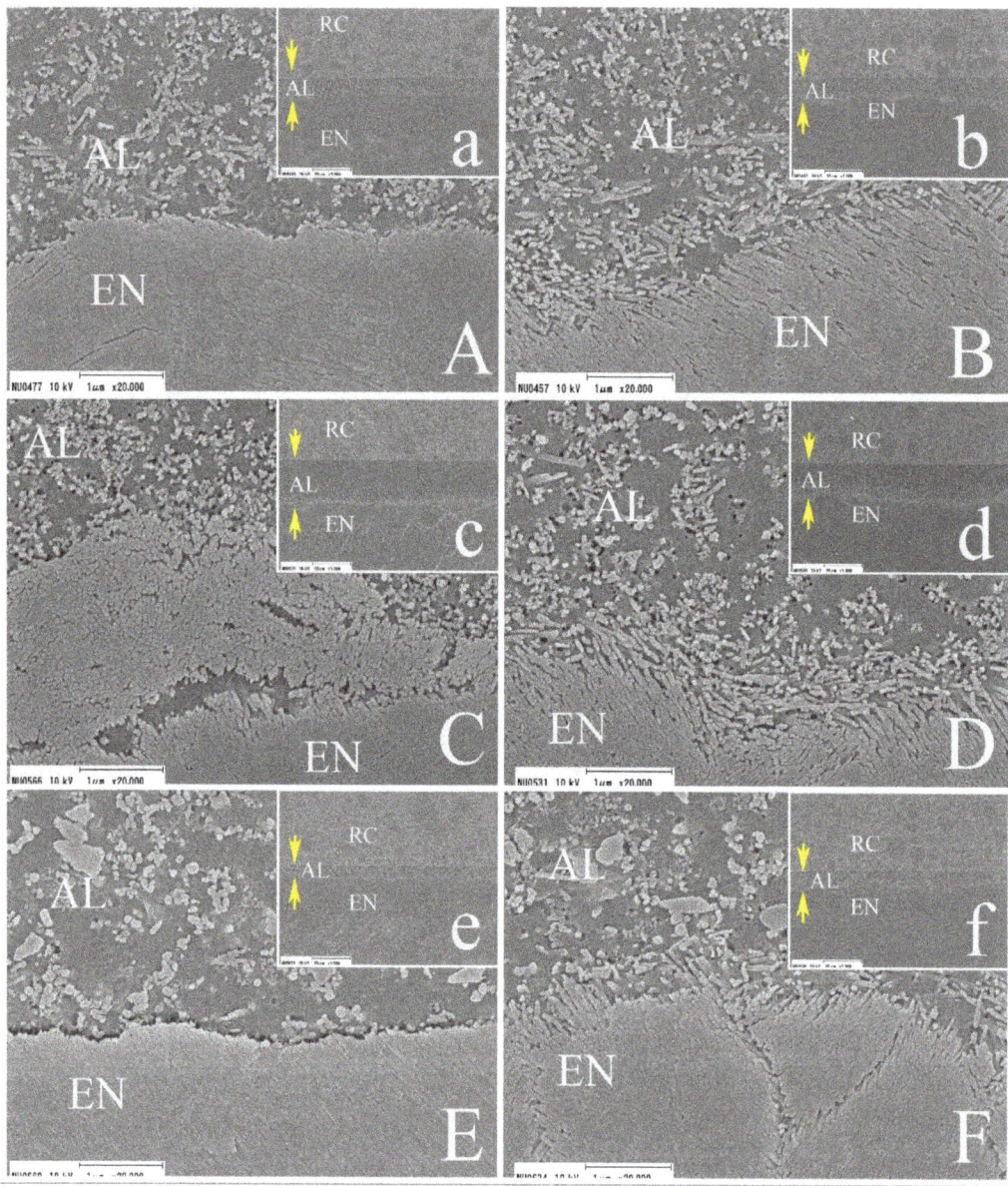

Figure 7. Representative SEM images of resin/enamel interfaces (Group I). (**A**) CS in SE mode (×20,000, ×1000). (**B**) CS in ER mode (×20,000, ×1000). (**C**) GU in SE mode (×20,000, ×1000). (**D**) GU in ER mode (×20,000, ×1000). (**E**) OX in SE mode (×20,000, ×1000). (**F**) OX in ER mode (×20,000, ×1000). AL: adhesive layer, EN: enamel, RC: resin composite. The yellow arrows indicate the adhesive layer.

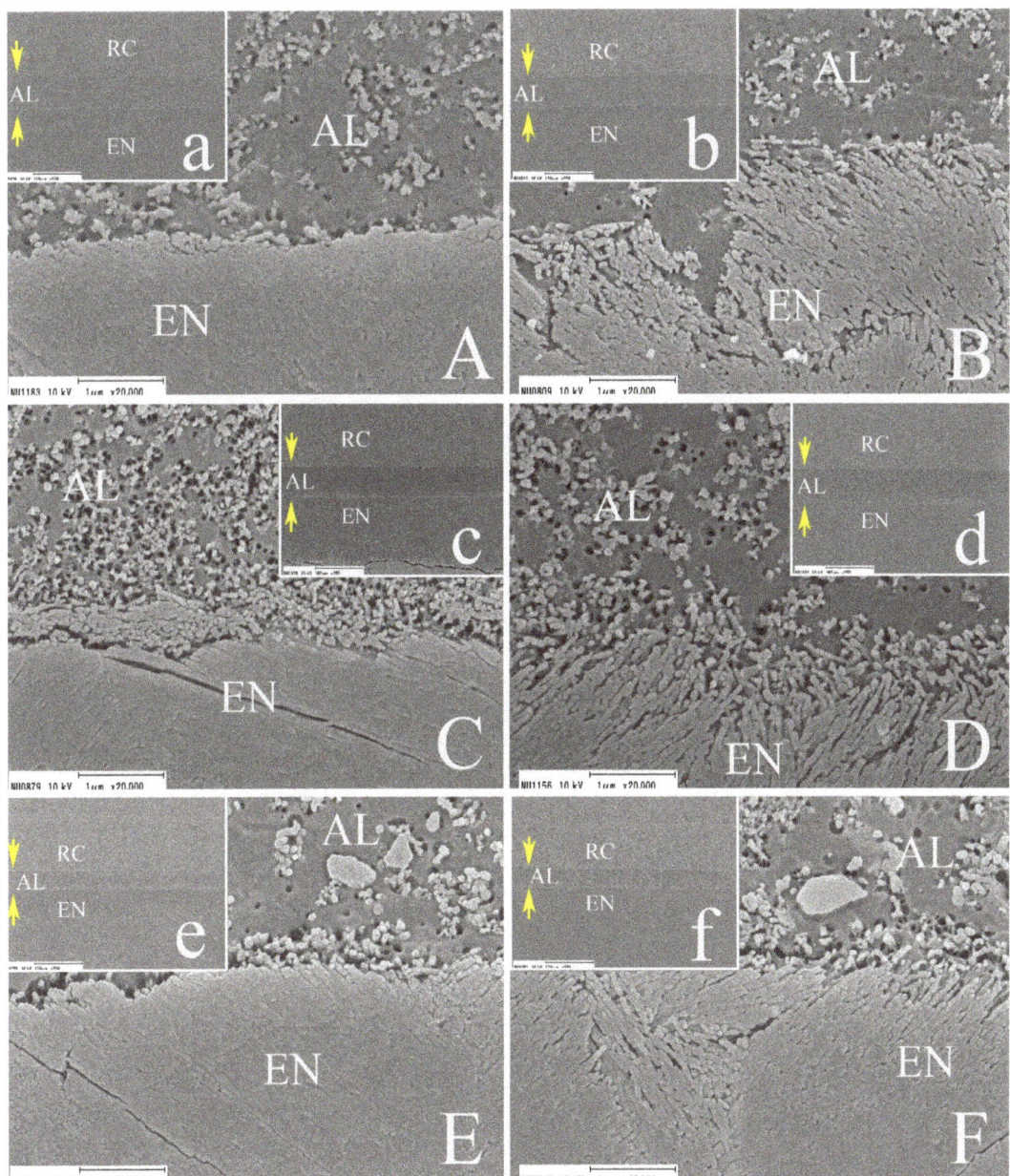

Figure 8. Representative SEM images of resin/enamel interfaces (Group II). (**A**) CS in SE mode (×20,000, ×1000). (**B**) CS in ER mode (×20,000, ×1000). (**C**) GU in SE mode (×20,000, ×1000). (**D**) GU in ER mode (×20,000, ×1000). (**E**) OX in SE mode (×20,000, ×1000). (**F**) OX in ER mode (×20,000, ×1000). AL: adhesive layer, EN: enamel, RC: resin composite. The yellow arrows indicate the adhesive layer.

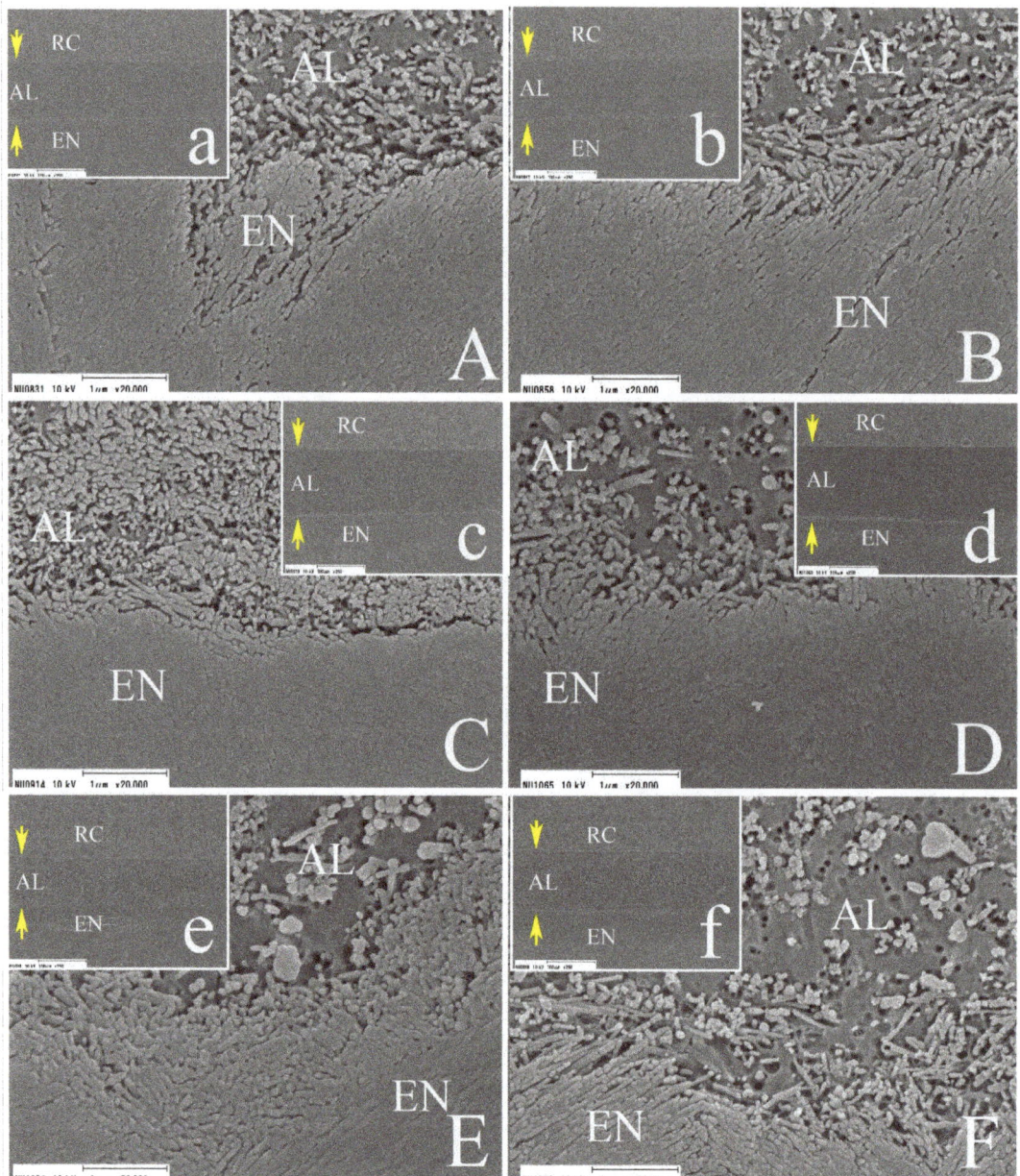

Figure 9. Representative SEM images of resin/enamel interfaces (Group III). (**A**) CS in SE mode (×20,000, ×1000). (**B**) CS in ER mode (×20,000, ×1000). (**C**) GU in SE mode (×20,000, ×1000). (**D**) GU in ER mode (×20,000, ×1000). (**E**) OX in SE mode (×20,000, ×1000). (**F**) OX in ER mode (×20,000, ×1000). AL: adhesive layer, EN: enamel, RC: resin composite. The yellow arrows indicate the adhesive layer.

4. Discussion

This study aimed to determine the influence of the thickness of the adhesive layer formed by different application modes on the immediate enamel bond performance and bond durability of a new-generation two-step adhesive system and to compare it with those of conventional two-step SE adhesive systems. A major concern regarding the experimental protocol was the standardization and reproduction of an adhesive layer of similar thickness with each bonded specimen. It is practically difficult to reproduce the same thickness with a limited error range of a few micrometers, and the adhesive thickness cannot be monitored in each bonded specimen during the SBS test. The different application methods used in this study produced adhesive layers of different thicknesses within a certain range, which were clinically accepted bonding procedures. Although the CV was dependent on the method of application, significant differences in film thickness were observed among the three groups. GU showed thicker films than the other adhesive systems; additionally, a significant difference in thickness was observed between GU and the other adhesives in Group I. This can be explained by the components of the primer and bonding agent in GU. The primer contains nanofillers and functional monomers that resemble universal adhesives. On the other hand, the bonding agent in GU does not contain any functional monomers, solvent, or HEMA. These factors might influence the viscosity of the primer and bonding agent and the polymerization performance of the resin monomer. In particular, the nanofillers in the primer in GU remained on the enamel surface and increased the thickness of the adhesive layer even when a strong stream of air was applied in Group I [16]. Therefore, the adhesive layer of GU in Group I might have been thicker than those in the other adhesive systems.

The bond performances of all the tested adhesive systems were dependent on the application method used. Therefore, the first null hypothesis, that the enamel bond durability of the new two-step adhesive system under thermal stress would not differ with the different application methods used, was rejected. All the adhesives in Group II showed superior immediate and durable bond performances to those in Groups I and III, regardless of the etching mode. Therefore, the optimal adhesive thickness for the effectiveness of the enamel bond in the tested two-step adhesive systems might be similar to that seen in Group II (approximately 40 to 60 μm).

In the 24 h group, all the adhesives showed significantly lower SBS values in Group I when compared to those in Group II in both etching modes. A thicker adhesive layer might act as an elastic buffer zone during the polymerization process of the resin composite [18,19]. Additionally, the stress distribution at the interface might be better, owing to the increase in the size of the plastic zone and the improved elasticity [20,21]. During bond strength testing, load stress might generate cracks and create plastic deformation zones near the ends of these cracks. Crack propagation and fracture are thought to be related to the size of the plastic deformation zone [20,21]. Therefore, the thicker adhesive layer in Group II allows for a plastic deformation zone that is larger than that in Group I; thus, the stress distribution at the interface might be more dispersed. Furthermore, the thickness of the adhesive in the oxygen inhibition layer in Group I is much higher than those in the other groups; thus, the thinner oxygen layer might prove to be weak under load stress [22].

There are only a few studies on the effect of the thickness of the adhesive layer on the enamel bond performance, in contrast to similar work on the dentin. Moreover, the efficacy of the double-layer technique and an extra layer of hydrophobic resin on the enamel bond performances of two-step adhesive systems is still controversial. Albuquerque et al. [19] reported that double application and the placement of an additional hydrophobic resin layer had a negative impact on the μ-TBS of the enamel when using Clearfil SE Bond. On the other hand, Hirokane et al. [8] found no significant difference in the SBS between the single and double-layer application methods when using Clearfil SE Bond. Fujiwara et al. [7] reported no significant change in the SBS between the single- and double-layer application methods with OptiBond XTR. In the present study, although CS did not show any significant differences between groups II and III in SBS regardless of etching mode, the other adhesives showed lower SBS values in group III than group II. Additionally, the proportion of adhesive failure was higher in all the adhesives in Group III when compared to those in Group II. Thus, it can be inferred that an excessively thick adhesive layer might be more prone to defects and voids leading to increased residual stress after polymerization [23]. This might have a negative impact on the mechanical-physical properties of the resin composite restoration when using the two-step adhesive system [24].

In Group I, although no significant differences were observed between the TC groups and the 24 h Group in CS, GU and OX presented with significantly higher SBS values in the TC groups in both etching modes. In particular, a drastic increase in SBS after TC was observed in GU when compared to those in the other adhesives. This might be attributed to a possible delay in the post-polymerization reaction in the adhesive layer in Group I when compared to those in Groups II and III. In the case of GU in Group I, the remnant water and solvent derived from the primer might inhibit the polymerization of the bonding agent during the early phase. Thus, the second null hypothesis that the trend in the durability of the enamel bond during the different application methods was similar among the tested two-step adhesive systems was rejected.

Most of the application groups and adhesive systems demonstrated significantly higher SBS values in the ER mode than in the SE mode. This was in line with previous studies, which showed that phosphoric acid pre-etching before the application of a primer contributes to enhanced immediate and durable enamel bond performance [25,26]. However, none of the adhesives in Group III after TC showed any significant differences in SBS between the ER and SE modes, apart from GU at TC 10,000. For all the adhesives in Group III, the proportion of adhesive failure tended to increase after TC, even in those subjected to the ER mode. This finding suggested that although a strong mechanical interlocking between the etched enamel substrate and the adhesive layer might have been achieved in Group III, the deterioration of the adhesive layer might have been accelerated by both thermal stress and hydrolytic degradation during TC. Additionally, the stress distribution might be different because of the different mechanical properties of each adhesive layer. In particular, the HEMA-, solvent-, and functional monomer-free bonding agent in GU is thought to create a hydrophobic adhesive layer, which might have higher mechanical properties than those formed in the other adhesives [15,16]. This might explain why GU was the only adhesive to show a significantly higher SBS in the ER mode than that in the SE mode at TC 10,000 in Group III.

Among the tested adhesive systems, the new-generation two-step adhesive GU, which utilizes a universal adhesive-derived primer, showed SBS values equal to or higher than the other conventional two-step adhesive systems, regardless of the application mode, etching mode, or bonded specimen storage period. In particular, GU in Group II (similar to the manufacturer's recommended bonding procedures) showed superior immediate and durable enamel bond performances to the other adhesives. Alternatively, GU did not demonstrate any significant differences in SBS under TC between Groups I and II. Hence, although an excessively thick adhesive layer appeared to have a negative impact on the immediate and durable bond performance in all the adhesives, GU appeared to be more tolerant of a thin adhesive layer than did the other materials, regardless of the etching mode.

In clinical situations, a thicker adhesive layer at the enamel margin can cause discoloration and gap formation in resin composite restorations. Additionally, it is likely to form the thicker adhesive layer at the corner of cavities. Thus, it is important to limit the thickness of the bonding agent when using a two-step adhesive system.

5. Conclusions

From the results of this study, we can draw the following conclusions.

1. All the factors (adhesive application method, TC period, and adhesive system) significantly influenced the SBS values in SE mode ($p < 0.001$).

2. All the factors (adhesive application method, TC period, and adhesive system) significantly influenced the SBS values in ER mode ($p < 0.001$).
3. Although the application method and adhesive systems significantly influenced the thickness of the adhesive layer ($p < 0.001$), the etching mode did not have any influence ($p = 0.974$).
4. Although GU and OX showed significantly higher SBS values in ER mode than in SE mode at 24 h, no significant differences in the SBS values of the three adhesives were observed between the SE and ER modes at TC 30,000 in Group III.
5. The application method in Group II, which conformed to the manufacturers' recommendations, resulted in an adhesive layer that was approximately 40–60 μm in thickness and appeared to be optimal for effective enamel bonding, regardless of the type of adhesive system or etching mode.
6. Within the limitations of this study, the new-generation two-step SE adhesive, which adopts a universal adhesive-derived primer and a hydrophobic bonding agent, showed superior bond performance to the conventional two-step adhesive systems.

Author Contributions: T.T. and M.M. conceived and designed the experiments; M.Y., K.S. and A.T. conducted the experiments; S.S. analyzed the data; T.T. wrote the paper; M.A.L. and W.W.B. proofread the manuscript and contributed to the discussion. All authors have read and agreed to the published version of the manuscript.

Funding: This work was supported in part by Grants-in-Aid for Scientific Research, Nos. 19K10158, 21K16975, 21K16977, and 21K09900 from the Japan Society for the Promotion of Science. This project was also supported in part by the Sato Fund (2021) and by a grant from the Dental Research Center of the Nihon University School of Dentistry (2021), Japan.

Conflicts of Interest: The authors of this manuscript certify that they have no proprietary, financial, or other personal interest of any nature or kind in any product, service, and/or company that is presented in this article.

References

1. Perdigão, J.; Muñoz, M.A.; Sezinando, A.; Luque-Martinez, I.V.; Staichak, R.; Reis, A.; Loguercio, A.D. Immediate adhesive properties to dentin and enamel of a universal adhesive associated with a hydrophobic resin coat. *Oper. Dent.* **2014**, *39*, 489–499. [CrossRef] [PubMed]
2. Saikaew, P.; Chowdhury, A.F.M.A.; Fukuyama, M.; Kakuda, S.; Carvalho, R.M.; Sano, H. The effect of dentine surface preparation and reduced application time of adhesive on bonding strength. *J. Dent.* **2016**, *47*, 63–70. [CrossRef]
3. Shiratsuchi, K.; Tsujimoto, A.; Takamizawa, T.; Furuichi, T.; Tsubota, K.; Kurokawa, H.; Miyazaki, M. Influence of warm air-drying on enamel bond strength and surface free-energy of self-etch adhesives. *Eur. J. Oral. Sci.* **2013**, *121*, 370–376. [CrossRef]
4. Takamizawa, T.; Barkmeier, W.W.; Tsujimoto, A.; Scheidel, D.D.; Erickson, R.L.; Latta, M.A.; Miyazaki, M. Effect of phosphoric acid pre-etching on fatigue limits of self-etching adhesives. *Oper. Dent.* **2015**, *40*, 379–395. [CrossRef]
5. Imai, A.; Takamizawa, T.; Sai, K.; Tsujimoto, A.; Nojiri, K.; Endo, H.; Barkmeier, W.W.; Latta, M.A.; Miyazaki, M. Influence of application method on surface free energy and bond strength of universal adhesive systems to enamel. *Eur. J. Oral Sci.* **2017**, *125*, 385–395. [CrossRef]
6. Moritake, N.; Takamizawa, T.; Ishii, R.; Tsujimoto, A.; Barkmeier, W.W.; Latta, M.A.; Miyazaki, M. Effect of active application on bond durability of universal adhesives. *Oper. Dent.* **2019**, *44*, 188–199. [CrossRef]
7. Fujiwara, S.; Takamizawa, T.; Barkmeier, W.W.; Tsujimoto, A.; Imai, A.; Watanabe, H.; Erickson, R.L.; Latta, M.A.; Nakatsuka, T.; Miyazaki, M. Effect of double-layer application on bond quality of adhesive systems. *J. Mech. Behav. Biomed. Mater.* **2018**, *77*, 501–509. [CrossRef]
8. Hirokane, E.; Takamizawa, T.; Kasahara, Y.; Ishii, R.; Tsujimoto, A.; Barkmeier, W.W.; Latta, M.A.; Miyazaki, M. Effect of double-layer application on the early enamel bond strength of universal adhesives. *Clin. Oral. Investig.* **2021**, *25*, 907–921. [CrossRef]
9. Yokoyama, M.; Takamizawa, T.; Tamura, Y.; Namura, Y.; Tsujimoto, A.; Barkmeier, W.W.; Latta, M.A.; Miyazaki, M. Influence of different application methods on the bonding effectiveness of universal adhesives to the dentin in the early phase. *J. Adhes. Dent.* **2021**, in press.
10. Shirai, K.; De Munk, J.; Yoshida, Y.; Inoue, S.; Lambrechts, P.; Suzuki, K.; Shintani, H.; Van Meerbeek, B. Effect of cavity configuration and aging on the bonding effectiveness of six adhesives to dentin. *Dent. Mater.* **2005**, *21*, 110–124. [CrossRef]

11. Cunha, L.G.; Alonso, R.C.B.; Pfeifer, C.S.C.; Correr-Sobrinho, L.; Ferracane, J.L.; Shihoreti, M.A.C. Contraction stress and physical properties development of a resin-based composite irradiated using modulated curing methods at two C-factor levels. *Dent. Mater.* **2008**, *24*, 392–398. [CrossRef]
12. Takamizawa, T.; Imai, A.; Hirokane, E.; Tsujimoto, A.; Barkmeier, W.W.; Erickson, R.L.; Latta, M.A.; Miyazaki, M. SEM observation of novel characteristic of the dentin bond interfaces of universal adhesives. *Dent. Mater.* **2019**, *35*, 1791–1804. [CrossRef]
13. Hashimoto, M.; Sano, H.; Yoshida, E.; Hori, M.; Kaga, M.; Oguchi, H.; Pashely, D.H. Effects of multiple adhesive coatings on dentin bonding. *Oper. Dent.* **2004**, *29*, 416–423.
14. Takamizawa, T.; Barkmeier, W.W.; Tsujimoto, A.; Endo, H.; Tsuchiya, K.; Erickson, R.L.; Latta, M.A.; Miyazaki, M. Influence of pre-etching times on fatigue strength of self-etch adhesives to enamel. *J. Adhes. Dent.* **2016**, *18*, 501–511. [CrossRef]
15. Yamanaka, A.; Mine, A.; Matsumoto, M.; Hagino, R.; Yumitate, M.; Ban, S.; Ishida, M.; Miura, J.; Van Meerbeek, B.; Yatani, H. Back to the multi-step adhesive system: A next-generation two-step system with hydrophobic bonding agent improves bonding effectiveness. *Dent. Mater. J.* **2021**. [CrossRef]
16. Tamura, T.; Takamizawa, T.; Ishii, R.; Hirokane, E.; Tsujimoto, A.; Barkmeier, W.W.; Latta, M.A.; Miyazaki, M. Influence of a primer resembling universal adhesive on the bonding effectiveness of an experimental two-step self-etch adhesive. *J. Adhes. Dent.* **2020**, *22*, 635–646. [CrossRef]
17. International Organization for Standardization. *Dentistry—Adhesion—Notched-Edge Shear Bond Strength Test*; ISO 29022 TR: Geneva, Switzerland, 2013.
18. Ausiello, P.; Apicella, A.; Davidson, C.L. Effect of adhesive layer properties on stress distribution in composite restorations-a 3D finite element analysis. *Dent. Mater.* **2002**, *18*, 295–303. [CrossRef]
19. Albuquerque, M.; Pegoraro, M.; Mattei, G.; Loguercio, A.D. Effect of double-application or the application of a hydrophobic layer for improved efficacy of one-step self-etch systems in enamel and dentin. *Oper. Dent.* **2008**, *33*, 564–570. [CrossRef]
20. Wakasa, K.; Yamaki, M.; Matsui, A. Calculation models for average stress and plastic deformation zone size of bonding area in dentine bonding systems. *Dent. Mater. J.* **1995**, *14*, 152–165. [CrossRef] [PubMed]
21. Chowdhury, A.F.M.A.; Saikaew, P.; Alam, A.; Sun, J.; Carvalho, R.M.; Sano, H. Effects of double application of contemporary self-etch adhesives on their bonding performance to dentin with clinically relevant smear layers. *J. Adhes. Dent.* **2019**, *21*, 59–66. [CrossRef] [PubMed]
22. Osorio, R.; Osorio, E.; Aguilera, F.S.; Tay, F.R.; Pinto, A.; Toledano, M. Influence of application parameters on bond strength of an "all in one" water-based self-etching primer/adhesive after 6 and 12 months of water aging. *Odontology* **2010**, *98*, 117–125. [CrossRef]
23. De Neves, A.A.; Coutinho, E.; Poitevin, A.; Van der Sloten, J.; Van Meerbeek, B.; Van Oostereyck, H. Influence of joint component mechanical properties and adhesive layer thickness on stress distribution in micro-tensile bond strength specimens. *Dent. Mater.* **2009**, *25*, 4–12. [CrossRef]
24. D'Arcangelo, C.; Vanini, L.; Prosperi, G.D.; Di Bussolo, G.; De Angelis, F.; D'Amario, M.; Caputi, S. The influence of adhesive thickness on the microtensile bond strength of three adhesive systems. *J. Adhes. Dent.* **2009**, *11*, 109–115. [CrossRef]
25. Ermis, R.B.; Temel, U.B.; Cellik, E.U.; Kam, O. Clinical performance of a two-step self-etch adhesive with additional enamel etching in Class III cavities. *Oper. Dent.* **2010**, *35*, 147–155. [CrossRef] [PubMed]
26. Suzuki, M.; Takamizawa, T.; Hirokane, E.; Ishii, R.; Tsujimoto, A.; Barkmeier, W.W.; Latta, M.A.; Miyazaki, M. Bond durability of universal adhesives to intact enamel surface in different etching modes. *Eur. J. Oral. Sci.* **2021**, *129*, e12768. [CrossRef]

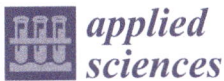

Article

Characterization of Heat-Polymerized Monomer Formulations for Dental Infiltrated Ceramic Networks

Janine Tiu, Renan Belli and Ulrich Lohbauer *

Research Laboratory for Dental Biomaterials, Dental Clinic 1—Operative Dentistry and Periodontology, University of Erlangen-Nuremberg, Glueckstrasse 11, 91054 Erlangen, Germany; janine.tiu@gmail.com (J.T.); renan.belli@fau.de (R.B.)
* Correspondence: ulrich.lohbauer@fau.de; Tel.: +49-9131-8543-740; Fax: +49-9131-8534-207

Abstract: (1) Objectives: This work examined properties of dental monomer formulations of an aromatic dimethacylate (BisGMA), aliphatic urethane dimethacrylate (UDMA), and triethylene glycol dimethacrylate (TEGDMA). The monomers were combined in different ratio formulations and heat-polymerized containing the initiator benzoyl peroxide (BPO) specifically for the purpose of infiltration into polymer-infiltrated composite structures. (2) Methods: The monomers were combined in different weight ratios and underwent rheological analysis (viscosity and temperature dependence), degree of conversion, and mechanical properties (elastic modulus, hardness, fracture toughness). (3) Results: Rheological properties showed Newtonian behavior for monomers with a large dependence on temperature. The addition of BPO allowed for gelation in the range of 72.0–75.9 °C. Degree of conversion was found between 74% and 87% DC, unaffected by an increase of TEGDMA (up to 70 wt%). Elastic modulus, hardness, and fracture toughness were inversely proportional to an increase in TEGDMA. Elastic modulus and hardness were found slightly increased for UDMA versus BisGMA formulations, while fracture toughness ranged between 0.26 and 0.93 MPa·m$^{0.5}$ for UDMA- and 0.18 and 0.68 MPa·m$^{0.5}$ for BisGMA-based formulations. (4) Significance: Heat-polymerization allows for greater range of monomer formulations based on viscosity and degree of conversion when selecting for infiltrated composite structures. Therefore, selection should be based on mechanical properties. The measured data for fracture toughness combined with the reduced viscosity at higher UDMA:TEGDMA ratios favor such formulations over BisGMA:TEGDMA mixtures.

Keywords: methacrylate monomer; heat polymerization; mechanical properties; resin infiltration

Citation: Tiu, J.; Belli, R.; Lohbauer, U. Characterization of Heat-Polymerized Monomer Formulations for Dental Infiltrated Ceramic Networks. *Appl. Sci.* **2021**, *11*, 7370. https://doi.org/10.3390/app11167370

Academic Editor: Mitsuru Motoyoshi

Received: 16 July 2021
Accepted: 9 August 2021
Published: 11 August 2021

Publisher's Note: MDPI stays neutral with regard to jurisdictional claims in published maps and institutional affiliations.

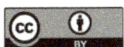

Copyright: © 2021 by the authors. Licensee MDPI, Basel, Switzerland. This article is an open access article distributed under the terms and conditions of the Creative Commons Attribution (CC BY) license (https://creativecommons.org/licenses/by/4.0/).

1. Introduction

Resin composites are successful and versatile in dental restorative applications. The assembled constituents of organic polymers, inorganic fillers, and silane coupling agent [1,2] result in an expansive array of mechanical and structural properties. By developing towards biomimetic design in dental materials, the expanded use of dental monomers comes into focus. In particular, several groups have challenged convention and moved towards composites with continuous and interconnected rigid and pliable constituents [3–17]. Additionally, known as polymer infiltrated ceramic networks (PICN), these materials must be preprocessed as CAD/CAM (computer aided design/computer aided manufacturing) blocks or discs. The conditions for infiltration through a rigid porous structure differ from the mixing of conventional particle reinforced structures [18,19]. The infiltration process can be represented by Darcy's Law, which describes fluid flow through a porous medium [20]. Besides geometry, the determining factors are the pressure gradient, the permeability of the porous medium, and the viscous behavior of the fluid. In the case of PICN composites, the pressure gradient is determined by the vacuum pressure exerted in impregnation machines, the permeability is determined from the geometry of porosity (i.e., size of ceramic particles and partial sintering conditions), and the viscosity is of the monomer.

The conventional dental base monomers in composite formulations include Bisphenol A diglycidyl ether dimethacrylate (BisGMA), urethane dimethacrylate (UDMA), and triethyleneglycol dimethacrylate (TEGDMA) [21], the last of which is used as a diluent and therefore dictates viscosity based on ratio formulations. The chemical structures of the monomers are shown in Figure 1.

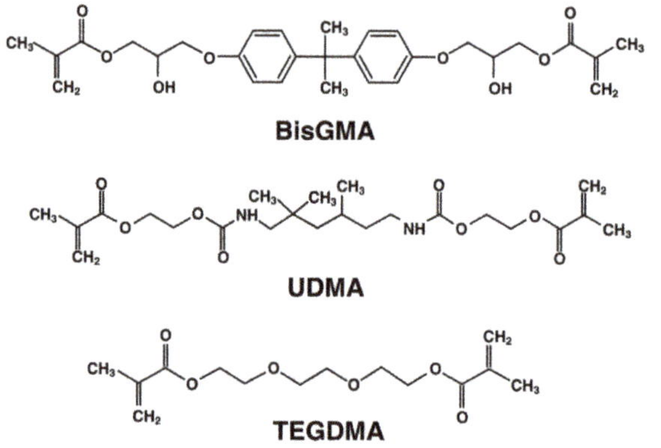

Figure 1. Molecular structure of dental monomers.

BisGMA is advantageous in that it has a high molecular weight and presents lower polymerization shrinkage. The stiff Bisphenol A core and two pendant hydroxyl groups allow for strong hydrogen bonds to be formed and have the largest and lowest concentration of double bonds [22]. On the other hand, UDMA has a flexible aliphatic core with two urethane links [23]. It is smaller than BisGMA and has a higher concentration of double bonds. TEGDMA is the smallest in size, has a high concentration of double bonds, but in turn has the greatest shrinkage. These three monomers in differing formulations comprise the majority of resin matrices used in dental composites.

For photo-polymerized resins under ambient temperatures, the double bond conversion is rapid [24]. As the resin turns glassy and vitrifies, mobility is reduced, continued monomer conversion is hindered, and reaction rate slows [25,26]. Mobility is greatly reduced to the extent that photo-polymerization will always lead to incomplete conversion. Photo-polymerized composites are guided by principles to maximize the degree of conversion as insufficient conversion could lead to color instability and material degradation [27–31]. Conversely, heat polymerization as used by PICN materials allows the consistent input requirements of heat energy to continue the reaction which results in a higher degree of conversion. Numerous studies have reported on mechanical property characterizations of photo-polymerized unfilled dental resins, including degree of conversion [32–34], elastic modulus [35], hardness [34,36,37], and fracture toughness [38]. In comparison, few studies report on mechanical properties of heat-polymerized unfilled dental resins. Nguyen [39] and colleagues found significant differences in strength between photo-polymerized and heat-polymerized UDMA, with significant increases with increased temperature and pressure. It is unclear how monomer formulations and differences in heat-polymerization protocols affect mechanical properties.

To establish a starting baseline, relevant research groups producing experimental dental PICN materials are summarized in Table 1. Here, information on the monomer formulations, the initiator type, and the polymerization protocol are extracted and presented as given. Common formulations are UDMA:TEGDMA and BisGMA:TEGDMA, both in a 1:1 weight ratio, and the most common initiator is 1 wt% Benzoyl Peroxide (BPO). Furthermore, heating protocols vary between groups. The minimum temperature for formulations with the heat initiator BPO is 70 °C increasing up to 110 °C, the holding time also differs from 2 h to 24 h, and some groups polymerize under high pressure. While it is possible that the choices made using heat-polymerization procedures are optimal, there has been no indication as to whether these monomer formulations are ideal and how they contribute to the mechanical properties of the PICN. Indeed, with experimental composites, characterizing base constituents must be pursued if the ideal PICN composite is to be constructed.

Table 1. Literature review on relevant monomer formulations for resin infiltration of porous ceramic networks.

Reference	Year	Rigid Network	Monomer/s	Initiator	Polymerization Protocol	Pressure (If Applicable)
Coldea et al. [4]	2013	Feldspar	UDMA:TEGDMA	BPO		
Petrini et al. [14]	2013	Alumina	Epoxy		40 °C 24 h	
Steier et al. [15]	2013	Alumina	UDMA:TEGDMA 1:1	0.3 vol% BPO	100 °C 2 h	280 MPa
Li et al. [12]	2013	ZrO2	MMA	BPO		
Li et al. [11]	2014	Yzr	PMMA	BPO	85 °C, 20 h	
Nguyen et al. [13]	2014	Albite glass	UDMA	0.5 wt% di-tert-amyl peroxide	180 °C	300 MPa
Cui et al. [7]	2016	Feldspar (potassium, sodium, calcium)	BisGMA:TEGDMA 1:1	BPO	70 °C 8 h, 110 °C 8 h	
Wang et al. [17]	2017	Sodium aluminium silicate	BisGMA:TEGDMA 1:1	1 wt% BPO	70 °C 16 h	
Li and Sun [40]	2017	Zirconia	UDMA:TEGDMA 1:1		180 °C	300 MPa
Li et al. [10]	2017	3Y-TZP	BisGMA:TEGDMA 1:1	BPO	70 °C 10 h	
Cui et al. [5]	2017	Sodium aluminium silicate	BisGMA:TEGDMA 1:1	1 wt% BPO	70 °C 8 h, 110 °C 8 h	
Eldafrawy et al. [9]	2018	Albite glass	UDMA	0.5 wt% di-tert-amyl peroxide	180 °C	300 MPa
Al-Jawoosh et al. [3]	2018	Alumina	UDMA:TEGDMA 1:1	1 vol% BPO	50 °C 2 h, 60 °C 3 h, 70 °C 6 h, 90 °C 12 h	
Cui et al. [8]	2019	Potassium aluminosilicate	BisGMA:TEGDMA 1:1	1 wt% BPO	70 °C 8 h, 110 °C 8 h	
Wang et al. [16]	2019	Silicon nitride	MMA	1 wt% BPO		
Cui et al. [6]	2020	Sodium aluminium silicate nanohydroxyapatitie	BisGMA:TEGDMA 1:1	1 wt% BPO	70 °C 8 h, 110 °C 8 h	

PICN composites attempt to combine favorable properties of two rather contrasting materials [18]. While the rigid constituent of PICN composites can be almost any type of dental grade ceramic, from porcelain [7,13,17] to high strength alumina [3,14,15] and zirconia [10–12], the monomer constituent is more limiting. A wide range of mechanical performances results from any number of rigid and pliable material combinations. Without a foundational understanding of the monomer constituent, development of experimental heat-polymerized dental composites is limited. The focus of this study was to elucidate specific properties of the heat-polymerized monomer matrix, especially significant in experimental material design. Although the mechanical properties of the PICN may well differ from its constituent materials, optimized properties and efficient composite design culminate from our understanding of the basic constituents. This is not an exhaustive report but a continued contribution in monomer formulation selection. Rheological analysis, degree of conversion, and selected mechanical properties measurements were employed. Therefore, the aim of this study is the characterization of heat-polymerized dental monomer formulations.

2. Experimental

2.1. Materials

The dental monomers BisGMA, UDMA, and TEGDMA and heat-initiator benzoyl peroxide (BPO) were used as provided by a dental manufacturer (VOCO, Germany). While volume percentage or mole fraction would be chemical convention, the study refers to them in weight percentage as this is the measure given in all experimental PICN studies. BPO was kept constant at 1 wt%. Different weight ratio mixtures of BisGMA:TEGDMA were 9:1 (89.43 vol%:10.57 vol%), 8:2 (79.00 vol%:21.00 vol%), 7:3 (68.70 vol%:31.30 vol%), 6:4 (58.5 vol%:41.48 vol%), 5:5 (48.47 vol%:51.53 vol%), 4:6 (38.54 vol%:61.46 vol%), 3:7

(28.73 vol%:71.27 vol%), 2:8 (19.04 vol%:80.96 vol%), and 1:9 (9.46 vol%:90.54 vol%). Weight ratios mixtures of UDMA:TEGDMA were 9:1 (89.85 vol%:10.15 vol%), 8:2 (79.74 vol%:20.26 vol%), 7:3 (69.66 vol%:30.34 vol%), 6:4 (59.61 vol%:40.39 vol%), 5:5 (49.59 vol%:50.41 vol%), 4:6 (39.61 vol%:60.39 vol%), 3:7 (29.66 vol%:70.34 vol%), 2:8 (19.74 vol%:80.26 vol%), and 1:9 (9.85 vol%:90.15 vol%).

2.2. Viscosity

Monomer mixtures were weighed and measured into small plastic containers (4 g) and premixed by hand with a small bamboo stick. Containers were placed into a dual asymmetric centrifuge (SpeedMixer™ DAC 150 SP, Hauschild, Germany) at 3000 rpm until the mixtures were consistent (up to 4 min). Mixtures were stored at 40 °C for at least 24 h. Viscosity measurements were performed using a rheometer (MCR 301, Anton Paar, Austria) with a 25 mm parallel aluminum disk and plate geometry with gap size between 0.3 and 0.5 mm. Rotational shear sweep test was performed at 25 °C with shear rates of 0.001–100 (1/s). Forty points were recorded, each test was repeated 3 times, and means were calculated. Rotational temperature sweep tests were performed on monomer mixes with viscosity > 0.01 Pa·s (25 °C). Temperature was increased from 20 °C to 45 °C at 1 °C/min with a constant shear rate of 10 1/s. Twenty-five data points were collected and plotted with complex viscosity (η^*). Data were analyzed using statistical software (SPSS ver, IBM Corp, Armonk, NY, USA) at $p < 0.05$ significance level. One-way ANOVA was used to compare the viscosity at each temperature (20 °C and 45 °C).

2.3. Temperature-Dependent Behavior

Mixing and resting protocol was the same for viscosity with the initial step of TEGDMA mixed together with 1.0 wt% BPO until dissolved, before BisGMA or UDMA were added according to the monomer mixes. Temperature-dependent behavior was performed on the mixtures (UDMA:TEGDMA, 2:8, 5:5, 8:2; BisGMA:TEGDMA, 2:8, 5:5, 8:2) using a rheometer (MCR 301, Anton Paar, Austria) with a 15mm parallel aluminium disk and plate geometry with gap size 0.5 mm. Oscillatory tests with angular frequency of 10 rad/s, amplitude of 5%, and temperature rate of 1 °C/min were performed with temperatures starting from 24 °C to 90 °C. Storage modulus (G') and loss modulus (G'') were plotted, and the sol/gel transition (T_{sg}) temperature (phase transition when $G' = G''$, equivalent to loss factor δ) was the point determining when the monomer became solid/polymerized.

2.4. Mechanical Properties

Mixing and resting protocol was the same for temperature-dependent behavior tests. Monomer mixtures were placed into custom silicon molds and allowed to sit overnight before the heating protocol. Specimens were heated from room temperature to 60 °C for 1 h (5 °C/min), raised until the final temperature (80 °C, 100 °C, and 120 °C), and held for 8 h. An 8 h maximum was chosen according to the limitations of the laboratory working hours. The oven was switched off and specimens were allowed to slow cool overnight. Polymers were cut into bar specimens (25 mm × 5 mm × 2.5 mm) using a precision sectioning saw (IsoMet™ Low Speed Saw, Buehler, Plymouth, MN, USA) and polished (up to 4000 grit). Fracture toughness specimens requiring a precrack (*a*) were created using a 1mm thick diamond disk to length 0.5mm using a custom notching machine. A razor blade was inserted into the shallow cut and a short tap created a notch with a sharp tip into the specimen. Precrack length was measured using an optical stereomicroscope (SteREO Discovery.V8, Zeiss, Oberkochen, Germany) with camera (AxioCam, Zeiss, Germany) and measuring software (Zen Core 2.7, Zeiss, Germany).

Specimens were tested in a universal testing machine (Z2.5, Zwick/Roell, Ulm, Germany) in a 3-point bending set-up (3-PB), with span (*S*) 20 mm, and crosshead speed of 0.01 mm/min. Specimens without notches were used for Young's modulus ($n = 6$) and pre-cracked specimens were used for fracture toughness ($n = 6$). Displacement was captured using an attached laser extensometer (laserXtens, Zwick/Roell, Germany) and recorded on software (testXpert III, Zwick/Roell, Germany). Mean and corresponding standard deviations as a measure of variability were calculated for each group.

Fracture toughness (K_{IC}) calculated according to ASTM E1820 given by the equation

$$K_{IC} = \left[\frac{PS}{BW^{3/2}}\right] f\left(\frac{a}{W}\right)$$

where P is the load, B is the width of the specimen, W is the height of the specimen, and $f\left(\frac{a}{W}\right)$ for 3-PB is given by

$$f\left(\frac{a}{W}\right) = \frac{3\left(\frac{a}{W}\right)^{1/2}\left[1.99 - \left(\frac{a}{W}\right)\left(1 - \frac{a}{W}\right)\left(2.15 - 3.93\frac{a}{W} + 2.7\left(\frac{a}{W}\right)^2\right)\right]}{2\left(1 + 2\frac{a}{W}\right)\left(1 - \frac{a}{W}\right)^{3/2}}$$

Hardness was measured using the Vickers hardness test using the standard DIN EN ISO 6507-1 and VDI/VDE 2626 part 2 as a guide. A diamond indenter with the applied force of 500 g was held for 30 s in an analogue materials testing machine (ZHV10, Zwick, Ulm, Germany). Three indentation points per specimen ($n = 3$, A = surface area of an indent measured from the diagonal dimensions d) were measured using an upright confocal microscope (Leica DMRXE, Leica Microsystems, Wetzlar, Germany), with an attached camera (AxioCam, Zeiss, Germany) and measuring software (Zen 2, Zeiss, Germany). The hardness value was calculated using the following equation:

$$HV = \frac{P}{A} = \frac{1.8544 F}{d^2}$$

2.5. Monomer Conversion

Monomer conversion was measured using Fourier transform infrared spectrometry (FTIR). Spectra was collected in absorbance with 42 scans at resolution 4 cm^{-1} over a wavenumber range of 400–4000 cm^{-1} using an FTIR spectrometer (IRAffinity-1S, Shimadzu, Duisburg, Germany) in conjunction with an ATR (attenuated total reflection) sampling algorithm. Degree of conversion (%DC) was determined by measuring the remaining proportlion peak intensity of the aliphatic C = C double bonds (at absorption band 1638 cm^{-1}) in the polymerized specimen relative to the total C = C double bonds in the monomer mixture. Unaffected by the polymerization reaction, aromatic C ... C absorption at 1609 cm^{-1} was used as an internal standard for BisGMA mixtures, while N ... H peak at 1537 cm^{-1} was used as the internal standard for UDMA [41]. Baseline was determined by connecting points taken in the depressions adjacent to each peak, and intensity was measured by maximum peak height relative to the baseline. %DC is given by the following equation:

$$\%DC = \left[1 - \frac{\left(\frac{1638\ cm^{-1}\ or\ 1537\ cm^{-1}}{1609\ cm^{-1}}\right) polymer}{\left(\frac{1638\ cm^{-1}\ or\ 1537\ cm^{-1}}{1609\ cm^{-1}}\right) monomer}\right] \times 100$$

3. Results and Discussion

3.1. Viscosity

Viscosity is the material property describing the resistance to flow, which is affected by intermolecular interactions. Figure 2 shows the average viscosity of each monomer formulation from a rotational shear sweep test. As the shear stress rate had no effect on viscosity, all formulations showed Newtonian rheological behavior. BisGMA showed the greatest viscosity at 520 Pa·s at 25 °C, attributed to its high molecular weight and the strong hydrogen bonding from its two pendant hydroxyl groups [42,43]. The viscosity of TEGDMA, attributed to its low molecular weight [44], is relatively low (0.0084 Pa·s), which naturally decreases the viscosity of the monomer formulations as percentage weight increases in accordance with other studies [45,46].

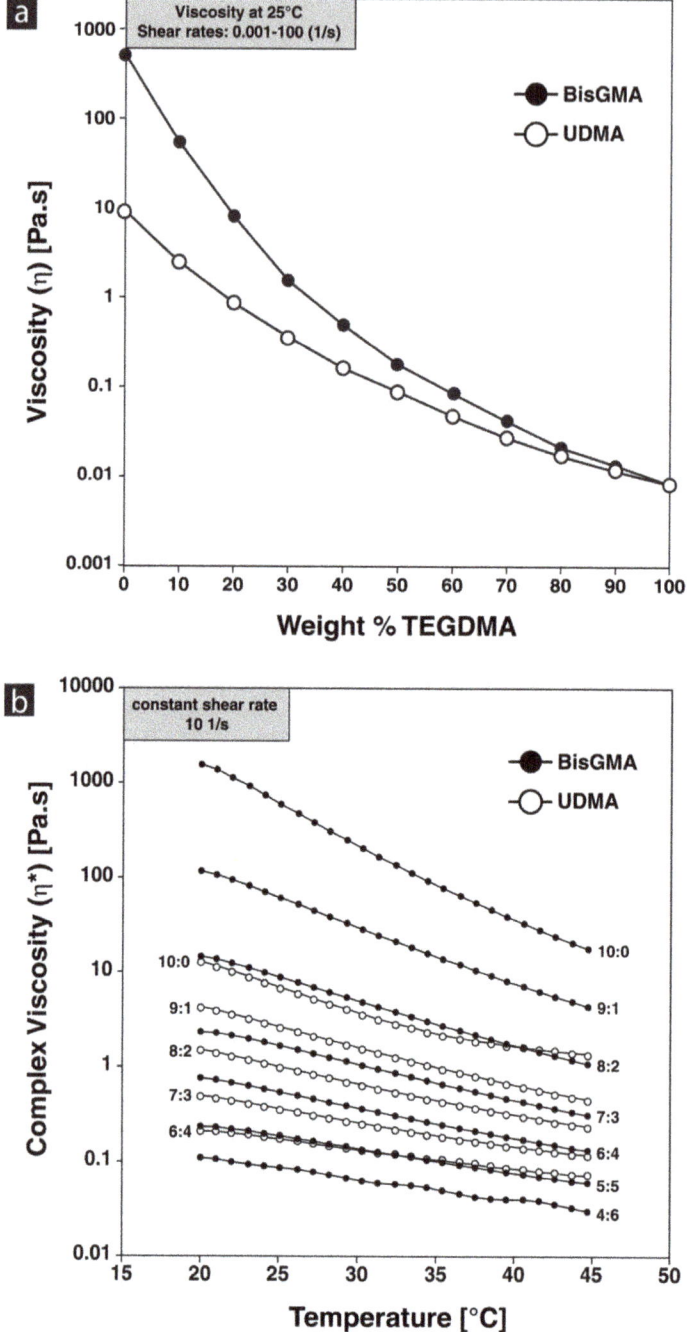

Figure 2. Viscosity of monomer formulations. (**a**) Shear sweep of monomer formulations at 25 °C; (**b**) temperature sweep of monomer formulations.

According to Darcy's law, the viscosity affects the fluid flow behavior into a porous substrate. Lower viscosity is needed for ease of flow, while a higher viscosity affects infiltration rate and pressure. One group [9] used pure UDMA for their PICN material, which at 10 Pa·s, is several magnitudes greater than the 5:5 wt% BisGMA:TEGDMA (0.181 Pa·s), and UDMA:TEGDMA (0.090 Pa·s) commonly used by others. Monomer formulations greater than 10 Pa·s would be difficult for infiltration; therefore, with regard to viscosity, the formulations of BisGMA:TEGDMA 9:1 and 8:2 would fall out of this range. Viscosity is significantly influenced by changes in temperature; Figure 2b shows complex viscosity with increasing temperature. Monomer formulations with viscosity less than 0.1 Pa·s were excluded from the temperature sweep. Temperature has such a pronounced effect on viscosity it is able to reduce viscosity by orders of magnitude. Therefore, most monomer formulations can reach low viscosities suitable for infiltration.

BisGMA in general shows higher viscosities compared to UDMA formulations, due to the differences in chain length of the used monomers. As consequence, the effect diminishes at higher TEGDMA ratios. A target viscosity for infiltration purposes should meet the criteria of sufficient flowability/penetrability into the network by retaining a minimum polymerization shrinkage and shrinkage stress at network interfaces. For BisGMA:TEGDMA, the optimum ratio is thus found between 7:3 and 5:5, while for UDMA:TEGDMA formulations, the window of applicability might be found between 9:1 and 6:4.

3.2. Temperature Dependency

Increasing temperature allows for many monomer formulations to reach a lower viscosity threshold for infiltration; however, there is a maximum limit placed on the temperature. Using free radical polymerization with the use of an initiator, Figure 3 shows temperature-dependent behavior of different monomer formulations. A greater difference between G'' and G' showing strong interaction forces is seen in formulations (2:8) and (5:5) for both UDMA:TEGDMA and BisGMA:TEGDMA, as opposed to formulations (8:2) for both UDMA:TEGDMA and BisGMA:TEGDMA, both showing a higher loss modulus (G'') over storage modulus (G') indicating weaker unlinked molecules. This hypothesis is based on observations in Figure 3, not accounting for differences in the chain structure of BisGMA versus UDMA with a higher concentration of crosslinking double bonds in UDMA. Sol/gel transition temperature T_{SG} lies between 72.0 and 75.9 °C for all formulations. All formulations with heat initiator BPO begin reactions around this temperature range. These values are in the range of temperatures selected for experimental PICN using BPO.

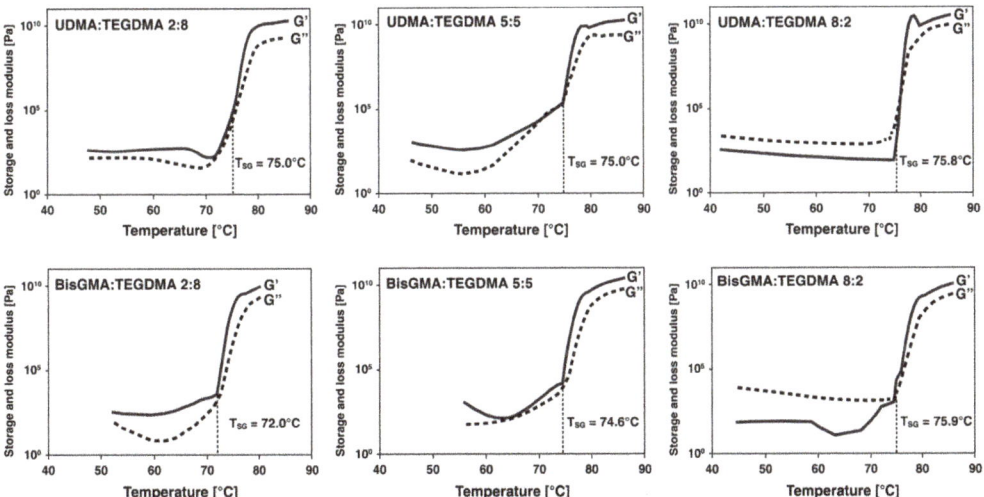

Figure 3. Temperature dependency of selected monomer formulations.

3.3. Degree of Conversion

The degrees of conversion of the different monomer formulations cured at different temperatures using FTIR spectroscopy are shown in Figure 4. The conversion for BisGMA formulations ranged from 81.6 to 87.3%. The UDMA formulations ranged from 74.2 to 86.4%, with the exception being BisGMA:TEGDMA 2:8 and 1:9, which has significant amounts of TEGDMA (80–90 wt%) with a conversion of 65.9% and 22.8%, respectively. Pure TEGDMA is found to have low conversion [23]. The degree of conversion is analyzed in photo-polymerized resin as critically affecting mechanical properties. The BisGMA molecule has a stiff core, less degrees of freedom, and reduced mobility resulting in kinematically a low degree of conversion. Coupled with low viscosity TEGDMA, the network forms cross-links, which also reduces mobility as the reaction progresses. However, when the monomer formulations undergo heat-polymerization, there is no clear correlation with increasing TEGDMA seen in photo-polymerized monomer formulations. The difference is that heat-polymerization allows the continual required energy input to improve the mobility and reactivity. As a result, degree of conversion is independent of the amount of TEGDMA (as long as this is over 30 wt% when formulated with BisGMA). A study by Cui et al. showed comparable monomer conversion of 81.9%DC for BisGMA:TEGDMA (5:5) and 81.7%DC for UDMA:TEGDMA (8:2) mixtures [47]. This study used comparable experimental settings as they heat-polymerized with 1 wt% BPO at 70 °C for 8 h.

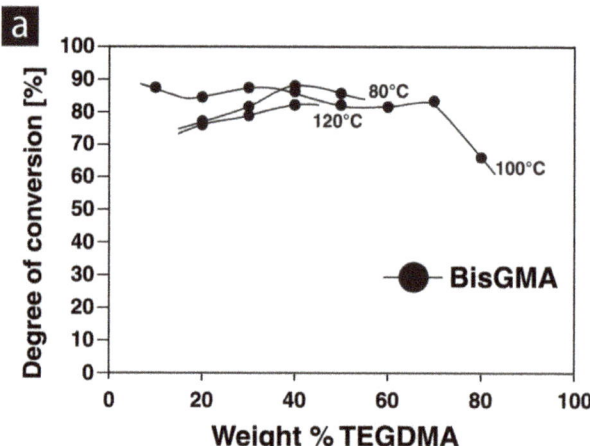

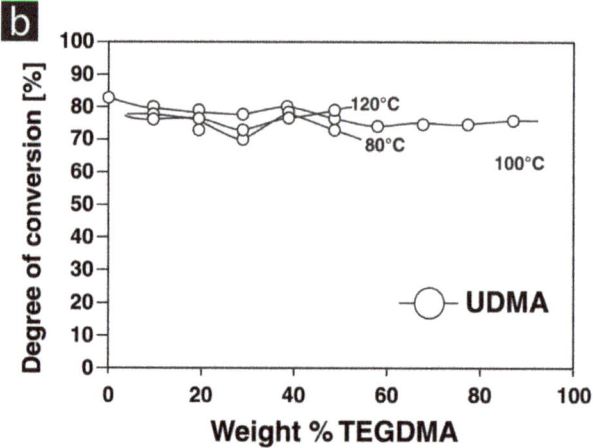

Figure 4. Degree of conversion of BisGMA:TEGDMA (**a**) and UDMA:TEGDMA (**b**) formulations.

3.4. Mechanical Properties

Figure 5a,b shows the elastic modulus and hardness of the monomer formulations cured at different temperatures and weight percentages of TEGDMA, respectively. There is a clear inverse correlation with the increase of TEGDMA in hardness, elastic modulus, and fracture toughness. The highest values for elastic modulus were seen in BisGMA:TEGDMA 8:2 (3.03 GPa) cured at 120 °C, and the lowest was UDMA:TEGDMA 1.9 (0.63 GPa) cured at 100 °C. The temperature did not affect UDMA:TEGDMA formulations. The highest hardness values were seen in the BisGMA:TEGDMA 9:1 formulation (249.07 ± 8.47 MPa), and the lowest in UDMA:TEGDMA 1:9 (33.81 ± 13.88 MPa). TEGDMA, with its low molecular weight, increases the flexibility of the polymer with an increase in weight ratio. This can be explained by the TEGMDA molecule's ability to coil under load and rotate about its ether linkages [37].

These properties are essential when considering dental restorations. Elastic properties and hardness should be as close as possible to the properties of our human teeth to replicate and establish the biomechanical functions and demands. A high hardness and elastic modulus can damage and abrade the opposing teeth, while the inverse would damage the restoration. Comparable damage tolerance is needed to absorb the loading energy and provide the essential durability and robustness for clinical success. In the case of high strength ceramics of alumina and zirconia, these strong and incredibly stiff ceramics can be made more compliant with the addition of monomers in PICN materials. Relative success in property matching has been seen in commercial dental PICN materials [4,48].

Cui et al. used similar formulations for infiltration of silica-based ceramic networks [47]. They measured an elastic modulus for the final PICN material of 18.7 GPa for BisGMA:TEGDMA (5:5) and 18.9 GPa for UDMA:TEGDMA (8:2) formulations, both values closely matching the dentin elasticity.

Figure 5c shows fracture toughness of the monomer formulations cured at different temperatures and weight percentages of TEGDMA. Basically, the fracture toughness was found considerably higher for UDMA- versus BisGMA-based formulations. Fracture toughness linearly decreased with increasing TEGDMA content. The highest values were seen in UDMA:TEGDMA formulations which ranged from 0.262 ± 0.078 MPa·m$^{0.5}$ (1:9) to 0.931 ± 0.159 MPa·m$^{0.5}$ (9:1). UDMA cured at 100 °C was 0.756 ± 0.082 MPa·m$^{0.5}$, and BisGMA:TEGDMA formulations ranged from 0.179 ± 0.043 MPa·m$^{0.5}$ (1:9) to 0.683 ± 0.113 MPa·m$^{0.5}$ (9:1). Fracture toughness is the ability of a material to resist crack growth from a pre-existing crack. In terms of clinical relevance, this mechanical property offers greater understanding of failure over elasticity. A resin formulation for infiltration purposes should hence exhibit a high fracture toughness with preference for UDMA-based mixtures at higher UDMA:TEGDMA ratios.

Clinical fractures often originate from existing flaws, and fracture toughness gives us a measure of the load needed to propagate the crack. The interpenetrating nature of PICN materials distinctly separates both material constituents; therefore, any advancing cracks are strongly subject to a variety of toughening mechanisms. When materials are effective in arresting developing cracks and absorb enough crack advancing forces, an increased input of energy is required to further propagate the crack, leading to a rising resistance curve (R-curve). Fracture toughness of a material is contributed to by intrinsic toughening mechanisms such as the inherent plasticity of the material working ahead of the crack tip [49]. As polymers are covalently bonded networks, at a critical shear strain, molecules are susceptible of sliding with respect to each other [50]. Having a low elastic modulus increases the amount of work done during flexure and in turn increases the strain energy release rate. These energy consuming processes inevitably increase the plastic zone around the crack tip leading to increased toughness.

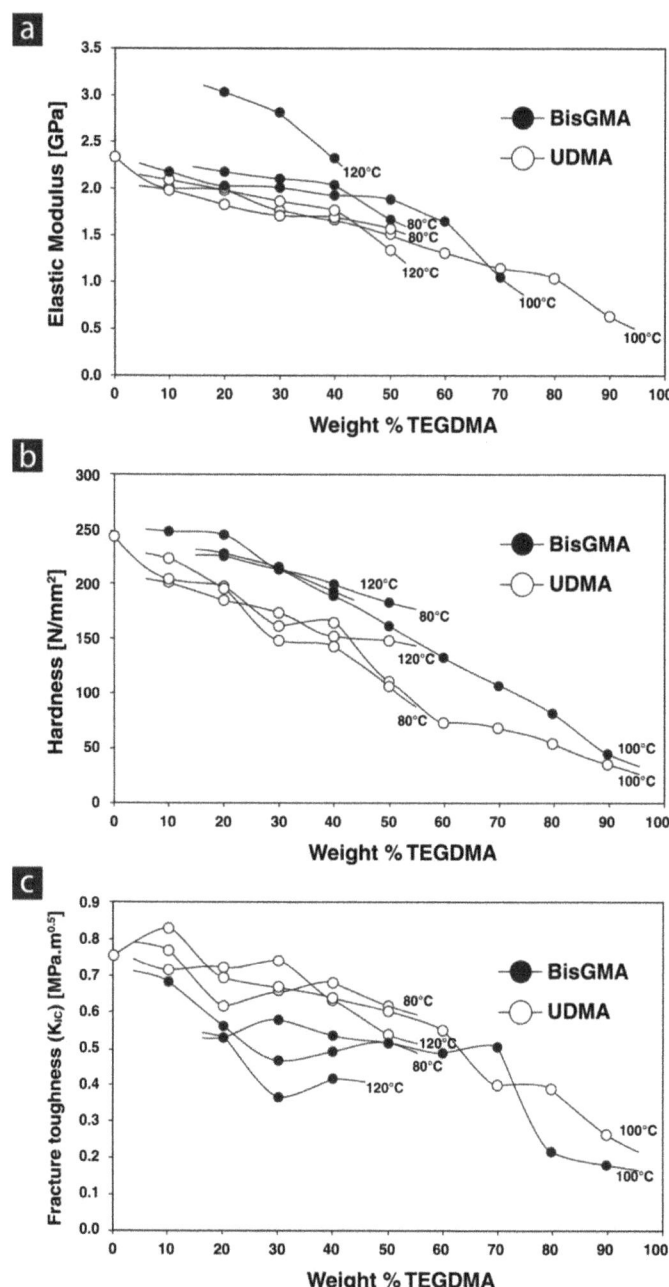

Figure 5. Mechanical properties of monomer formulations cured at different temperatures. Elastic modulus (**a**), hardness (**b**), and fracture toughness (**c**).

Conversely, extrinsic toughening mechanisms work outside of the inherent material property and inflict energy consuming processes working behind the crack tip such as crack bridging. The increasing R-curve is seen in interpenetrating networks of metals and ceramics where the metal acts as the compliant phase, and its ductility leads to bridging effects behind the crack tip [51]. Ceramics themselves are brittle in nature, meaning that at a certain load, cracks occur catastrophically. In the case of dental PICN materials, the monomer resin acts as the compliant phase and would be responsible for extrinsic toughening mechanisms if any were to exist. To our knowledge, significant rising R-curve behavior has not been seen in commercial dental PICN materials, but that is not to say that it is an impossible feat. With a slow enough loading rate, localized deformation leading to crazing will form in glassy polymers. With crack advancement, fibrils are left at the trailing edge [50]. Interpenetrating composites outside of dentistry using ceramic and polymers have indicated the potential of bridging polymer fibrils or ligaments using 6-Nylon infiltrated into porous hydroxyapatite leading to a rising R-curve [48,52]. Fibril bridging effects were also seen in calcium phosphate scaffolds with Poly (e-caprolactone) [53]. Going forward with experimental dental PICN materials, increasing the fracture toughness and inducing the favored R-curve effect in dental PICN materials require a proper understanding of the resin matrix and if the possibility of polymer fibrils exists.

It is difficult to compare the property differences between studies using dental monomer formulations. The composition and polymerization method can result in markedly different properties. However, based on information as outlined in Table 1, monomer compositions can be tailored to specific properties and applications. Selection of heat-polymerized monomer formulations must consider many variables. The infiltration of monomers relies on an appropriate viscosity; however, the temperamental response to temperature demonstrate that ideal viscosity can be achieved in most monomer formulations. With the addition of chemical initiator BPO, the monomer formulations need to achieve temperatures of at least 72.0–75.9 °C to reach gelation and begin the reaction. By keeping the heating procedure as a constant variable, it was demonstrated that the degree of conversion is also unaffected by monomer formulations. These factors are important to consider with photo-polymerized composites but become inconsequential with heat-polymerized monomers. Instead, a pivotal consideration for resin matrix selection is assigned to the mechanical performance. It becomes clear how the relative concentration of monomers affects the contribution to mechanical performance. Increasing the TEGDMA ratio reduces elastic modulus, hardness, and fracture toughness. This could be due to the stronger hydrogen bonds in BisGMA and UDMA restricting the sliding of the molecules relative to each other over TEGDMA, with a pronounced effect due to concentration.

The importance for the selection of appropriate resin monomer formulations with specific chemical and physical properties is not just limited to infiltration purposes. The use of similar formulations with comparable relations between various properties has already been applied to 3D printing technologies. A study by Hodasova et al. has shown the performance of BisGMA:TEGDMA (4:6) formulations for infiltration of 3D-printed zirconia (3Y-TZP) networks [54]. Based on rapidly advancing additive manufacturing technologies, the importance of selecting appropriate resin formulations with specific properties for, e.g., simultaneous and multi-material printing techniques further increases.

4. Conclusions

Viscosity, temperature dependency, degree of conversion, and mechanical tests were performed on BisGMA:TEGDMA- versus UDMA:TEGDMA-based monomer formulations. The viscosity of UDMA was generally lower compared to BisGMA formulations, allowing for a higher UDMA:TEGDMA ratio. Both combinations heat-polymerized at 70 °C for 8 h using 1 wt% BPO proved a high degree of conversion of approximately 74–87% with a higher crosslinking density for BisGMA formulations. Elastic modulus and hardness were found slightly higher for BisGMA versus UDMA mixtures, linearly decreasing for both materials with increasing TEGDMA content. The fracture toughness as an ultimate measure of fracture resistance and hence reinforcing stability was considerably higher for UDMA versus BisGMA formulations, also linearly decreasing for higher TEGDMA mixtures. Taking into account the reduced viscosity of UDMA versus BisGMA thus allows for a higher UDMA:TEGDMA ratio, which is in turn beneficial for further expanding the window of applicability.

Author Contributions: Conceptualization, J.T., R.B. and U.L.; methodology, J.T. and U.L.; software, J.T.; validation, R.B. and U.L.; formal analysis, J.T.; investigation, J.T.; resources, U.L.; data curation, J.T.; writing—original draft preparation, J.T.; writing—review and editing, U.L.; visualization, R.B.; supervision, U.L.; project administration, U.L.; funding acquisition, J.T. and U.L. All authors have read and agreed to the published version of the manuscript.

Funding: This research received external funding in the frame of a postdoctoral research fellowship from the Alexander-von-Humboldt Foundation for J.T.

Institutional Review Board Statement: Not applicable.

Informed Consent Statement: Not applicable.

Conflicts of Interest: The authors declare no conflict of interest.

References

1. Ferracane, J.L. Resin composite—State of the art. *Dent. Mater.* **2011**, *27*, 29–38. [CrossRef]
2. Cramer, N.; Stansbury, J.; Bowman, C. Recent Advances and Developments in Composite Dental Restorative Materials. *J. Dent. Res.* **2010**, *90*, 402–416. [CrossRef]
3. Al-Jawoosh, S.; Ireland, A.; Su, B. Fabrication and characterisation of a novel biomimetic anisotropic ceramic/polymer-infiltrated composite material. *Dent. Mater.* **2018**, *34*, 994–1002. [CrossRef]
4. Coldea, A.; Swain, M.; Thiel, N. Mechanical properties of polymer-infiltrated-ceramic-network materials. *Dent. Mater.* **2013**, *29*, 419–426. [CrossRef]
5. Cui, B.; Li, J.; Wang, H.; Lin, Y.; Shen, Y.; Li, M.; Deng, X.; Nan, C. Mechanical properties of polymer-infiltrated-ceramic (sodium aluminum silicate) composites for dental restoration. *J. Dent.* **2017**, *62*, 91–97. [CrossRef] [PubMed]
6. Cui, B.; Zhang, R.; Sun, F.; Ding, Q.; Lin, Y.; Zhang, L.; Nan, C. Mechanical and biocompatible properties of polymer-infiltrated-ceramic-network materials for dental restoration. *J. Adv. Ceram.* **2020**, *9*, 123–128. [CrossRef]
7. Cui, B.C.; Li, J.; Wang, H.N.; Lin, Y.H.; Shen, Y.; Nan, C.W. Mechanical Properties of Polymer-Infiltrated-Feldspar for Restorative Composite CAD/CAM Blocks. *Key Eng. Mater.* **2016**, *697*, 648–651. [CrossRef]
8. Cui, B.-C.; Li, J.; Lin, Y.-H.; Shen, Y.; Li, M.; Deng, X.-L.; Nan, C.-W. Polymer-infiltrated layered silicates for dental restorative materials. *Rare Met.* **2019**, *38*, 1003–1014. [CrossRef]
9. Eldafrawy, M.; Nguyen, J.; Mainjot, A.; Sadoun, M. A Functionally Graded PICN Material for Biomimetic CAD-CAM Blocks. *J. Dent. Res.* **2018**, *97*, 1324–1330. [CrossRef]
10. Li, J.; Zhang, X.-H.; Cui, B.-C.; Lin, Y.-H.; Deng, X.-L.; Li, M.; Nan, C.-W. Mechanical performance of polymer-infiltrated zirconia ceramics. *J. Dent.* **2017**, *58*, 60–66. [CrossRef] [PubMed]
11. Li, S.; Zhao, Y.; Zhang, J.-F.; Xie, C.; Zhao, X. Machinability of poly(methyl methacrylate) infiltrated zirconia hybrid composites. *Mater. Lett.* **2014**, *131*, 347–349. [CrossRef]
12. Li, S.B.; Zhao, Y.M.; Zhang, J.F.; Xie, C.; Li, D.M.; Tang, L.H.; Zhao, X.Y. Mechanical properties and microstructure of PMMA-ZrO2 nanocomposites for dental CAD/CAM Blocks. *Adv. Mater. Res.* **2013**, *785*, 533–536. [CrossRef]
13. Nguyen, J.; Ruse, N.D.; Phan, A.; Sadoun, M. High-temperature-pressure Polymerized Resin-infiltrated Ceramic Networks. *J. Dent. Res.* **2014**, *93*, 62–67. [CrossRef] [PubMed]
14. Petrini, M.; Ferrante, M.; Su, B. Fabrication and characterization of biomimetic ceramic/polymer composite materials for dental restoration. *Dent. Mater.* **2013**, *29*, 375–381. [CrossRef]
15. Steier, V.F.; Koplin, C.; Kailer, A. Influence of pressure-assisted polymerization on the microstructure and strength of polymer-infiltrated ceramics. *J. Mater. Sci.* **2013**, *48*, 3239–3247. [CrossRef]
16. Wang, F.; Guo, J.; Li, K.; Sun, J.; Zeng, Y.; Ning, C. High strength polymer/silicon nitride composites for dental restorations. *Dent. Mater.* **2019**, *35*, 1254–1263. [CrossRef] [PubMed]
17. Wang, H.; Cui, B.; Li, J.; Li, S.; Lin, Y.; Liu, D.; Li, M. Mechanical properties and biocompatibility of polymer infiltrated sodium aluminum silicate restorative composites. *J. Adv. Ceram.* **2017**, *6*, 73–79. [CrossRef]
18. Swain, M.; Coldea, A.; Bilkhair, A.; Guess, P. Interpenetrating network ceramic-resin composite dental restorative materials. *Dent. Mater.* **2016**, *32*, 34–42. [CrossRef]
19. Ruse, N.; Sadoun, M. Resin-composite Blocks for Dental CAD/CAM Applications. *J. Dent. Res.* **2014**, *93*, 1232–1234. [CrossRef]
20. Whitaker, S. Flow in porous media I: A theoretical derivation of Darcy's law. *Transp. Porous Media* **1986**, *1*, 3–25. [CrossRef]
21. Peutzfeldt, A. Resin composites in dentistry: The monomer systems. *Eur. J. Oral Sci.* **1997**, *105*, 97–116. [CrossRef]
22. Venhoven, B. De Gee, A.; Davidson, C. Polymerization contraction and conversion of light-curing BisGMA-based methacrylate resins. *Biomaterials* **1993**, *14*, 871–875. [CrossRef]
23. Floyd, C.J.; Dickens, S.H. Network structure of Bis-GMA- and UDMA-based resin systems. *Dent. Mater.* **2006**, *22*, 1143–1149. [CrossRef]
24. Stansbury, J.W.; Dickens, S.H. Network formation and compositional drift during photo-initiated copolymerization of dimethacrylate monomers. *Polymer* **2001**, *42*, 6363–6369. [CrossRef]
25. Dickens, S.H.; Stansbury, J.; Choi, K.; Floyd, C. Photopolymerization kinetics of methacrylate dental resins. *Macromolecules* **2003**, *36*, 6043–6053. [CrossRef]

26. Lovell, L.G.; Berchtold, K.A.; Elliott, J.E.; Lu, H.; Bowman, C.N. Understanding the kinetics and network formation of dimethacrylate dental resins. *Polym. Adv. Technol.* **2001**, *12*, 335–345. [CrossRef]
27. Van Landuyt, K.L.; Nawrot, T.; Geebelen, B.; De Munck, J.; Snauwaert, J.; Yoshihara, K.; Scheers, H.; Godderis, L.; Hoet, P.; Van Meerbeek, B.; et al. How much do resin-based dental materials release? A meta-analytical approach. *Dent. Mater.* **2011**, *27*, 723–747. [CrossRef]
28. Mohsen, N.; Craig, R.G.; Hanks, C. Cytotoxicity of urethane dimethacrylate composites before and after aging and leaching. *J. Biomed. Mater. Res.* **1998**, *39*, 252–260. [CrossRef]
29. Rathbun, M.A.; Craig, R.G.; Hanks, C.T.; Filisko, F.E. Cytotoxicity of a BIS-GMA dental composite before and after leaching in organic solvents. *J. Biomed. Mater. Res.* **1991**, *25*, 443–457. [CrossRef]
30. Tanaka, K.; Taira, M.; Shintani, H.; Wakasa, K.; Yamaki, M. Residual monomers (TEGDMA and Bis-GMA) of a set visible-light-cured dental composite resin when immersed in water. *J. Oral Rehabilitation* **1991**, *18*, 353–362. [CrossRef] [PubMed]
31. Söderholm, K.-J.; Mariotti, A. BIS-GMA–based resins in dentistry: Are they safe? *J. Am. Dent. Assoc.* **1999**, *130*, 201–209. [CrossRef] [PubMed]
32. Schroeder, W.; Vallo, C. Effect of different photoinitiator systems on conversion profiles of a model unfilled light-cured resin. *Dent. Mater.* **2007**, *23*, 1313–1321. [CrossRef] [PubMed]
33. Sideridou, I.; Tserki, V.; Papanastasiou, G. Effect of chemical structure on degree of conversion in light-cured dimethacrylate-based dental resins. *Biomaterials* **2002**, *23*, 1819–1829. [CrossRef]
34. Furuse, A.Y.; Mondelli, J.; Watts, D. Network structures of Bis-GMA/TEGDMA resins differ in DC, shrinkage-strain, hardness and optical properties as a function of reducing agent. *Dent. Mater.* **2011**, *27*, 497–506. [CrossRef] [PubMed]
35. Asmussen, E.; Peutzfeldt, A. Influence of UEDMA, BisGMA and TEGDMA on selected mechanical properties of experimental resin composites. *Dent. Mater.* **1998**, *14*, 51–56. [CrossRef]
36. Barszczewska-Rybarek, I.M. Structure–property relationships in dimethacrylate networks based on Bis-GMA, UDMA and TEGDMA. *Dent. Mater.* **2009**, *25*, 1082–1089. [CrossRef]
37. Beatty, M.; Swartz, M.L.; Moore, B.K.; Phillips, R.W.; Roberts, T.A. Effect of crosslinking agent content, monomer functionality, and repeat unit chemistry on properties of unfilled resins. *J. Biomed. Mater. Res.* **1993**, *27*, 403–413. [CrossRef]
38. Pfeifer, C.S.; Silva, L.R.; Kawano, Y.; Braga, R.R. Bis-GMA co-polymerizations: Influence on conversion, flexural properties, fracture toughness and susceptibility to ethanol degradation of experimental composites. *Dent. Mater.* **2009**, *25*, 1136–1141. [CrossRef]
39. Phan, A.C.; Tang, M.-L.; Nguyen, J.-F.; Ruse, N.D.; Sadoun, M. High-temperature high-pressure polymerized urethane dimethacrylate—Mechanical properties and monomer release. *Dent. Mater.* **2014**, *30*, 350–356. [CrossRef] [PubMed]
40. Li, W.; Sun, J. Effects of Ceramic Density and Sintering Temperature on the Mechanical Properties of a Novel Polymer-Infiltrated Ceramic-Network Zirconia Dental Restorative (Filling) Material. *Med Sci. Monit.* **2018**, *24*, 3068–3076. [CrossRef] [PubMed]
41. Guerra, R.M.; Duran, I.; Ortiz, P. FTIR monomer conversion analysis of UDMA-based dental resins. *J. Oral Rehabil.* **2008**, *23*, 632–637. [CrossRef] [PubMed]
42. Charton, C.; Falk, V.; Marchal, P.; Pla, F.; Colon, P. Influence of Tg, viscosity and chemical structure of monomers on shrinkage stress in light-cured dimethacrylate-based dental resins. *Dent. Mater.* **2007**, *23*, 1447–1459. [CrossRef]
43. Lemon, M.T.; Jones, M.S.; Stansbury, J.W. Hydrogen bonding interactions in methacrylate monomers and polymers. *J. Biomed. Mater. Res.* **2007**, *83*, 734–746. [CrossRef]
44. Moszner, N.; Salz, U. New developments of polymeric dental composites. *Prog. Polym. Sci.* **2001**, *26*, 535–576. [CrossRef]
45. Lee, J.-H.; Um, C.-M.; Lee, I.-B. Rheological properties of resin composites according to variations in monomer and filler composition. *Dent. Mater.* **2006**, *22*, 515–526. [CrossRef] [PubMed]
46. Beun, S.; Bailly, C.; Dabin, A.; Vreven, J.; Devaux, J.; Leloup, G. Rheological properties of experimental Bis-GMA/TEGDMA flowable resin composites with various macrofiller/microfiller ratio. *Dent. Mater.* **2009**, *25*, 198–205. [CrossRef] [PubMed]
47. Cui, B.; Sun, F.; Ding, Q.; Wang, H.; Lin, Y.; Shen, Y.; Li, M.; Deng, X.; Zhang, L.; Nan, C. Preparation and Characterization of Sodium Aluminum Silicate-Polymer Composites and Effects of Surface Roughness and Scratch Directions on Their Flexural Strengths. *Front. Mater.* **2021**, *8*, 655156. [CrossRef]
48. Nakahira, A.; Tamai, M.; Miki, S.; Pezzotti, G. Fracture behavior and biocompatibility evaluation of nylon-infiltrated porous hydroxyapatite. *J. Mater. Sci.* **2002**, *37*, 4425–4430. [CrossRef]
49. Ritchie, R.O. The conflicts between strength and toughness. *Nat. Mater.* **2011**, *10*, 817–822. [CrossRef]
50. Launey, M.E.; Ritchie, R.O. On the Fracture Toughness of Advanced Materials. *Adv. Mater.* **2009**, *21*, 2103–2110. [CrossRef]
51. Prielipp, H.; Knechtel, M.; Claussen, N.; Streiffer, S.; Müllejans, H.; Rühle, M.; Rödel, J. Strength and fracture toughness of aluminum/alumina composites with interpenetrating networks. *Mater. Sci. Eng. A* **1995**, *197*, 19–30. [CrossRef]
52. Pezzotti, G.; Asmus, S. Fracture behavior of hydroxyapatite/polymer interpenetrating network composites prepared by in situ polymerization process. *Mater. Sci. Eng. A* **2001**, *316*, 231–237. [CrossRef]
53. Peroglio, M.; Gremillard, L.; Gauthier, C.; Chazeau, L.; Verrier, S.; Alini, M.; Chevalier, J. Mechanical properties and cytocompatibility of poly(ε-caprolactone)-infiltrated biphasic calcium phosphate scaffolds with bimodal pore distribution. *Acta Biomater.* **2010**, *6*, 4369–4379. [CrossRef] [PubMed]
54. Hodásová, L.; Sans, J.; Molina, B.G.; Alemán, C.; Llanes, L.; Fargas, G.; Armelin, E. Polymer infiltrated ceramic networks with biocompatible adhesive and 3D-printed highly porous scaffolds. *Addit. Manuf.* **2021**, *39*, 101850.

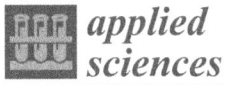

Article

Effects of Composite Resin on the Enamel after Debonding: An In Vitro Study—Metal Brackets vs. Ceramic Brackets

Alexandru Vlasa [1], Eugen Silviu Bud [1,*], Mariana Păcurar [1], Luminița Lazăr [1], Laura Streiche [1], Sorana Maria Bucur [2,*], Dorin Ioan Cocoș [2] and Anamaria Bud [1]

[1] Faculty of Dental Medicine, University of Medicine and Pharmacy, Science and Tehnology, 38 Gheorghe Marinescu Str., 540139 Târgu Mureș, Romania; alexandru.vlasa@gmail.com (A.V.); marianapac@yahoo.com (M.P.); Luminita.lazar@umfst.ro (L.L.); laura.streiche@gmail.com (L.S.); anamaria.bud@umfst.ro (A.B.)
[2] Faculty of Medicine, Dimitrie Cantemir University of Târgu Mureș, 3-5 Bodoni Sandor Str., 540545 Târgu Mureș, Romania; cdorin1123@gmail.com
* Correspondence: eugen.bud@umfst.ro (E.S.B.); bucursoranamaria@gmail.com (S.M.B.); Tel./Fax: +407-4443-7661 (E.S.B.); +407-5375-6551 (S.M.B.)

Abstract: Fixed orthodontic therapies include several procedures that can affect the enamel surface. The aim of this study was to assess the action of composite resin on the surface of the tooth through variation of enamel changes after debonding metal and ceramic brackets, by means of scanning electron microscopy. An in vitro study was conducted on 48 human premolar specimens, which were extracted within a period of two months for orthodontic purposes. On half of them, metal brackets were bonded, and on the other half, ceramic brackets (Al_2O_3) were bonded, using light cure adhesive paste and a two-step, etch-and-bonding technique. The brackets were debonded after 24 h using a straight debonding plier. The adhesive remnant index (ARI) was determined by visual observation of the specimen. Post-debonding scans were aligned with the baseline, and the surfaces' changes were quantified. A quantitative analysis was made on the debonded brackets to determine the presence or absence of enamel on the base pad. Evaluation of pre-bonded and post-clean-up enamel surface revealed no crack and increased roughness in both ceramic and metal brackets, which was higher for the ceramic ones. The enameled band (perikymata), artificial caries, or the superficial fissures revealed in the pretreatment stage were replaced with the loss of the prismatic structure and the presence of remnant adhesive. No enamel substance was found on the base pad. The ARI_{tooth} was higher for metallic brackets than for ceramic ones. Metallic brackets and ceramic brackets have undergone mechanical changes by showing fractures in their structure. According to our present investigation, we can conclude that the adhesive composite resin is safe for use on both metal and ceramic brackets in orthodontic treatments, with no iatrogenic enamel damages.

Keywords: bracket debonding; dental enamel; scanning electron microscopy; orthodontics

Citation: Vlasa, A.; Bud, E.S.; Păcurar, M.; Lazăr, L.; Streiche, L.; Bucur, S.M.; Cocoș, D.I.; Bud, A. Effects of Composite Resin on the Enamel after Debonding: An In Vitro Study—Metal Brackets vs. Ceramic Brackets. *Appl. Sci.* **2021**, *11*, 7353. https://doi.org/10.3390/app11167353

Academic Editor: Mitsuru Motoyoshi

Received: 30 June 2021
Accepted: 9 August 2021
Published: 10 August 2021

Publisher's Note: MDPI stays neutral with regard to jurisdictional claims in published maps and institutional affiliations.

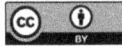

Copyright: © 2021 by the authors. Licensee MDPI, Basel, Switzerland. This article is an open access article distributed under the terms and conditions of the Creative Commons Attribution (CC BY) license (https://creativecommons.org/licenses/by/4.0/).

1. Introduction

The concept of biomaterials, which is widely used nowadays, could include everything from metal to ceramic, plastic, and any other material that is well tolerated by the human body. In the field of fixed orthodontics, brackets are used very often during the treatment. These appliances are mostly made of metal alloys, polycarbonate, ceramic, zirconia [1,2], different kind of wires, and various bonding materials. Although the materials from which the brackets were made have significantly evolved, the metallic ones are still widely used due to their mechanical and chemical properties [3]. Intense research over the years on these materials has led to a great diversity of ferroalloys used for brackets, wires, bands, and other orthodontic accessories, such as cobalt–chromium alloy (Cr–Co), stainless steel, and titanium alloys, all of which have nickel (Ni) as one of the main components [4].

Ceramic brackets began to be used in the late 1980s, and nowadays, they are commonly used for orthodontic fixed therapy [5]. They were designed in an attempt to satisfy the esthetic requirements of the patients with fixed orthodontic appliances. These translucent brackets are made from aluminum oxide (alumina) particles and are available in the monocrystalline and polycrystalline form [5]. Aluminum oxide is an inert crystalline powder, insoluble in water and odorless [6].

Aluminum oxide has a chemical formula Al_2O_3. It is amphoteric in nature and has been used in various chemical, industrial, and commercial applications. It is considered an indirect additive used in food contact substances by the FDA [6]. The crystal structure of aluminum oxide is illustrative of the principles involved with ceramics having a substantial ionic bonding character. The crystal structure [7] consists of a nearly hcp arrangement of the larger oxygen anions (O^{2-}), with the smaller aluminum cations (Al^{3+}) located in two-thirds of the octahedral interstitial sites in the hcp structure. The layers in the structure provide the maximum separation of the Al^{3+} ions. These octahedral sites have sixfold coordination, i.e., each aluminum ion is surrounded by six oxygen ions. The crystal structure is determined by the ratio of the radii of the aluminum and oxygen ions, and the requirement of an electrically neutral unit cell.

Both physical and chemical characteristics of aluminum oxide products vary depending on the processing method that leads to changes in the crystal structure. The variety formed at very high temperatures is quite inert chemically [5,6].

Concern about enamel damage occurs especially when ceramic brackets are used. The first generations of ceramic brackets resulted in a major alteration of the enamel. Thus far, they have undergone significant improvements. The purpose of debracketing is to remove brackets and adhesive material from the tooth, giving it the initial appearance and contour, and minimizing the loss of iatrogenic hard tissue during this maneuver [8]. The manufacturers of the new generations of ceramic brackets assure that their use in orthodontic treatment is safe, due to the design of the base. Technological evolution allows researchers to quantitatively measure the surface of the enamel, which can be reduced after debracketing. The use of metal brackets registers the presence of the remaining adhesive material and leads to a loss of hard tooth substance of 20–50 μm after their removal [6,8].

The objective of this in vitro study was to compare the changes in the enamel surface following the removal of ceramic and metal brackets, namely, the appearance of new cracks or the deepening of the existing ones. Quantitative analysis was performed using dispersive X-ray spectroscopy in the base of the brackets, and the ARI_{tooth} score [9] is retained.

2. Materials and Methods

For analysis, a number of 174 freshly extracted premolars for orthodontic purposes were collected. After extraction, teeth were kept at room temperature in 10% formalin solution for a period of 7 days, which was subsequently replaced by saline solution (NaCl 0.9%) and was changed daily for 10 more days. After storage, teeth were examined and inspected. Teeth that showed signs of enamel degradation, caries, tartar, or fillings on the vestibular surface, as well as fluorosis or hypoplasia, were excluded from the study. On the subsequent stage of the study, 147 premolars with intact vestibular surfaces were analyzed. Teeth from the study group underwent periodontal ligament removal using a Gracey™ 5–6 curette and then were polished with Depural Neo™ Spofa Dental, Jičín, Czech Republic, and stored back in the saline solution.

Later in the study, an S-3400N electron microscope, Hitachi, Chiyoda, Tōkyō, Japan, was used to analyze the enamel surface pretreatment (Figure 1). Data were recorded and used as a benchmark later in the study for comparison with the images obtained post treatment.

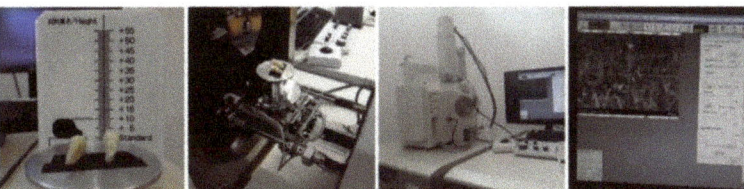

Figure 1. The steps taken to view the samples at SEM.

The samples did not require prior preparation because the microscope has a vacuum function that allows the observation of nonconductive specimens at a working distance of 9 mm, without the need to apply any conductive layer. The acceleration voltage of the microscope was operated at 15 kV. The only intervention on the enamel surface was to draw an indicative perimeter of the future base of the bracket for an easier investigation of the surface. For this purpose, we used a round disk of 0.10 mm diameter.

After the preliminary analysis using SEM, the study group was divided into 2 sub-groups as follows:

- Study sub-group 1 consisted of 72 premolars, in which we applied metal Gemini™ brackets (3M Unitec™, USA) with the following chemical composition: Ni 83.98%, Si 6.46%, Fe 5.90%, and Cr 3.52%;
- Study subgroup 2 consisted of 75 premolars, in which we applied ceramic brackets Forestadent™, Germany (Al_2O_3).

The enamel's surface was dried for 10 s using the air spray, and 37% phosphoric acid (Unitek Etching Gel System from 3M Unitek) was applied for 30 s. The acid was removed by a jet of water applied for 10 s, followed by a jet of air from the unit's spray for 10 s. To promote adhesion, a primer Transbond XT™ from 3M Unitek was used; the primer was applied with a micro brush by circular movements on the previously prepared surface then it was photo-polymerized for 20 s by using a high-power led lamp Elipar S10™, 3M ESPE, with the tip of the lamp curing tube placed 1 mm away from the vestibular surface of the tooth. The bracket's base was loaded with the adhesive paste Transbond ™ from 3M Unitek, then placed very similar to and following the positioning bonding rules described by Armstrong et al. [10] in the center of the vestibular surface. After correct positioning, brackets were pressed to 300 g using an orthodontic dynamometer. Excess composite resin was removed prior to light curing with a dental probe. The polymerization was performed mesially and distally from the bracket for 10 s on each side. After 24 h, the brackets were removed using straight take-off pliers and acting directly on the brackets' bases. The adhesive material was removed with a high-speed multi-laminated tungsten carbide burr. The cleaning process was continued until the adhesive material was no longer visible to the visual inspection and the enamel became smooth, without roughness detectable on examination with the dental probe.

After the brackets were removed, the teeth were stored in saline solution at room temperature until the second analysis at SEM, when the samples were analyzed at the same parameters as before treatment, and possible irregularities and cracks in the enamel surface were monitored. In the next step of the study a quantitative analysis, the energy-dispersive X-ray spectroscopy (EDX) was also performed on the entire surface of the brackets' soles to detect any traces of enamel. For analysis, we used APEX™, EDAX, Unterschleissheim Germany software for Windows™ (Figure 2) that helped us identify the chemical elements and provided information on the quantitative composition of the sample.

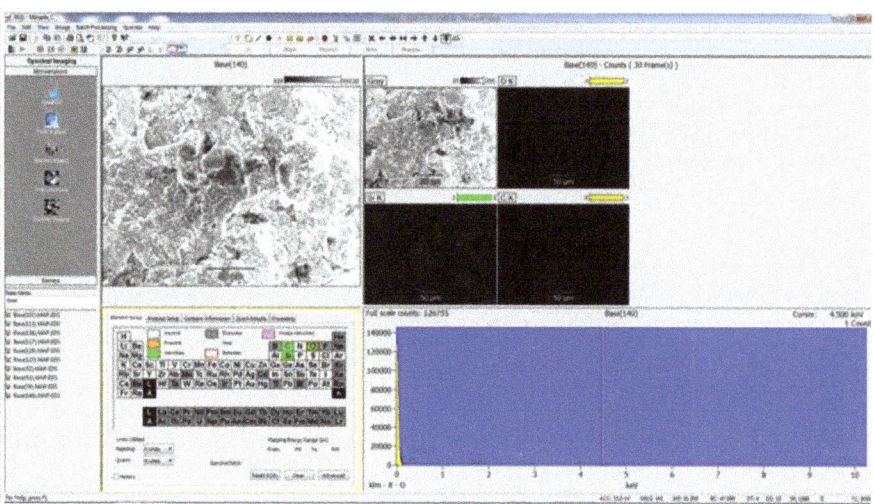

Figure 2. Software used to perform EDX analysis.

ARI Score

After the second SEM analysis was performed, the adhesive remnant index (ARI) was evaluated. ARI score records the amount of residual adhesive located on the tooth or bracket sole. For analysis, we chose to evaluate the amount of adhesive present on the enamel surface after removing the brackets using the values that were proposed by Artün and Bergland in 1984 [11].

- Score 0—without adhesive on the tooth surface;
- Score 1—less than 50% adhesive present on the tooth surface;
- Score 2—more than 50% adhesive present on the tooth surface;
- Score 3—all the adhesive present on the tooth surface.

Statistical processing was performed using GraphPad Prism™ V6.01 software for Windows™. The D'Agostino and Pearson omnibus normality test was used to determine the normality of the data. The chosen significance threshold was $alpha = 0.05$, considering p significant when $p < 0.05$.

3. Results

3.1. Appearance of the Enamel

When comparing pre- and posttreatment data, there was no evidence of new cracks in the enamel. An increase in the roughness of the enamel was observed using both types of brackets (Figures 3–5).

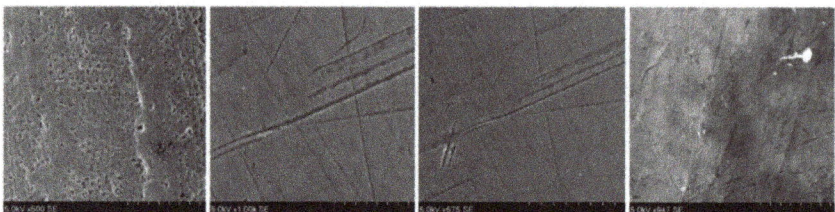

Figure 3. Microscopic appearance of the enamel before treatment 6.0 kV.

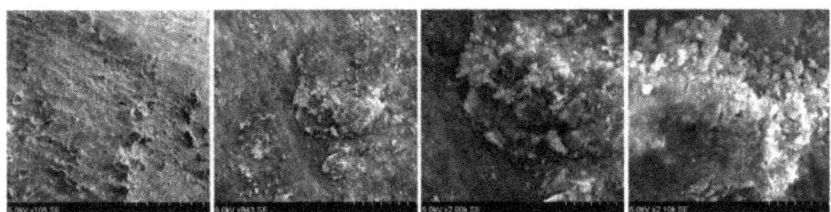

Figure 4. Microscopic appearance of enamel after removal of metal brackets 6.0 kV.

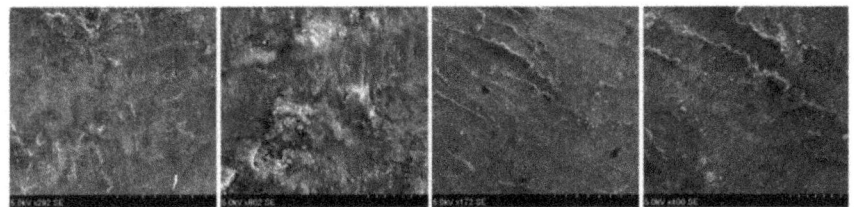

Figure 5. Microscopic appearance of the enamel after removal of the ceramic brackets 6.0 kV.

No statistically significant differences were found regarding the ARI score between metallic and ceramic brackets in the study groups (Figure 6).

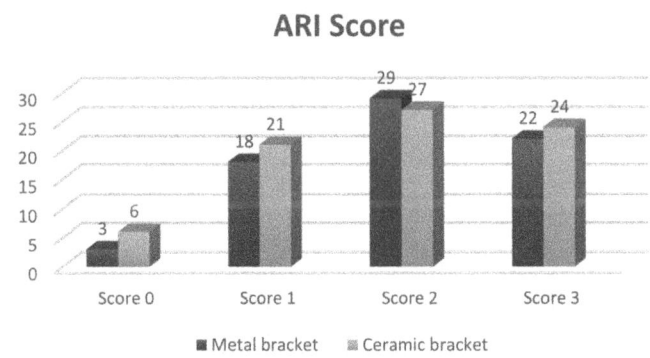

Figure 6. Graphical representation of ARI scores.

3.2. EDX Analysis

Quantitative EDX analysis was performed on the detached brackets to determine the absence or the presence of enamel on the brackets' soles. According to the tables below, the presence of carbon, oxygen, and silicon, which are all constituents of the adhesive material, could be observed. There were no traces of calcium or phosphorus, which are the main constituents of the enamel (Figures 7–11).

Element Line	Net Counts	Weight %	Atom %
C K	106	41.29	51.99
O K	123	40.31	38.10
Si K	262	18.40	9.91
Total		100.00	100.00

Figure 7. EDX result of metal bracket.

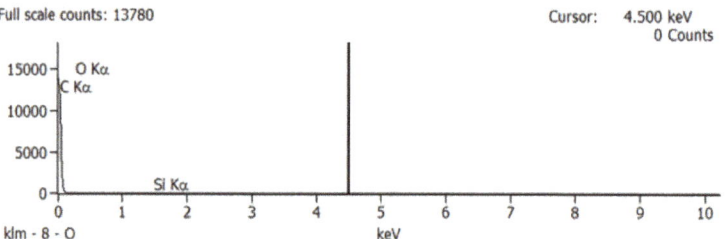

Figure 8. Graphical representation of the EDX analysis presented above.

Element Line	Net Counts	Weight %	Atom %
C K	88	44.35	55.25
O K	82	37.54	35.11
Si K	191	18.11	9.65
Total		100.00	100.00

Figure 9. EDX result of ceramic bracket.

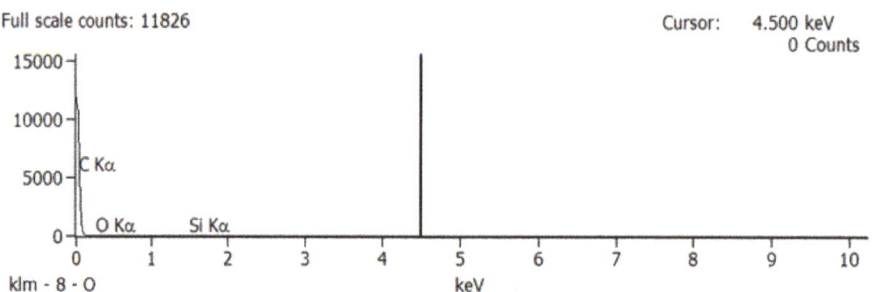

Figure 10. Graphical representation of the EDX analysis presented above.

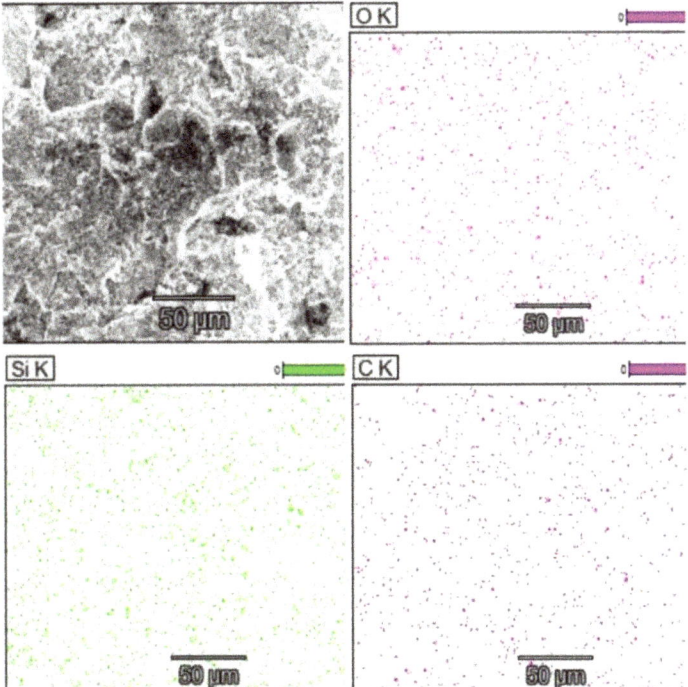

Figure 11. Density of the elements O, Si, and C on an area of 50 microns.

3.3. Condition of Brackets after Removal from Teeth

The metal brackets were removed from teeth without breaking; however, macroscopic signs of structural damage, such as mechanical deformation of the bracket, were noticeable on all the metallic brackets used in the study. Regarding the ceramic brackets, 63% of the brackets presented, from a macroscopic point of view, fractured structure or fissures in the mass of the bracket, while 37% remained intact after debonding.

4. Discussion

In this paper, the debracketing technique was used by positioning the pliers at the base of the bracket and the presence of enamel was not identified either at the level of the ceramic or metal brackets.

Artun and Bergland found that all brackets analyzed with EDX contain calcium, and by default enamel, in the form of a thin layer, fragments, or even in those where no trace of residual material is visible. The debracketing was performed in this experiment by positioning the pliers at the level of the wings [11]. Further studies that analyzed the presence of calcium on ceramic, metal (SS), and self-ligating brackets confirm that the highest amount of calcium was recorded in ceramic (4%), followed by metal (1.44%), and finally, self-ligating (1.42%). In this study, the debracketing was performed by positioning the pliers at the base of the bracket [12,13].

Furthermore, in another study comparing the two methods of debracketing metal brackets, i.e., wings and soles, it was found that the $ARI_{bracket}$ score is similar (WM = 66.7%, BM = 68.7%), which assumes that the rupture occurred at either the adhesive–adhesive or adhesive–enamel interface [14]. The two debracketing techniques were expected to result in different ARI scores. However, the ARI score and the presence of calcium were similar in the two methods, despite the difference in force applied, which was previously measured [15]. The explanation for this dichotomy is that the crack is probably initiated at the level of the adhesive layer and propagated at the bracket–adhesive or adhesive–enamel interface. It should also be taken into account the fact that metal brackets cast with light-curable material have an initially lower adhesion strength at the bracket–adhesive interface than the enamel–adhesive interface because the light-cured resin under the sole of the bracket has reflected light. This is supported by a short-term study that showed that the rupture occurs at the bracket–adhesive interface [16]. Further recent studies [14,15] demonstrated that after a longer period of time, 24 months, the composite is completely polymerized with a strong adhesion force. Another aspect to consider is that the enamel under the sole of the bracket may be affected by decalcification resulting from food debris and poor hygiene that damages the enamel–adhesive bond. The authors claimed that regardless of the method of debracketing chosen, the rupture occurred at the adhesive–enamel interface [15,16]. Türkkahraman et al. [17] reported that the biggest part of brackets' failures occurred within the adhesive layer.

An analysis of photoelastic stress showed that the force applied to the outer wings of the bracket transfers less stress to the enamel, compared to the force applied to the base of the bracket and the adhesion area, which creates a region of stress concentration in the enamel, thus leading to a separation at the adhesive–enamel interface. Nevertheless, Brosh et al. [14] did not find any significant difference between the two possibilities of applying the forceps (on the wings/at the base of the bracket) in terms of calcium score.

In this situation, a question arises: is there a correlation between the ARI score and the presence of calcium on the sole of the bracket?

One study claims that a thin layer of enamel is removed when the bracket is cut out [18]. This is due to acid etching and the fact that the adhesive material penetrates the micropores produced by this process. Most likely, the partially demineralized enamel around the pores detaches more easily from the tooth and remains adhered to the adhesive material during debracketing. The study was performed in vivo with a treatment duration of 24 months +/− 3 months. The bracket–adhesive interface is considered to be the most favorable for debracketing, thus leaving most of the adhesive on the tooth surface, as happens at an ARI_{tooth} score of 2 and 3 [19–21].

Because partial demineralization of the enamel may occur, some authors suggested the use of nano-hydroxyapatite in demineralized enamel before orthodontic bonding of brackets [22]. Scribante et al. [22], in their study, showed that a great visual remineralization effect can be noticed already after the second application cycle of biomimetic nano-hydroxyapatite. On the other hand, there are studies that demonstrated that the use of pre-orthodontic treatment fluoride lacquer or varnish develops lower bond strengths, which is likely to result in a higher frequency of premature detachment of the bracket [23]. More recently, Bącela J et al. [24], in their study regarding coating the orthodontic devices, as well as modifying their surface with additives, showed that this method improves their mechanical properties and can minimize bacterial adhesion on the surface. Appropriate coating techniques enable the reduction in corrosivity, wear and tear, and its delamination. The material used in the coating may accelerate orthodontic treatment. The analysis of additives such as TiO_2, ZnO, Ag, and silver nanoparticles, as well as uncoated arches, can compare antimicrobial activity and environmental resistance. The layer thickness of coatings applied to the archwires is also relevant for the antibacterial effect.

After bracketing, it is recommended to preserve the integrity of the enamel layer; in the meantime, the persistence of the adhesive material on the tooth is an objective to be pursued. This goal was achieved in this study, as the ARI scores obtained were 2 and 3 for most of the ceramic and metal brackets.

4.1. Roughness

The degree of roughness depends on the tools used to remove the adhesive material.

It has been shown that by assessing the roughness before and after debracketing, it is increased in all cases at the end of treatment [25]. Goel et al. claim that using the Sof-Lex disc and the self-etching primer achieves a degree of roughness in the enamel surface similar to the pretreated one; this is followed by the combination of using the self-etching primer and the tungsten carbide burr [19].

Further studies state that the best results were obtained with the help of the tungsten carbide burr operated at low speed. The study compared low-speed tungsten carbide burr, tungsten carbide burr, and ultrafine diamond burr, both at high speed, together with cooling and Er: YAG laser instrument, with a wavelength of 2940 nm [20].

Another recent study reports that the most efficient is the high-speed multifilament tungsten carbide cutter, followed by the low-speed multifilament tungsten carbide cutter. The fiberglass cutter is inefficient, leaving a large amount of adhesive behind [21].

4.2. Integrity of Brackets after Debonding

Over 60% of the ceramic brackets were broken during debonding, while the metal brackets remained intact. This is due to the increased adhesion force of the ceramic brackets. The adhesion force of metal brackets is lower than that of ceramic brackets with mechanical retention, which indicates a higher risk of enamel degradation while debracketing [26].

The study conducted by Ciocan et al. stated that the increased adhesion strength of ceramic brackets may be due to the design of the bracket sole, which provides strong bonding and requires special debracketing procedures recommended by the manufacturer [27].

Several studies indicated that the design of the base can influence the adhesion force and can play a role in the absorption of stress by the enamel and producing iatrogenic effects at this level [28,29].

When evaluating the results of these studies, it should be borne in mind that clinical debonding may differ from in vitro conditions. Debracketing forces can be applied slightly differently, while temperature, humidity, and other oral factors can affect the adhesion force and therefore damage to the enamel. Patients should be informed of the possible side effects of the removal of the brackets on enamel [29]. The extracted teeth used during the studies may have undetectable cracks in the surface, due to forceps, amplifying the degradation of the enamel. However, the results of in vitro studies remain very relevant [8].

It should be noted that in this study, the teeth were subjected to a pretreatment analysis, the debracketing technique consisted in applying the pliers at the base of the bracket, and the study was performed in vitro. These are the factors that contribute to the identification of the enamel on the sole of the bracket in the conditions of the examination of the samples collected from the patients. Other in vitro studies performed debracketing after 24 h [16,30] as we did in this scientific paper, and the difficulty with which the brackets were removed, both metal and ceramic, did not confirm the hypothesis of insufficient polymerization of the adhesive material.

5. Conclusions

Unfortunately, debracketing may lead to bracket fracture. Bracket fragments may detach (loose fragments) or remain attached to the enamel surface. Low-speed or high-speed grinding of the bracket fragments with no water coolant may bring forth permanent damage and necrosis of the dental pulps. Therefore, water cooling is absolutely necessary during the grinding/removal of ceramic bracket fragments. Analyzing the pretreatment and posttreatment results, no crack was observed in the enamel, only increased roughness in both types of brackets. The sole of the bracket did not show traces of calcium to confirm the loss of substance.

The persistence of the adhesive material on the tooth is a goal to be pursued, and the placement of the straight orthodontic plier at the base of the bracket makes this possible, thus preserving the integrity of the enamel. Although more brittle and prone to breakage, ceramic brackets did not favor the loss of enamel, similar to the metallic ones.

Author Contributions: All authors contributed equally to this research. E.S.B., M.P. and A.B. designed and performed the in vitro phase; L.L., S.M.B. and D.I.C. derived the models and analyzed the data; A.V., E.S.B. and M.P. assisted with measurements and helped carry out the statistical analysis; A.V., L.L., S.M.B. and D.I.C. produced the manuscript in consultation with E.S.B., L.S., M.P. and A.B.;

M.P. and L.L. techno-redacted the text and gave final expert approval. All authors have read and agreed to the published version of the manuscript.

Funding: This research received no external funding.

Institutional Review Board Statement: The study was conducted according to the guidelines of the Declaration of Helsinki, and approved by the Institutional Review Board of SC Algocalm SRL, private medical center, Targu-Mures, Romania (906/05.01.2021).

Informed Consent Statement: Informed consent was obtained from all subjects involved in the study.

Data Availability Statement: Not applicable.

Conflicts of Interest: The authors declare no conflict of interest.

References

1. Matasa, C.G. Tendances dans les biomatériaux orthodontiques: Métaux et céramiques [Trends in orthodontic biomaterials: Metals and ceramics]. *L'Orthodontie Française* **2000**, *71*, 335–341. [CrossRef]
2. Kilponen, L.; Varrela, J.; Vallittu, P.K. Priming and bonding metal, ceramic and polycarbonate brackets. *Biomater. Investig. Dent.* **2019**, *6*, 61–72. [CrossRef]
3. Ogiński, T.; Kawala, B.; Mikulewicz, M.; Antoszewska-Smith, J. A Clinical Comparison of Failure Rates of Metallic and Ceramic Brackets: A Twelve-Month Study. *Biomed Res. Int.* **2020**, *2020*, 9725101. [CrossRef]
4. Wendl, B.; Wiltsche, H.; Lankmayr, E.; Winsauer, H.; Walter, A.; Muchitsch, A.; Jakse, N.; Wendl, M.; Wendl, T. Metal release profiles of orthodontic bands, brackets, and wires: An in vitro study. *J. Orofac. Orthop.* **2017**, *78*, 494–503. [CrossRef]
5. Khatri, J.M.; Sawant, S.S.; Naidu, N.R.; Vispute, S.S.; Patankar, K.A. An update on orthodontic brackets—A review. *Int. J. Orthod. Rehabil.* **2020**, *11*, 136–144.
6. National Center for Biotechnology Information. PubChem Compound Summary for CID 9989226, Aluminum Oxide. Available online: https://pubchem.ncbi.nlm.nih.gov/compound/Aluminum-oxide (accessed on 13 June 2021).
7. Shtyka, O.; Maniukiewicz, W.; Ciesielski, R.; Kedziora, A.; Shatsila, V.; Sierański, T.; Maniecki, T. The Formation of Cr-Al Spinel under a Reductive Atmosphere. *Materials* **2021**, *14*, 3218. [CrossRef] [PubMed]
8. Suliman, S.N.; Trojan, T.M.; Tantbirojn, D.; Versluis, A. Enamel loss following ceramic bracket debonding: A quantitative analysis in vitro. *Angle Orthod.* **2015**, *85*, 651–656. [CrossRef] [PubMed]
9. Electronic Microscope. Available online: https://ro.wikipedia.org/wiki/Microscop_electronic (accessed on 26 January 2021).
10. Armstrong, D.; Shen, G.; Petocz, P.; Darendeliler, M.A. A comparison of accuracy in bracket positioning between two techniques—Localizing the centre of the clinical crown and measuring the distance from the incisal edge. *Eur. J. Orthod.* **2007**, *29*, 430–436. [CrossRef]
11. Artun, J.; Bergland, S. Clinical trials with crystal growth conditioning as an alternative to acid-etch enamepretreatment. *Am. J. Orthod.* **1984**, *85*, 333–340. [CrossRef]
12. Reimann, S.; Bourauel, C.; Weber, A.; Dirk, C.; Lietz, T. Friction behavior of ceramic injection-molded (CIM) brackets. *J. Orofac. Orthop.* **2016**, *77*, 262–271. [CrossRef]
13. Zanarinia, M.; Gracobb, A.; Latucacc, M. Bracket base remnants after orthodontic debonding. *Angle Orthod.* **2013**, *83*, 889–890. [CrossRef]
14. Brosh, T.; Kaufman, A.; Balabanovsky, A.; Vardimon, A.D. In vivo debonding strength and enamel damage in two orthodontic debonding methods. *J. Biomech.* **2005**, *38*, 1107–1113. [CrossRef]
15. Radhakrishnan, P.D.; Sapna Varma, N.K.; Ajith, V.V. Assessment of Bracket Surface Morphology and Dimensional Change. *Contemp. Clin. Dent.* **2017**, *8*, 71–80. [CrossRef]
16. Delavarian, M.; Rahimi, F.; Mohammadi, R.; Imani, M.M. Shear bond strength of ceramic and metal brackets bonded to enamel using color-change adhesive. *Dent. Res. J.* **2019**, *16*, 233–238.
17. Türkkahraman, H.; Adanir, N.; Gungor, A.Y.; Alkis, H. In Vitro evaluation of shear bond strengths of colour change adhesives. *Eur. J. Orthod.* **2010**, *32*, 571–574. [CrossRef] [PubMed]
18. Henkin, F.S.; Macêdo, É.O.; Santos, K.D.; Schwarzbach, M.; Samuel, S.M.; Mundstock, K.S. In Vitro analysis of shear bond strength and adhesive remnant index of different metal brackets. *Dent. Press J. Orthod.* **2016**, *21*, 67–73. [CrossRef] [PubMed]
19. Goel, A.; Singh, A.; Grupta, T.G. Evaluation of surface roughness of enamel ater various bonding and clean-up procedures on enamel bonded with three different bonding agents: An in-vitro study. *J. Clin. Exp. Dent.* **2017**, *9*, 608–616.
20. Ahrari, F.; Akbari, M.; Akbari, J. Enamel Surface Roughness after Debonding of Orthodontic Brackets and Various Clean-Up Techniques. *J. Dent.* **2013**, *10*, 82–93.
21. Claudino, D.; Kuga, M.C.; Belizário, L.; Pereira, J.R. Enamel evaluation by scanning electron microscopy after debonding brackets and removal of adhesive remnants. *J. Clin. Exp. Dent.* **2018**, *10*, 248–251. [CrossRef] [PubMed]
22. Scribante, A.; Dermenaki Farahani, M.R.; Marino, G.; Matera, C.; Rodriguez YBaena, R.; Lanteri, V.; Butera, A. Biomimetic Effect of Nano-Hydroxyapatite in Demineralized Enamel before Orthodontic Bonding of Brackets and Attachments: Visual, Adhesion Strength, and Hardness in In Vitro Tests. *Biomed. Res. Int.* **2020**, *30*, 6747498. [CrossRef] [PubMed]

23. Lanteri, V.; Segu, M.; Doldi, J.; Butera, A. Pre-bonding prophylaxis and brackets detachment: An experimental comparison of different methods. *Int. J. Clin. Dent.* **2014**, *7*, 191–197.
24. Bącela, J.; Łabowska, M.B.; Detyna, J.; Zięty, A.; Michalak, I. Functional Coatings for Orthodontic Archwires—A Review. *Materials* **2020**, *13*, 3257. [CrossRef] [PubMed]
25. Bishara, S.E.; Laffoon, J.F.; Vonwald, L.; Warren, J.J. The effect of repeated bonding on the shear bond strength of different orthodontic adhesives. *Am. J. Orthod. Dentofac. Orthop.* **2002**, *121*, 521–525. [CrossRef] [PubMed]
26. Bishara, S.E.; Oonsombat, C.; Soliman, M.M.; Warren, J.J.; Laffoon, J.F.; Ajlouni, R. Comparison of bonding time and shear bond strength between a conventional and a new integrated bonding system. *Angle Orthod.* **2005**, *75*, 237–242. [PubMed]
27. Ciocan, D.I.; Stanciu, D.; Popescu, M.A.; Miculescu, F.; Plotog, I.; Vărzaru, G.; Ciocan, L.T. Electron microscopy analysis of different orthodontic brackets and their adhesion to the tooth enamel. *Rom. J. Morphol. Embryol.* **2014**, *55*, 591–596. [PubMed]
28. Ahangar Atashi, M.H.; Sadr Haghighi, A.H.; Nastarin, P.; Ahangar Atashi, S. Variations in enamel damage after debonding of two different bracket base design: An in vitro study. *J. Dent. Res. Dent. Clin. Dent. Prospects* **2018**, *12*, 56–62. [CrossRef] [PubMed]
29. Vaida, L.; Mutiu, G.; Tara, I.G.; Bodog, F. An Algorithm of Ethical Approach to The Orthodontic Patient. *Iran. J. Public Health* **2015**, *44*, 1296–1298.
30. Yamamoto, A.; Yoshida, T.; Tsubota, K.; Takamizawa, T.; Kurokawa, H.; Miyazaki, M. Orthodontic bracket bonding: Enamel bond strength vs time. *Am. J. Orthod. Dentofac. Orthop.* **2006**, *130*, 435. [CrossRef]

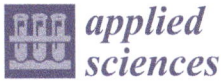

Article

Occlusal Splint Therapy Followed by Orthodontic Molar Intrusion as an Effective Treatment Method to Treat Patients with Temporomandibular Disorder: A Retrospective Study

Bálint Nemes [1], Dorottya Frank [2,*], Andreu Puigdollers [3] and Domingo Martín [4]

1. Department of Paediatric Dentistry and Orthodontics, Faculty of Dentistry, Semmelweis University, 1085 Budapest, Hungary; nemesbalintdr@gmail.com
2. Department of Dentistry, Oral and Maxillofacial Surgery, University of Pécs, 7622 Pécs, Hungary
3. Department of Orthodontics and Dentofacial Orthopaedics, Faculty of Dentistry, International University of Catalunya, 08017 Barcelona, Spain; apuigdollersp@gmail.com
4. Private Practice Martin-Goenaga, 20005 San Sebastián, Spain; domingomartin@domingomartin.com
* Correspondence: frank.dorottya@pte.hu; Tel.: +36-72-535-920

Abstract: Our goal is to show that temporomandibular disorder (TMD) patients with orthopaedic instability can be effectively treated by the combination of occlusal splint therapy and molar intrusion. Diagnostic records of 18 patients reporting previous TMD and treated with splint therapy were evaluated. Postsplint anterior open bite was treated by skeletally anchored molar intrusion. Changes in overjet (OJ), overbite (OB) were measured on articulator mounted models: initially in maximal intercuspidation (MI), centric "de jour", postsplint centric relation (CR) and postintrusion CR. Changes in ANB (A point-Nasion-B point) angle, mandibular plane–palatal plane angle and facial axis angle were assessed on lateral cephalograms. Morphological changes of the condyle were detected on pre-and posttreatment CBCT images. When compared screening mountings to MI models, significant differences were found in OJ and OB. Following splint wear, there was a significant increase in lower facial height and significant decrease in facial axis angle, which in turn increased ANB angle. OB and OJ showed a significant change on the postsplint mountings when compared to MI. After intrusion, mandible exhibited counterclockwise rotation, which decreased lower facial height, increased OB and facial axis angle and decreased ANB and OJ. Posttreatment CBCTs confirmed improved condylar morphology. Occlusal splint therapy followed by orthodontic molar intrusion provides MI-CR harmony, therefore, it seems to be an effective method for treating TMD patients.

Keywords: molar intrusion; orthodontic treatment; temporomandibular disorder; occlusal splint; centric relation

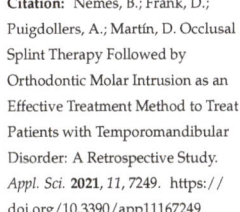

1. Introduction

Orthodontic treatment of patients with temporomandibular disorder (TMD) due to orthopaedic instability has always been challenging. Many clinicians advocate that the ideal occlusion should be related to an ideal condyle-disk-fossa relationship, what they refer to as centric relation (CR) [1]. TMD patients often show shift between maximal intercuspidation (MI) and CR [1,2]. Moreover the degree of CR-MI discrepancy has been shown to strongly correlate with the severity of the symptoms and signs of temporomandibular disorder (TMD) and therefore, it was proposed to be a contributory factor to the development of TMD [3]. Dawson and Roth were the first to explain how CR-MI discrepancy may lead to the development of TMD [4–6]. They declared that if CR interference exist during jaw closure, the inferior lateral pterygoid muscle is non-physiologically contracted in order to achieve MI. The contraction of the muscle distracts the condyle out of CR position resulting in hyperactivation of the elevator muscles. Imbalance between the elevator and depressor muscles can lead to consequent masticatory muscle spasm and pain [4,5]. As stated by Okeson; positional stability of the joint is determined by the muscles that pull across the joint and prevent separation of the articular surfaces. The muscles' directional forces determine the optimum, orthopedically stable joint position [7]. The continuous existence of occlusal interferences can contribute to chronic muscle hyperactivity, articular disc derangement and disc displacement which causes temporomandibular joint (TMJ) clicking and further progression will result in intracapsular disorders [4–6]. Over the years, the most preferably and commonly used therapy for treating patients with TMD with orthopaedic instability has been the occlusal stabilization splint [8]. Due to its design, it can reposition the mandible to CR and switch off the neuromuscular adaptation to MI by relaxing the muscles and achieve orthopaedic stability. Therefore, in orthodontic patients reporting TMD due to orthopaedic instability these stabilization splints are recommended prior to orthodontic therapy. During the splint wear, condyle is passively seated in the fossa, resulting in altered dental occlusion; contact on the most posterior teeth and anterior open bite (AOB) will develop [9,10]. Before the era of temporary anchorage devices (TADs), possible therapeutic solutions for adult AOB patients were camouflage treatment by extruding the anterior teeth, extraction, surgical maxillary impaction [11] and intrusion of posterior teeth by either intermaxillary [12] or extraoral appliances [13]. Shellhart [14] was the first who used dental implants for intruding molars. In 1996, Melsen and Fiorelli [15] demonstrated that significant amount of true orthodontic molar intrusion can be achieved which can largely facilitate the prosthetic reconstruction of partially edentulous patients and in the absence of gingival inflammation, it can improve periodontal health as well [16–18]. Since then, many techniques have been introduced for skeletally anchored posterior teeth intrusion [19–25]. Although, in many of these articles, intrusion mechanics, force magnitudes and treatment details are precisely described, not too much attention has been paid towards the real condyle position so far. Besides, far less is mentioned about the shape and position of the condyle seen in 3D as in CBCT images. In turn, treatment started from and ended in CR-where the condyle is centered in the fossa and the disc position is correct–with orthopaedic stability, can be one of the assurances for long-term occlusal stability and temporomandibular joint (TMJ) health. Accordingly, not considering CR in these patients may query even the real start-, and endpoint of the treatment and the stability as well. Therefore, the aim of the present study is to present the results of a series of 18 consecutive cases with orthopaedic instability treated with occlusal splint therapy followed by skeletally anchored molar intrusion, and studied by pre and posttreatment articulator mounting, lateral cephs and CBCT.

2. Materials and Methods

2.1. Subjects

In our study, pre-and posttreatment diagnostic records of 47 orthodontic patients with TMD (18 men, 29 women, mean age: 35.3 years) treated at a private praxis between 2008–2018 were evaluated. Table 1 summarizes the age and gender distribution of the subjects.

All of the patients were diagnosed with orthopaedic instability and had complaint of muscle pain (masseter, temporal, medial pterygoid and/or suboccipital), 31 subjects had reversible disc dislocation (13 unilateral, 18 bilateral) and 16 patients had disc displacement without reduction and therefore, were treated with full-coverage hard acrylic occlusal splints. After achieving an orthopaedic stability and the elimination of TMD, postsplint AOB was treated by non-surgical orthodontic approach. From the original 47 patients, only 18 patients (2 men, 16 women; mean age 28.7 years) were included in the study. 29 were excluded due to missing diagnostic records, no use of skeletal anchors, lack of proper compliance in full-time splint wear and because of moving to another location. Molars were intruded by buccal zygomatic miniplates with combination of either palatal miniscrews or transpalatal bars. In two cases where dental implants were present, these implants were used to facilitate intrusion (Figure 1a–f).

Table 1. Age and gender distribution of the subjects.

	Gender	
	Men	Women
Number of subjects	18	29
Mean age (years)	35.42	35.27
Age range (years)		
10–20	0	2
21–30	8	8
31–40	6	12
41–50	2	3
51–60	0	3
61–70	2	1

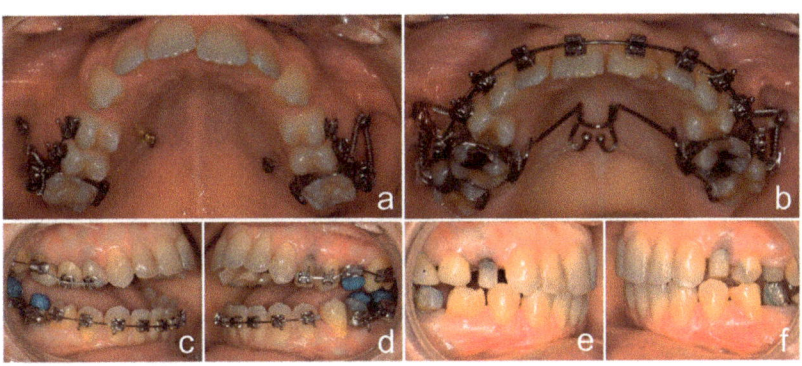

Figure 1. Skeletally anchored molar intrusion. Buccal miniplates combined palatal miniscrews (**a**) or with transpalatal bar (**b**) or bilateral molar dental implants (**c**–**f**) were used for orthodontic molar intrusion following occlusal splint therapy.

Occlusal bite blocks were used to enhance intrusion and maintain CR position. Average intrusion was 1.95 ± 0.58 mm and following intrusion the maxillary molars were ligature tied to the TADs. The average treatment time was 22 ± 2.5 months. The study was conducted in accordance with the Declaration of Helsinki Ethical Principles and Good Clinical Practices and was approved by the Clinical Research Ethics Committee of the University Hospital Sta.Universitario Mª del Rosel, Areas II and VIII of Health of the Murcian Health Service (El ID: EO 19/52. Intrusion molar ortodoncia).

2.2. Model Analysis

Panadent articulators (IML GmbH, Germany) were used for all mounting processes. Overjet (OJ) and overbite (OB) were evaluated on the pre-and posttreatment articulator mounted models in four positions by using a Pittsburg digital caliper (Harbor Freight Tools, Calabasas, CA, USA):

$T0^{MI}$. Initially in MI and $T0^{CR}$. in centric "de jour"

T1. In CR after 3–12 months of full-time splint wear with a stable joint position

T2. In CR after molar intrusion

Changes in OJ and OB were then calculated between the mounted positions ($T0^{MI}$ vs. $T0^{CR}$, $T0^{MI}$ vs. T1, T1 vs. T2). The criteria of stable CR position were the followings: No signs and symptoms of TMD (muscle tenderness, pain, clicking, locked joint), no change regarding the contact points on the splint for at least 3 appointments (12 weeks) and easy manipulation of the mandible by the clinician.

2.3. Centric Relation Registrations

All CR registrations were performed with dual wax bite method. The registrations were taken with hard wax (Almore, Beaverton, OR, USA) in two sections; anterior and posterior. The anterior section consisted of a 4-layer softened wax and included both upper and lower anteriors (canine to canine). First, patients were instructed to close gently on the arc of mandibular closure without protrusion, until approximately 2 mm of space remained between posterior-most teeth. In order to remove the wax without distorsion, patients were instructed to hold this position until wax was cooled and hardened. Following, a posterior 2-layer-thick softened wax was inserted together with the previously obtained hard anterior wax and then mandible was slightly guided into CR. At the end, subjects were instructed to close firmly and hold until the posterior section cooled and hardened as well.

2.4. Cepahlometric Measurements

Initial presplint (T0), postsplint (T1) and final posttreatment (T2) lateral cephalograms of the subjects were evaluated. T0 cephs were taken in MI position. For T1 cephs, wax bites were prepared (Beauty Pink Wax X, Miltex, York, PA, USA) based on the stable CR position achieved via splint wear. Wax bites were constructed in the CR mounted articulator with first contact on the most posterior teeth. Postintrusion T2 cephs were captured in MI position which was equivalent (MI-CR discrepancy less than 0.5 mm) with CR as checked on the mounted casts. As described in Table 2, ANB angle, vertical jaw relationship (Mandibular plane–Palatal plane angle) and Facial axis angle by Ricketts were evaluated on the lateral cephalograms.

Table 2. Definitions of cephalometric measurements used in this study.

Measurement	Definition
ANB angle	A point–Nasion–B point angle
Palatal plane–Mandibular plane angle	Angle between Posterior nasal spine–Anterior nasal spine and Gonion-Menton
Facial Axis angle by Ricketts	Angle between Nasion-Basion and the facial axis (Pterygomaxillare-Gnathion)

All tracings and superimpositions were performed digitally. Lateral cephs were superimposed by using cranial base and skull contours. Landmarks necessary for above mentioned measurements were marked and differences between T0 vs. T1 and T1 vs. T2 were evaluated.

2.5. Condylar Morphological Evaluation Using Bilateral CBCT Scans of TMJ

Pre-and posttreatment bilateral CBCT (NewTom, Verona, Italy) images of the TMJ were used to assess condylar position, detect any existing signs of internal derangement and monitor condylar morphological changes following the orthodontic treatment. Exposure parameters were identical for all subjects. CBCT data of all patients were evaluated in sagittal and coronal sections by two examiners blinded for the clinical diagnosis (neither knowing if the CBCTs were taken pre-or posttreatment). In case of disagreement a third examiner was asked in order to reach a final agreement. The most frequent osseous changes were examined in the CBCT images of the right and left TMJ areas according to criteria used in previous studies at [26,27]:

1. Flattening of the articular surface- loss of an even convexity of the joint (Figure 2a–d)
2. Surface erosion (decreased density of the cortical and adjacent bone) and/or condylar surface irregularity (loss of continuity of condylar cortex) (Figure 2b)
3. Absence of condylar anterosuperior position and/or apparent irregular TMJ joint space (Figure 2c)

4. Sclerosis (increased density of cortical bone extending into the bone marrow) (Figure 2d)

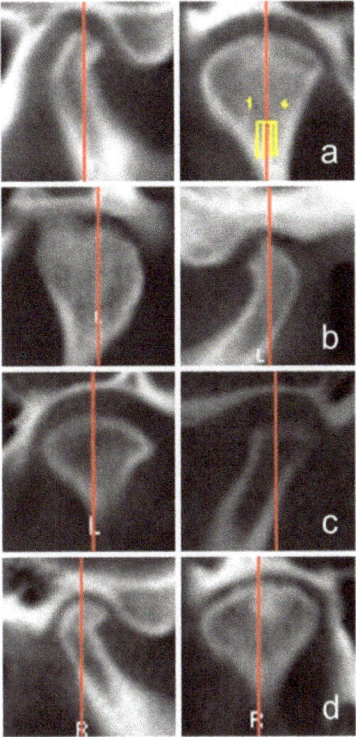

Figure 2. Representative CBCT images of the most frequent osseous changes of TMJ; flattening (**a**), surface erosion associated with surface irregularity (**b**), irregular TMJ joint space (**c**), sclerosis (**d**).

2.6. Statistical Analysis

All statistical analyses were performed using R Core Team (2018), R: A Language and Environment for Statistical Computing statistical software. Tracings of all lateral cephalograms were done by one examiner. To measure intraexaminer reliability, repeated tracings of all cephalograms and model measurements were done after 2 weeks. To determine the repeatability of measurements, mixed-effects model was used. In every examined variable, repetition had no significant effects on measure outcomes, supporting good intraexaminer reliability. To evaluate changes in OJ, OB and cephalometric parameters during the treatment multiple comparison correction was performed by repeated measures ANOVA followed by Turkey post hoc test. In order to verify differences in frequencies of pre-and posttreatment joint derangements McNemar's chi-square test was used with continuity correlation. Namely after the blinded examination, the pre- and posttreatment samples were re-paired again and as far as, there were no retrogression among the subjects, only those samples were included in the statistical analysis were pretreatment symptoms were detected. Statistically significant differences between groups were defined at p values <0.05.

3. Results

Table 3 represents the means, the lower (CI.l) and upper (CI.u) limits of 95% confidence interval of the changes between $T0^{MI}$ vs. $T0^{CR}$, $T0^{MI}$ vs. T1 and T1 vs. T2 mountings for OJ and OB and Table 4 changes between T0 vs. T1 and T1 vs. T2 lateral cephs for the selected cephalometric variables, respectively.

Table 3. Changes in OJ and OB (* $p < 0.05$).

		Mean	CI.l	CI.u	p Value
OB	T0^{MI} vs. T0^{CR}	−1.3333	−2.2082	−0.4585	0.0005 *
	T0^{MI} vs. T1	−3.1389	−4.0137	−2.2641	0.0000 *
	T1 vs. T2	4.0278	3.1529	4.9026	0.0000 *
OJ	T0^{MI} vs. T0^{CR}	1.2222	0.3367	2.1078	0.0022 *
	T0^{MI} vs. T1	2.5833	1.6978	3.4689	0.0000 *
	T1 vs. T2	−2.0556	−2.9411	−1.1700	0.0000 *

Table 4. Changes in Mandibular plane–Palatal plane angle, Facial axis angle by Ricketts and ANB angle (* $p < 0.05$).

		Mean	CI.l	CI.u	p Value
Mandibular plane–Palatal plane angle	T0 vs. T1	2.5778	1.776	3.3800	0.0000 *
	T1 vs. T2	−2.8333	−3.635	−2.0311	0.0000 *
Facial axis angle by Ricketts	T0 vs. T1	−1.6667	−2.684	−0.649	0.0004 *
	T1 vs. T2	2.3333	1.316	3.351	0.0000 *
ANB angle	T0 vs. T1	1.4722	0.8474	2.0971	0.0000 *
	T1 vs. T2	−1.6667	−2.2915	−1.0418	0.0000 *

When compared screening mountings to models in MI (T0^{MI} vs. T0^{CR}) significant differences were found in horizontal and vertical overlap of the incisors. OB decreased by 1.33 ± 0.73 mm ($p = 0.0005$) while OJ increased by 1.22 ± 0.69 mm ($p = 0.0022$).

Following full time acrylic splint wear (T0 vs. T1), there was a significant average increase (2.58° ± 0.93°) ($p = 0.0000$) in lower facial height (palatal plane-mandibular plane angle) and a significant decrease in facial axis angle (1.67° ± 1.54°) ($p = 0.0004$), which in turn had a sagittal effect as the ANB angle increased significantly by 1.47° ± 0.70° ($p = 0.0000$). Consequently, both OB and OJ showed a significant change on postsplint mountings when compared to centric occluded models (T0^{MI} vs. T1); OB had an average decrease of 3.14 ± 1.65 mm ($p = 0.0000$) and OJ an average increase of 2.58 ± 1.51 mm ($p = 0.0000$).

In every examined variable, molar intrusion (T1 vs. T2) resulted in statistically significant changes as well. After intrusion of the molars, mandible exhibited counterclockwise rotation, which was confirmed by decreased lower facial height and increased OB (4.03 ± 1.88 mm ($p = 0.0000$)), decreases in ANB and OJ. The palatal plane-mandibular plane angle decreased by 2.83° ± 1.78° ($p = 0.0000$), the ANB angle by 1.67° ± 1.12° ($p = 0.0000$) and the OJ by 2.06 ± 2.13 mm ($p = 0.0000$). The mean change in facial axis angle was + 2.33° ± 2.08° ($p = 0.0000$).

Figure 3a shows representative superimpositions of T0 vs. T1 and Figure 3b superimpositions of T1 vs. T2 lateral cephalographs, respectively.

When comparing pre -and posttreatment CBCT images of TMJ, the frequency of derangement was found to be different on the left and right sides. Table 5 summarizes the pre-and posttreatment frequencies of TMJ alterations. On the right side, flattening before the treatment was seen in 61.11% and 72.22% on the left side, which showed a significant improvement to 27.78% on the right and 38.89% on the left side following intrusion (posttreatment). Assessment of the CBCT findings of surface erosion and irregular condylar surface showed 72.22% on the right and 55.56% on the left side which significantly decreased to 22.22% on both posttreatment sides. Irregular TMJ space and/or absence of anterosuperior position of the condyle was 66.67% on the right and 61.11% on the left side, which significantly improved, as only 16.67% of the patients showed still nonideal posttreatment condylar position. No pre-and posttreatment differences were found in sclerosis, as the frequency remained 22.22% of the right and 11.11% of the left TMJ.

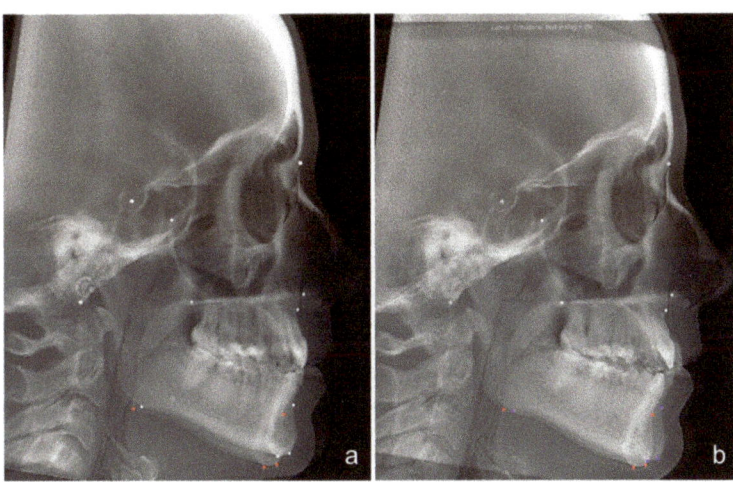

Figure 3. Representative superimpositions of presplint (T1) vs. postsplint (T2) (**a**) and postsplint (T2) vs. postintrusion (T3) (**b**) lateral cephalograms. Following splint wear (**a**), there was a significant increase in lower facial height and significant decrease in facial axis angle, which in turn increased ANB angle. After intrusion (**b**), mandible exhibited counterclockwise rotation, which was confirmed by decreased lower facial height, increased OB and facial axis angle and decreases in ANB.

Table 5. Frequency of osseous changes before and after therapy (* $p < 0.05$).

Morphological Signs	Pretreatment Right	Posttreatment Right	p Value	Pretreatment Left	Posttreatment Left	p Value
Flattening	61.11%	27.78%	0.0412 *	72.22%	38.89%	0.0412 *
Surface erosion, surface irregularities	72.22%	22.22%	0.0077 *	55.56%	22.22%	0.0412 *
Irregular TMJ space	66.67%	16.67%	0.0077 *	61.11%	16.67%	0.0133 *
Sclerosis	22.22%	22.22%	1	11.11%	11.11%	1

4. Discussion

Treatment of orthodontic patients with TMD due to orthopaedic instability has always been challenging especially as one of the desired outcomes of the orthodontic therapy is the achievement of an orthopaedic stability with an ideal harmony between occlusal functions and TMJ [1]. Many case studies are available demonstrating TMD patients treated with stabilization splint and/or molar intrusion [5,22,23,28–30]. But, so far a series of larger number of TMD orthodontic subjects, treated by stabilization splint followed by molar intrusion, with the main focus on TMJ health and CR-MI harmony have not been examined so extensively and studies have not been published yet. The aim of our study was to investigate and demonstrate that TMD patients with an orthopaedic instability can be effectively treated by the occlusal splint therapy followed by skeletally anchored molar intrusion.

TMD is by far a complex disease and the nature of it is not completely understood [31,32]. Most common signs and symptoms are masticatory muscle pain, TMJ sounds, limited movements (jaw opening capacity and deviations in mandibular movements), which tend to fluctuate with temporary remissions [33,34]. It has been generally accepted that

TMD has a multifactorial origin [28]. There is still a debate, whether occlusion plays a role in the etiology of TMD, nevertheless, completely rejecting the role of it may be inappropriate [1,35]. It has been reported that TMD is closely associated with some type of malocclusions, such as open bite, deep bite and posterior cross bite [29]. Disharmony between CR-MI has been suggested to be a causative factor as well [2,5] and it has been showed that the degree of CR-MI discrepancy has a strong positive correlation with the severity of TMD signs and symptoms [3,5] and by achieving harmony between CR-MI during the orthodontic treatment decreases the risk of TMD. According to this, the mandible should seat ideally into MI during closure without condylar deflection from CR position caused by occlusal interferences [4,36,37]. Therefore, CR-MI harmony should be one of the major goals of the orthodontic treatment. In most of the published literature that have failed to prove an existing relationship between occlusion and TMD, several inadequacies are present; such as no instrumentation was used. Most of the studies used only questionnaires, clinical examinations and only dental cast [38,39]. In a review, McNamara, Seligman and Okeson have also found relative low association between TMD and occlusal factors, although in the studies they reviewed, the occlusions were evaluated only intraorally and by using chin-point evaluation [40]. No attempt has been made to examine the condylar position and the possible effect on the stability of the TMJ by means of articulator models or precise determination of condyle with 3D imaging. To assess both condylar and occlusal relationships, articulator mounted models are recommended [41–43]. In our study, all diagnostic cast were mounted into articulators at different stages of the treatment; initially in MI (T0^{MI}), in centric "de jour" (T0^{CR}), after splint wear in CR (T1) and following molar intrusion in CR (T2), therefore we could monitor condyle position. We found significant CR-MI disharmony between the screening mountings and the initial records. The discrepancy was even more expressed when we compared the initial models with the postsplint ones, where following deprogramming the neuromuscular avoidance patterns were not present making the condylar seating accurate. These results are in agreement with He et al., who investigated the relationship between CR-MI discrepancy and TMD have found that CR-MI shift is strongly correlated with the signs and symptoms of TMD [3]. For TMD treatment, various methods have been used, including physio- and relaxation therapy, pharmacological interventions, arthroscopic surgery, behavioral and educational counseling and occlusal splints as well [44,45]. Pharmacologic therapies mainly aim to reduce pain and inflammation. There is growing interest for the use of polyphenols, however their beneficial effects on modulation of oxidative stress and inflammation remain highly limited due to their low bioavailability and bio-transformation [46]. A recent network meta-analysis of randomized controlled trials showed that hard stabilization splints in conjunction with counselling therapy can produce maximum benefit for TMD patients, furthermore, hard stabilization splint is far superior in patients with myogenous TMD [47]. Recently, randomized clinical trials have indicated that stabilization splints are superior to other treatments for TMD due to orthopaedic instability [34,44]. These splints are made of hard acrylic material, which can eliminate occlusal interferences, reduce abnormal muscle activity and therefore provide good neuromuscular balance. Splint therapy has been shown to be effective in changing the occlusal pattern of the teeth and improving the function of the masticatory system [35,45,48]. All patients included in the present study received full coverage acrylic splint therapy prior to the orthodontic treatment, in order to eliminate the signs and symptoms. Patients were instructed to full-time splint wear, as strong association between wearing time and effectiveness had been previously reported [47]. Following the splint wear altered occlusal relationship; AOB develops, which should be corrected. Molar intrusion is one of the most valid treatment approaches used for open bite corrections [49]. It has a similar effect to surgery in that sense that the upward molar repositioning autorotates the mandible in counter-clockwise direction (up- and forwards) and as an indirect consequence the incisor relationships will improve as well. Compared to orthognathic surgery application of TADs requires no compliance, has low risk and morbidity, is less expensive and invasive and more acceptable by patients. Several studies investigated the biological processes involved in molar intrusion [50,51]. In animal studies, alveolar bone and nasal/sinus floor remodeling without pulp vitality loss and clinically significant root resorption have been found to occur during and following molar intrusion [50,51]. Furthermore, micro-CT studies of human teeth has also confirmed that root resorption following molar intrusion is clinically insignificant [19]. Moreover, Akan et al. [23] demonstrated that molar intrusion has no negative effect on TMJ and masticatory system. According to these, in all subjects, TADs were used in order to correct AOB developed after splint wear. In our study, after intruding molars, mandibular counterclockwise rotation occurred toward closing the bite, which in turn induced up-and forward displacement of the B point as well as reduction in the ANB, mandibular plane angle and anterior facial height. The average mandibular rotation seen in our patients was 2.8°, which is similar to others [19,22–25]. Regarding the dental changes, following molar intrusion we found an average increase in OB, which is similar change observed by others as well [22,52,53].

So far, numerous imagining techniques have been used to evaluate morphological changes of the TMJ. Panoramic radiographs have 2D limitations and low sensitivity due to structural distortion and superimposition of the zygomatic process [54]. For visualization of disc-condyle relationship Magnetic Resonance Imagining (MRI) technique has been used as the gold standard diagnostic method [55]. CT can be used to detect bony changes, however, besides its high diagnostic efficacy, CBCT has several advantages over it, such as; lower radiation dose, better accessibility, lower cost [56]. In this study we used CBCT to evaluate the pre-and posttreatment (following intrusion) condylar morphology. Among the 18 patients with orthopedic instability, flattening, surface erosion and surface irregularities were the most frequent pretreatment bony changes. This is in agreement with Shahidi et al., who found flattening in 73.3% of TMJ related symptomatic cases [27]. When comparing pretreatment and posttreatment joints, except the sclerosis, significant improvements were seen following treatment in the three examined variables on both sides; approximately 50% of the condylar surfaces regained their convexity, cortical bone continuity and condylar position improved by about 40%. In previous study, flattening was found to show positive correlation with TMD [26]. Those studies, where no correlation has been found between TMD and morphological changes, the high prevalence of bony changes in asymptomatic patients was explained by the adaptive and compensatory potential of the TMJ [57]. Furthermore, a systematic review pointed out a potential sample selection bias among the papers comparing morphological changes between TMD and non-TMD patients; namely, in most studies patients included in those studies were referred to TMD and facial pain services, meaning that only asymptomatic and not the healthy control group could have been assured [58]. In summary, our results highlighted that occlusal splint therapy followed by orthodontic molar intrusion has a positive impact on bony changes of the TMJ.

5. Conclusions

The results of this study showed that occlusal splint therapy followed by skeletally anchored molar intrusion is an effective treatment method for patients with TMD as it provides CR-MI harmony, therefore orthopaedic stability and favourable bony changes of the TMJ.

Author Contributions: B.N. contributed to data collection, performed all the measurements, statistical analysis and was involved in manuscript drafting. D.F. contributed to planning the study design was involved in data analysis and interpretation and was the major contributor to writing the manuscript. A.P. was involved in data analysis and manuscript writing. D.M. was the supervisor of the overall project, critically revised the final version of the manuscript and has the overall responsibility. All authors have read and agreed to the published version of the manuscript.

Funding: This research received no external funding.

Institutional Review Board Statement: The study was approved by the Clinical Research Ethics Committee of the University Hospital Sta.Universitario Mª del Rosel, Areas II and VIII of Health of the Murcian Health Service (El ID: EO 19/52. Intrusion molar ortodoncia).

Informed Consent Statement: Not applicable.

Data Availability Statement: Datasets used and/or analyzed during the current study are available from the corresponding author on reasonable request.

Conflicts of Interest: The authors declare no conflict of interest.

References

1. Alexander, S.R.; Moore, R.N.; DuBois, L.M. Mandibular condyle position: Comparison of articulator mountings and magnetic resonance imaging. *Am. J. Orthod Dentofac. Orthop.* **1993**, *104*, 230–239. [CrossRef]
2. Dawson, P.E. Centric relation. Its effect on occluso-muscle harmony. *Dent. Clin. N. Am.* **1979**, *23*, 169–180.
3. He, S.S.; Deng, X.; Wamalwa, P.; Chen, S. Correlation between centric relation-maximum intercuspation discrepancy and temporomandibular joint dysfunction. *Acta. Odontol. Scand* **2010**, *68*, 368–376. [CrossRef] [PubMed]
4. Roth, R.H. Functional occlusion for the orthodontist. *J. Clin. Orthod.* **1981**, *15*, 174–199. [PubMed]
5. Crawford, S.D. Condylar axis position, as determined by the occlusion and measured by the CPI instrument, and signs and symptoms of temporomandibular dysfunction. *Angle Orthod.* **1999**, *69*, 103–115. [PubMed]
6. Dawson, P.E. *Functional Occlusion: From TMJ to Smile Design*; Mosby: St Louis, MO, USA, 2007.
7. Okeson, J.P. Evolution of occlusion and temporomandibular disorder in orthodontics: Past, present, and future. *Am. J. Orthod. Dentofac. Orthop.* **2015**, *147*, S216–S223. [CrossRef] [PubMed]
8. Iwasa, A.; Horiuchi, S.; Kinouchi, N.; Izawa, T.; Hiasa, M.; Kawai, N.; Yasue, A.; Hassan, A.H.; Tanaka, E. Skeletal anchorage for intrusion of bimaxillary molars in a patient with skeletal open bite and temporomandibular disorders. *J. Orthod. Sci.* **2017**, *6*, 152–158.
9. Magdaleno, F.; Ginestal, E. Side effects of stabilization occlusal splints: A report of three cases and literature review. *CRANIO* **2010**, *28*, 128–135. [CrossRef]
10. Oh, J.W.; Ahn, Y.W.; Jeong, S.H.; Ju, H.M.; Song, B.S.; Ok, S.M. Prediction of anterior open-bite development after stabilization splint treatment in patients with temporomandibular disorder. *CRANIO* **2020**, *12*, 1–10. [CrossRef]
11. Kassem, H.E.; Marzouk, E.S. Prediction of changes due to mandibular autorotation following miniplate-anchored intrusion of maxillary posterior teeth in open bite cases. *Prog. Orthod.* **2018**, *19*, 1–7. [CrossRef]
12. Dellinger, E.L.; Dellinger, E.L. Active vertical corrector treatment-long-term follow-up of anterior open bite treated by the intrusion of posterior teeth. *Am. J. Orthod. Dentofac. Orthop.* **1996**, *110*, 145–154. [CrossRef]
13. Closs, L.; Pangrazio Kulbersh, V. Combination of bionator and high-pull headgear therapy in a skeletal open bite case. *Am. J. Orthod. Dentofac. Orthop.* **1996**, *109*, 341–347. [CrossRef]
14. Shellhart, W.C.; Moawad, M.; Lake, P. Case report: Implants as anchorage for molar uprighting and intrusion. *Angle Orthod.* **1996**, *66*, 169–172.
15. Melsen, B.; Fiorelli, G. Upper molar intrusion. *J. Clin. Orthod.* **1996**, *30*, 91–96.
16. Melsen, B.; Agerbaek, N.; Eriksen, J.; Terp, S. New attachment through periodontal treatment and orthodontic intrusion. *Am. J. Orthod. Dentofac. Orthop.* **1988**, *94*, 104–116. [CrossRef]
17. da Silva, V.C.; Cirelli, C.C.; Ribeiro, F.S.; Leite, F.R.; Benatti Neto, C.; Marcantonio, R.A.; Cirelli, J.A. Intrusion of teeth with class III furcation: A clinical, histologic and histometric study in dogs. *J. Clin. Periodontol* **2008**, *35*, 807–816. [CrossRef]
18. Bayani, S.; Heravi, F.; Radvar, M.; Anbiaee, N.; Madani, A.S. Periodontal changes following molar intrusion with miniscrews. *Dent. Res. J.* **2015**, *12*, 379–385. [CrossRef] [PubMed]
19. Carrillo, R.; Rossouw, P.E.; Franco, P.F.; Opperman, L.A.; Buschang, P.H. Intrusion of multiradicular teeth and related root resorption with mini-screw implant anchorage: A radiographic evaluation. *Am. J. Orthod. Dentofac. Orthop.* **2007**, *132*, 647–655. [CrossRef] [PubMed]
20. Sugawara, J.; Baik, U.B.; Umemori, M.; Takahashi, I.; Nagasaka, H.; Kawamura, H.; Mitani, H. Treatment and posttreatment dentoalveolar changes following intrusion of mandibular molars with application of a skeletal anchorage system (SAS) for open bite correction. *Int. J. Adult Orthodon. Orthognath. Surg.* **2002**, *17*, 243–253. [PubMed]
21. Kuroda, S.; Sakai, Y.; Tamamura, N.; Deguchi, T.; Takano-Yamamoto, T. Treatment of severe anterior open bite with skeletal anchorage in adults: Comparison with orthognathic surgery outcomes. *Am. J. Orthod. Dentofac. Orthop.* **2007**, *132*, 599–605. [CrossRef]
22. Erverdi, N.; Usumez, S.; Solak, A.; Koldas, T. Noncompliance open-bite treatment with zygomatic anchorage. *Angle Orthod.* **2007**, *77*, 986–990. [CrossRef] [PubMed]
23. Akan, S.; Kocadereli, I.; Aktas, A.; Tasar, F. Effects of maxillary molar intrusion with zygomatic anchorage on the stomatognathic system in anterior open bite patients. *Eur. J. Orthod.* **2013**, *35*, 93–102. [CrossRef]

24. Deguchi, T.; Kurosaka, H.; Oikawa, H.; Kuroda, S.; Takahashi, I.; Yamashiro, T.; Takano-Yamamoto, T. Comparison of orthodontic treatment outcomes in adults with skeletal open bite between conventional edgewise treatment and implant-anchored orthodontics. *Am. J. Orthod. Dentofac. Orthop.* **2011**, *139*, S60–S68. [CrossRef] [PubMed]
25. Buschang, P.H.; Carrillo, R.; Rossouw, P.E. Orthopedic correction of growing hyperdivergent, retrognathic patients with miniscrew implants. *J. Oral. Maxillofac. Surg.* **2011**, *69*, 754–762. [CrossRef]
26. Talaat, W.; Al Bayatti, S.; Al Kawas, S. CBCT analysis of bony changes associated with temporomandibular disorders. *CRANIO* **2016**, *34*, 88–94. [CrossRef] [PubMed]
27. Shahidi, S.; Salehi, P.; Abedi, P.; Dehbozorgi, M.; Hamedani, S.; Berahman, N. Comparison of the Bony Changes of TMJ in Patients With and Without TMD Complaints Using CBCT. *J. Dent.* **2018**, *19*, 142–149.
28. Song, F.; He, S.; Chen, S. Temporomandibular disorders with skeletal open bite treated with stabilization splint and zygomatic miniplate anchorage: A case report. *Angle Orthod.* **2015**, *85*, 335–347. [CrossRef]
29. Tanne, K.; Tanaka, E.; Sakuda, M. Association between malocclusion and temporomandibular disorders in orthodontic patients before treatment. *J. Orofac. Pain* **1993**, *7*, 156–162.
30. Tanaka, E.; Yamano, E.; Inubushi, T.; Kuroda, S. Management of acquired open bite associated with temporomandibular joint osteoarthritis using miniscrew anchorage. *Korean J. Orthod.* **2012**, *42*, 144–154. [CrossRef]
31. Fricton, J.R. Recent advances in orofacial pain and temporomandibular disorders. *J. Back Musculoskelet. Rehabil.* **1996**, *6*, 99–112. [CrossRef]
32. de Wijer, A.; Steenks, M.H.; de Leeuw, J.R.; Bosman, F.; Helders, P.J. Symptoms of the cervical spine in temporomandibular and cervical spine disorders. *J. Oral. Rehabil.* **1996**, *23*, 742–750. [CrossRef] [PubMed]
33. Alanen, P.; Kuttila, M.; Le Bell, Y. Fluctuation of temporomandibular disorders in accordance with two classifications: The Helkimo dysfunction index and treatment need grouping. *Acta. Odontol. Scand.* **1997**, *55*, 14–17. [CrossRef] [PubMed]
34. Ekberg, E.; Nilner, M. Treatment outcome of appliance therapy in temporomandibular disorder patients with myofascial pain after 6 and 12 months. *Acta. Odontol. Scand.* **2004**, *62*, 343–349. [CrossRef]
35. Mohlin, B.; Ingervall, B.; Thilander, B. Relation between malocclusion and mandibular dysfunction in Swedish men. *Eur. J. Orthod.* **1980**, *2*, 229–238. [CrossRef]
36. Williamson, E.H. Occlusion: Understanding or misunderstanding. *Angle. Orthod.* **1976**, *46*, 86–93.
37. Cordray, F.E. Centric relation treatment and articulator mountings in orthodontics. *Angle. Orthod.* **1996**, *66*, 153–158. [PubMed]
38. Pullinger, A.G.; Seligman, D.A.; Solberg, W.K. Temporomandibular disorders. Part II: Occlusal factors associated with temporomandibular joint tenderness and dysfunction. *J. Prosthet. Dent.* **1988**, *59*, 363–367. [CrossRef]
39. Seligman, D.A.; Pullinger, A.G.; Solberg, W.K. Temporomandibular disorders. Part III: Occlusal and articular factors associated with muscle tenderness. *J. Prosthet. Dent.* **1988**, *59*, 483–489. [CrossRef]
40. McNamara, J.J.A.; Seligman, D.A.; Okeson, J.P. Occlusion, Orthodontic treatment, and temporomandibular disorders: A review. *J. Orofac. Pain* **1995**, *9*, 73–90.
41. Roth, R.H. Temporomandibular pain-dysfunction and occlusal relationships. *Angle Orthod.* **1973**, *43*, 136–153.
42. Parker, W.S. Centric relation and centric occlusion–an orthodontic responsibility. *Am. J. Orthod.* **1978**, *74*, 481–500. [CrossRef]
43. Slavicek, R. Clinical and instrumental functional analysis and treatment planning. Part 4. Instrumental analysis of mandibular casts using the mandibular position indicator. *J. Clin. Orthod.* **1988**, *22*, 566–575.
44. Magnusson, T.; Adiels, A.M.; Nilsson, H.L.; Helkimo, M. Treatment effect on signs and symptoms of temporomandibular disorders-comparison between stabilisation splint and a new type of splint (NTI). A pilot study. *Swed. Dent. J.* **2004**, *28*, 11–20.
45. Okeson, J. *Management of Temporomandibular Disorders and Occlusion*; Elsevier: Amsterdam, The Netherlands, 2020.
46. Moccia, S.; Nucci, L.; Spagnuolo, C.; d'Apuzzo, F.; Piancino, M.G.; Minervini, G. Polyphenols as Potential Agents in the Management of Temporomandibular Disorders. *Appl. Sci.* **2020**, *10*, 305. [CrossRef]
47. Al-Moraissi, E.A.; Farea, R.; Qasem, K.A.; Al-Wadeai, M.S.; Al-Sabahi, M.E.; Al-Iryani, G.M. Effectiveness of occlusal splint therapy in the management of temporomandibular disorders: Network meta-analysis of randomized controlled trials. *Int. J. Oral. Maxillofac. Surg.* **2020**, *49*, 1042–1056. [CrossRef]
48. McLaughlin, R.P. Malocclusion and the temporomandibular joint-an historical perspective. *Angle Orthod.* **1988**, *58*, 185–191. [PubMed]
49. Alsafadi, A.S.; Alabdullah, M.M.; Saltaji, H.; Abdo, A.; Youssef, M. Effect of molar intrusion with temporary anchorage devices in patients with anterior open bite: A systematic review. *Prog. Orthod.* **2016**, *17*, 1–13. [CrossRef] [PubMed]
50. Ramirez-Echave, J.I.; Buschang, P.H.; Carrillo, R.; Rossouw, P.E.; Nagy, W.W.; Opperman, L.A. Histologic evaluation of root response to intrusion in mandibular teeth in beagle dogs. *Am. J. Orthod. Dentofac. Orthop.* **2011**, *139*, 60–69. [CrossRef] [PubMed]
51. Daimaruya, T.; Takahashi, I.; Nagasaka, H.; Umemori, M.; Sugawara, J.; Mitani, H. Effects of maxillary molar intrusion on the nasal floor and tooth root using the skeletal anchorage system in dogs. *Angle Orthod.* **2003**, *73*, 158–166.
52. Vela-Hernandez, A.; Lopez-Garcia, R.; Garcia-Sanz, V.; Paredes-Gallardo, V.; Lasagabaster-Latorre, F. Nonsurgical treatment of skeletal anterior open bite in adult patients: Posterior build-ups. *Angle Orthod.* **2017**, *87*, 33–40. [CrossRef]
53. Hart, T.R.; Cousley, R.R.; Fishman, L.S.; Tallents, R.H. Dentoskeletal changes following mini-implant molar intrusion in anterior open bite patients. *Angle Orthod.* **2015**, *85*, 941–948. [CrossRef]
54. Crow, H.C.; Parks, E.; Campbell, J.H.; Stucki, D.S.; Daggy, J. The utility of panoramic radiography in temporomandibular joint assessment. *Dentomaxillofac. Radiol.* **2005**, *34*, 91–95. [CrossRef] [PubMed]

55. d'Apuzzo, F.; Minervini, G.; Grassia, V.; Rotolo, R.P.; Perillo, L.; Nucci, L. Mandibular Coronoid Process Hypertrophy: Diagnosis and 20-Year Follow-Up with CBCT, MRI and EMG Evaluations. *Appl. Sci.* **2021**, *11*, 504. [CrossRef]
56. Barghan, S.; Tetradis, S.; Mallya, S. Application of cone beam computed tomography for assessment of the temporomandibular joints. *Aust. Dent. J.* **2012**, *57* (Suppl. S1), 109–118. [CrossRef] [PubMed]
57. Molinari, F.; Manicone, P.F.; Raffaelli, L.; Raffaelli, R.; Pirronti, T.; Bonomo, L. Temporomandibular joint soft-tissue pathology, I: Disc abnormalities. *Semin. Ultrasound CT MRI* **2007**, *28*, 192–204. [CrossRef] [PubMed]
58. Hilgenberg-Sydney, P.B.; Bonotto, D.V.; Stechman-Neto, J.; Zwir, L.F.; Pachêco-Pereira, C.; Canto, G.L.; Porporatti, A.L. Diagnostic validity of CT to assess degenerative temporomandibular joint disease: A systematic review. *Dentomaxillofac. Radiol.* **2018**, *47*, 20170389. [CrossRef] [PubMed]

Article

A Novel Dental Caries Model Replacing, Refining, and Reducing Animal Sacrifice

Amit Wolfoviz-Zilberman [1,2], Yael Houri-Haddad [1,†] and Nurit Beyth [1,*,†]

1 Department of Prosthodontics, Hadassah Medical Center, Faculty of Dental Medicine, Hebrew University of Jerusalem, Jerusalem 9112001, Israel; amit.wolfoviz@mail.huji.ac.il (A.W.-Z.); yaelho@ekmd.huji.ac.il (Y.H.-H.)
2 Institute of Dental Sciences, Hadassah Medical Center, Faculty of Dental Medicine, Hebrew University of Jerusalem, Jerusalem 9112001, Israel
* Correspondence: Nurit.Beyth@mail.huji.ac.il
† These authors contributed equally to this work.

Abstract: In vitro and in vivo models simulating the dental caries process enable the evaluation of anti-caries modalities for prevention and treatment. Animal experimentation remains important for improving human and animal health. Nonetheless, reducing animal sacrifice for research is desirable. The aim of the study was to establish a new reproducible in vitro caries model system and compare it to an in vivo model using similar conditions. Hemi-mandibles were extracted from previously euthanized healthy 10-week-old BALB/C female mice. Jaws were subjected to saliva, high-sucrose diet, and dental caries bacteria *Streptococcus mutans UA159* for 5 days. Similar caries induction protocol was used in vivo in fifteen BALB/c female mice (6–7 weeks old) and compared to the in vitro model. Caries lesions were assessed clinically by photographic analysis and μCT analysis, and bacterial growth was evaluated. Under in vitro experimental conditions, carious lesions evolved within 5 days, prominently in the depth of the occlusal fissures in the control group as depicted by photographic analysis, μCT analysis, and bacterial growth. The developed in vitro caries model presented in this study may be a novel animal sparing model for caries disease studies and can be used widely to evaluate the efficacy of different antibacterial dental materials.

Keywords: caries model; *Streptococcus mutans*; demineralization; dental caries

Citation: Wolfoviz-Zilberman, A.; Houri-Haddad, Y.; Beyth, N. A Novel Dental Caries Model Replacing, Refining, and Reducing Animal Sacrifice. *Appl. Sci.* **2021**, *11*, 7141. https://doi.org/10.3390/app11157141

Academic Editor: Mitsuru Motoyoshi

Received: 28 June 2021
Accepted: 30 July 2021
Published: 2 August 2021

Publisher's Note: MDPI stays neutral with regard to jurisdictional claims in published maps and institutional affiliations.

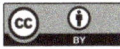

Copyright: © 2021 by the authors. Licensee MDPI, Basel, Switzerland. This article is an open access article distributed under the terms and conditions of the Creative Commons Attribution (CC BY) license (https://creativecommons.org/licenses/by/4.0/).

1. Introduction

Dental caries is a common infectious and transmissible disease. The basic mechanism is the demineralization of enamel and dentin via acid generated by bacterial biofilm. Oral bacteria metabolize carbohydrates, producing organic acid that diffuses into the enamel and dentin and dissolves minerals [1].

Although several studies have related the participation of other bacteria in the pathogenesis of dental caries [2–4], *Streptococcus mutans* plays a central role in the development of cariogenic biofilms [5]. The acidogenic and aciduric (associated with acid tolerance) properties of *S. mutans*, together with its ability to synthesize extracellular glucans, are the major factors for the development and establishment of cariogenic biofilms.

Caries models are valuable when trying to understand the complex process of the disease by addressing various questions related to biofilm formation, the process of caries development, and its prevention. Moreover, caries models are extremely valuable to determine prevention and treatment approaches prior to clinical application.

Various in vitro and in vivo techniques have been developed for caries simulation. Many of these studies focus on the evaluation of bacterial growth or biofilm composition rather than demineralization of the enamel [6–9]. Furthermore, most in vivo caries studies have been conducted using rats rather than mice and facilitated cariogenic bacteria by including oral shifting via desalivation and/or antibiotic treatment, which created a non-natural environment [10–15].

The rodent model has several advantages in mimicking human caries due to its similarity in genetics and hard tissues composition. Moreover, rodent caries models allow for a similar but accelerated caries development process: rodents have thinner layers of enamel and dentin, which may enhance the demineralization process. Previous in vivo studies in mice required 5–7 weeks of cariogenic bacteria inoculation for caries lesions development [10,16,17].

Animal experiments contribute essential knowledge to the medical and pharmaceutical research that cannot be achieved in vitro. Unfortunately, this knowledge requires millions of lab animals annually. The pain and death resulting from these experiments has been at the center of debate for a long time. Reducing animal sacrifice by developing alternative models without compromising the obtained knowledge is indeed required [18,19].

The objective of this study was to develop a new quantitative and reproducible in vitro caries model, using mice jaws of euthanized healthy mice that were sacrificed for other research purposes and are no longer used (for example control group mice). An in vivo caries model was designed to evaluate and verify the in vitro model's similarity and resemblance to the real oral conditions.

Preferably the combination of advantages of in vitro models with animal models may be beneficial for studying the caries disease. The ability to mimic the oral conditions in a controlled in vitro study using hard tissues that usually require a living host to model caries but without the animal sacrifice may be advantageous.

The null hypotheses of this study were that the development of an in vitro caries model using extracted jaws from euthanized healthy mice will mimic the common in vivo caries model and will introduce an alternative approach for dental research experiments.

2. Materials and Methods

2.1. Ethics Approval

Saliva was collected from 5 healthy volunteers, age range 22–67 (3 female, 2 men) (authorized by the institutional ethics committee #HMO-0706-16). All participants gave verbal and written assent to participate.

All animal experimental procedures were reviewed and approved by the IACUC of the Hadassah-Hebrew University Medical Center (MD-17-15315-3).

2.2. Bacterial Strains and Culture Conditions

Streptococcus mutans UA159 was grown overnight in brain–heart infusion (BHI) broth (Difco, Detroit, MI, USA) at 37 °C. Bacterial suspensions adjusted to total bacterial load of 10^8 CFU/mL. Viable counts using serial dilutions were used to assess bacterial concentration (CFU/mL).

2.3. Extracted Jaws Preparation

Ten sacrificed 10-week-old BALB/C female mice hemi-mandibles were obtained from previously euthanized healthy mice.

2.4. Saliva Sterilization

To simulate the oral cavity conditions, the samples were subjected to sterilized saliva according to Kalfas and Rnudegren [20] with a modification. Saliva was collected from healthy volunteers (authorized by the institutional ethics committee #HMO-0706-16). Dithiothreitol (DTT) 1M (Merck KGaA, Darmstadt, Germany) was added to saliva to reach 2.5 mM concentration. The saliva was cooled at 4 °C for 10 mins and then centrifuged for 15 mins. The upper fluid was discarded, and sterile double-distilled water (DDW) was added, adjusting to 25% saliva concentration. At last, the saliva was filtered using 0.22 µm filter and frozen for re-use.

2.5. Caries-Promoting Environment

Each sample was placed in a well in a 48-well flat-bottom microtiter plate (Nunclon, Nunc; Thermo Fisher Scientific Inc, Waltham, MA, USA) using a sterile tweezer. The samples were subjected to 50 µL sterilized saliva for 30 min. Then, 50 µL of bacterial suspension and 400 µL of brain–heart infusion (BHI) broth (Difco, Detroit, MI, USA) containing 5% sucrose and bacitracin (2.77 mg/mL) were added. BHI was replaced every 24 h for 5 days, after which the samples were analyzed. Five jaws were subjected to saliva, and BHI served as a control group. Figure 1 summarize schematically the in vitro caries model experiment course.

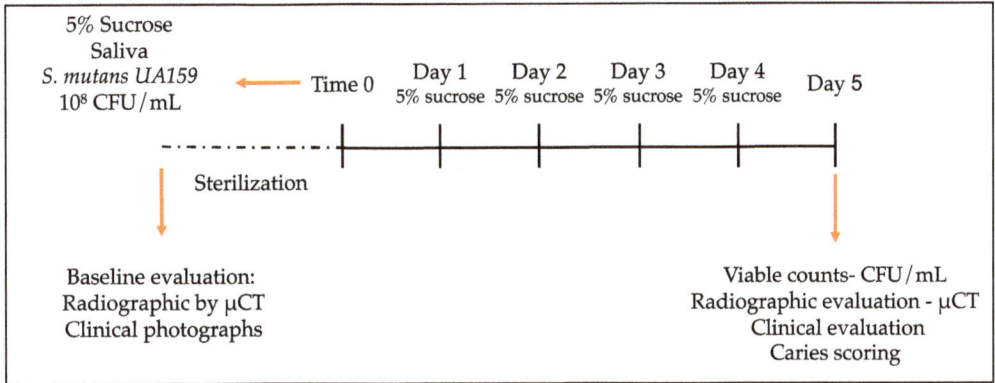

Figure 1. Schematic diagram summarized in vitro caries model over extracted jaws from healthy euthanized mice. Before subjecting the jaws to a caries-promoting environment, all jaws were photographed using an SMZ25 stereomicroscope (Nikon, Tokyo, Japan) and scanned using micro-computed tomography (µCT) (µCT 40, Scanco Medical, Switzerland). Then, all jaws were autoclaved. At time 0, jaws were subjected to saliva, bacterial infection by *S. mutans UA159*, and 5% sucrose growth media. Growth media was replaced every 24 h. A group of five jaws served as a control group without bacterial infection. After 5 days, microbiological samples were collected using a low-speed dental bur 0.25 mm (MDT, Israel) for viable counts evaluation. Then, hemi-mandibles were photographed again using SMZ25 stereomicroscope and scanned using µCT for demineralization quantification.

2.6. Photographic Depiction

Each jaw was photographed using an SMZ25 stereoscope (Nikon, Tokyo, Japan) before and after subjecting to caries-promoting conditions. A custom-made silicone stand was prepared for each jaw allowing a reproducible photographic capture taken in the similar conditions of light and resolution.

2.7. Carious Lesions Micro-Computed Tomography (MCT) Evaluation

Jaws underwent micro-computed tomography (µCT) (µCT 40, Scanco Medical, Switzerland) before and after experiment for demineralization quantification. Each jaw was placed in an Eppendorf tube containing 100 µL of phosphate-buffered saline (PBS) and autoclaved before experiment.

For quantitative 3-dimensional analysis of the mineral tissue loss, the hemi-mandibles were examined by a desktop µCT system (µCT 40, Scanco Medical, Switzerland) energy of 70 kV, intensity of 114 µA, and resolution of 6 µm^3 voxel size. Samples were placed in a cylindrical sample holder, and about 300 microtomographic slices were acquired covering the entire crown volume of each hemi-jaw. Sample scans, before and after experiment, were aligned as described by Goldman et al. [21]. In brief, three points of alignment in the first molar were chosen: the mesial apical constriction, the coronal part of the mesial canal, and the distal apical constriction. After alignment, a slice in which the coronal pulp, radicular pulp of both canals, and both apical foramens are presented was chosen (as demonstrated in

Figure 2). The total crown volume of first molar was marked as a rectangle from the mesial cemento-enamel junction and adjusted accordingly to all slices in which the crown's enamel was observed. Then, the marked total cubic volume was evaluated using a dedicated algorithm that gives the percentage of total volume for 6 selected ranges of density (by mgHA/ccm). Air and pulp have a similar radiographic density, which was examined and determined to 0–500 mgHA/ccm. The remaining five ranges have been standardized with respect to total volume. The caries density range is determined to 500–1500 mgHA/ccm, while healthy dentin and enamel were determined to 1500–3000 mgHA/ccm according to the respected density determined by the microCT machine.

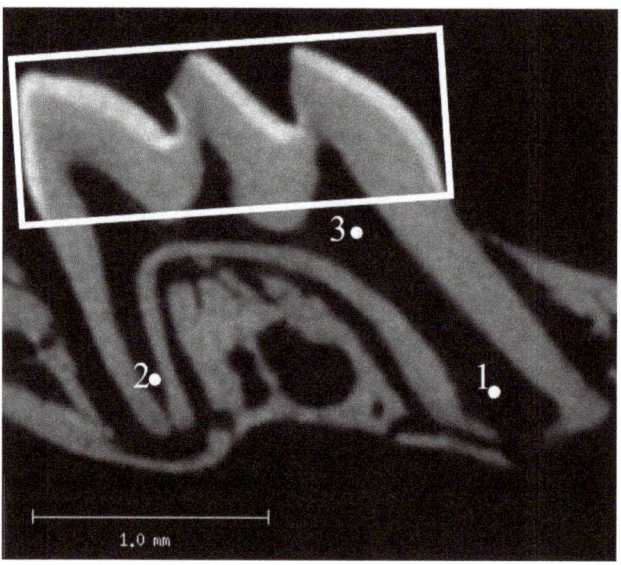

Figure 2. Standardized μCT analysis. μCT analysis included standardized alignment and selection of total crown cubic volume. μCT scans were aligned using three points in the first molar: 1—the mesial apical constriction, 2—the distal apical constriction, 3—coronal part of the mesial canal. Total crown volume from the mesial cemento-enamel junction was marked (white rectangle) over the slice in which the coronal pulp, radicular pulp of both canals, and both apical foramens are presented. Total crown cubic volume (mm^3) was determined by the marked rectangle over all slices in which crown enamel was observed.

The mean volumetric percentage of 500–1500 mgHA/ccm range of each group, which represent demineralized tissue, was compared.

2.8. Viable Count Evaluation

A low-speed dental bur 0.25 mm (MDT, Afula, Israel) was used to collect a hard tissue surface sample from the third molar. The bur was placed in an Eppendorf tube with 100 μL PBS and sonicated for 5 min to disrupt the biofilm (Bandelin sonopuls HD 2200, Berlin, Germany). Then, the tube was vortexed and plated on mitis salivarius agar plates (Difco, Detroit, MI, USA) for live bacterial count evaluation (CFU/mL).

2.9. Caries Scoring Using a Scoring Method over Hemi-Sectioned Molars

Caries lesions were evaluated using Keyes' caries scoring method with slight modification [14].

First, mandibular molars were hemi-sectioned along the mesiodistal sagittal plane using Super-Snap finishing and polishing disks (SHOFU inc., Kyoto, Japan).

Hemi-sectioned molars were photographed using an SMZ25 stereoscope (Nikon, Tokyo, Japan). The occlusal surface of the first molars was divided into eight surfaces; a vertical tangent for the tip of each cusp and the depth of each fissure was marked. The verticals divided the occlusal surface into eight units (as shown in Figure 3). Lesions were scored as the number of occlusal surfaces that were diagnosed with caries that have reached the cemento-enamel junction (CEJ).

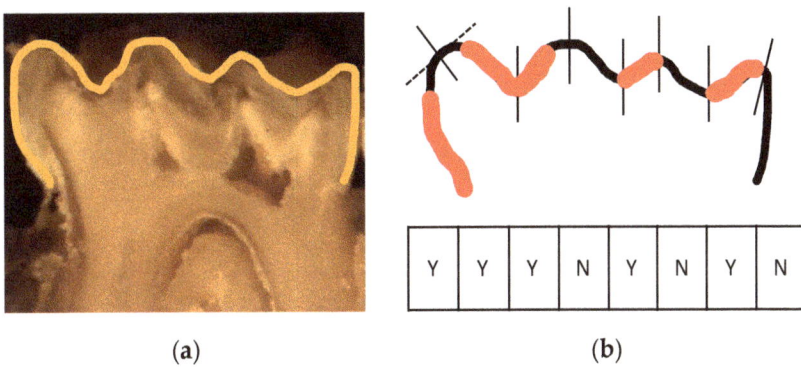

Figure 3. Caries scoring using hemi-sectioned molars. First mandibular molars were hemi-sectioned along the mesiodistal plane and photographed using an SMZ25 stereoscope. (a) Representative hemi-section of caries-infected mandibular molar with marked occlusal surface outline. (b) Occlusal surface was divided into eight surfaces; a vertical tangent for the tip of each cusp and the depth of each fissure was marked. The verticals divided the occlusal surface into eight units. Each unit was marked using the table below: Y = Caries was detected, N = No caries was detected. The units identified as caries infected were marked in red and were summed to numeric score.

2.10. Statistical Analysis

The results were analyzed as the mean ± standard error of the mean of 5 samples in each experimental group. Statistical significance was calculated by Student's t-test (significance level: $p < 0.01$).

2.11. In Vivo Dental Caries Promotion

2.11.1. Mice

Caries was induced according to Keyes et al. [13] with modifications, using mice rather than rats.

Fifteen BALB/c female mice (6–7 weeks old) were purchased from Harlan (Jerusalem, Israel). All the animals were housed in ventilated cages at room temperature under a 16 h light and 8 h dark cycle. Ten mice received 10% sucrose containing distilled water and cariogenic diet KEYES #2000 [13] ad libitum, while five mice served as a control group receiving distilled water and normal diet ad libitum. All animal experimental procedures were reviewed and approved by the IACUC of the Hadassah-Hebrew University Medical Center (MD-17-15315-3).

A group of five mice was subjected to bacterial infection; five mice received high-sucrose diet only while five mice served as a control group.

The time allotted for the experiment is 42 days, as in previous studies [10,16,17]; the lesions developed within 5–7 weeks.

2.11.2. Bacterial Infection

S. mutans UA159 was grown and adjusted to total bacterial load of 10^8 (CFU/mL) similarly as described above for in vitro experiments. Bacterial infection was performed every 48 h, using a 0.2 mL oral gavage of bacterial suspension with 2% carboxymethyl cellulose (CMC).

2.11.3. Bacterial Outgrowth Evaluation and Carious Lesions Assessment

After 42 days, microbiological samples were collected using an oral swab from the murine mouths for 20 s. Viable bacterial number was evaluated (CFU/ mL) on mitis salivarius for *S. mutans* and BHI agar plates for total bacterial count.

The experiment was terminated after 42 days. Mice were anesthetized and euthanized. Hemi-mandibula were harvested. All tests were carried similarly as in the in vitro experiments. The hemi-mandibula were photographed using an SMZ25 stereoscope (Nikon, Tokyo, Japan) and scanned using micro-computed tomography (μCT) (μCT 40, Scanco Medical, Switzerland) for demineralization quantification.

3. Results

3.1. Assessment of Caries Lesions in Extracted—Jaws from Dissected Healthy Mice

3.1.1. Clinical Evaluation

Caries lesions were detected clinically in the *UA159* bacterial infected group within 5 days. Representative images of an average lesion developed, before, and after bacterial infection, are shown in Figure 4(B1,B2), respectively. No carious lesions were observed in the non-infected hemi-mandibles, as shown in Figure 4(A1,A2).

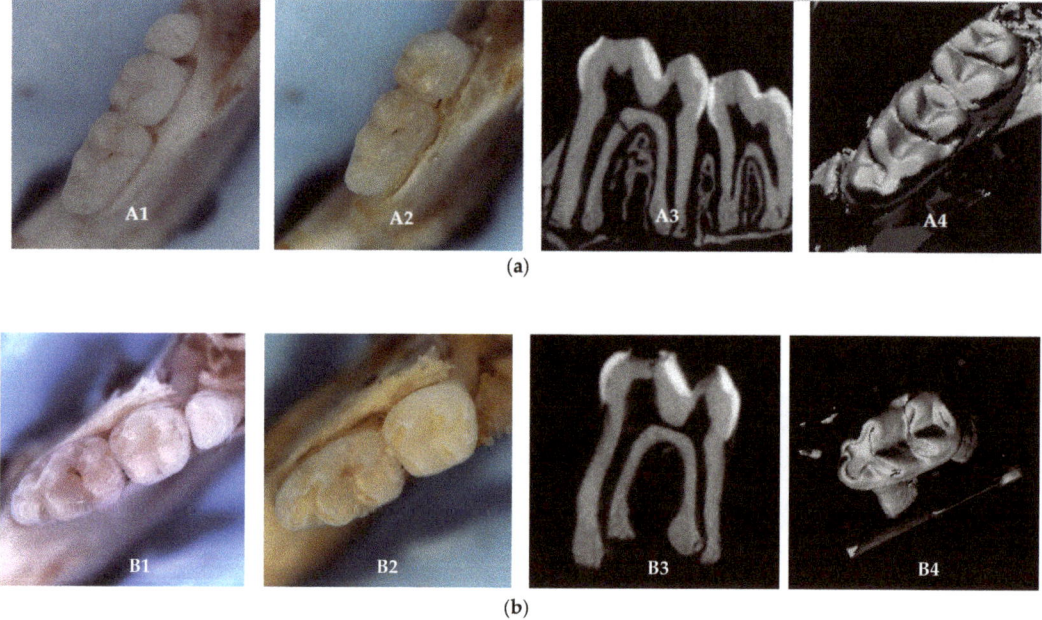

Figure 4. Evaluation of caries lesions, clinical and radiographic, after 5 days in a caries-promoting environment. Representative clinical and radiographic images. (**a**) represents the no bacteria group; (**b**) represents the *S. mutans* UA159 bacterial-infected group. Clinical photos were depicted before (**A1,B1**) and after (**A2,B2**) caries induction using high-sucrose media and cariogenic bacteria (*S. mutans UA159*) for 5 days. Radiographic (**A3,A4**) scans were used for demineralization evaluation and quantification; hemi-mandibles were segmented and reconstructed to acquire 3D images by the μCT (**A4,B4**).

3.1.2. Quantification of Demineralization

μCT scans demonstrated carious lesions in the bacterial-infected groups, while teeth in the control group remain intact, depending on the clinical appearance. Representative radiographic images after infection are shown in Figure 4(A3,B3).

In the *UA159* bacterial-infected group, the radiographic images demonstrate extensive dentin lesions in fissures (Figure 4(B3)), while the teeth in the control group remain intact (Figure 4(B4)).

Figure 5 shows the differences in the caries range before and after inducing caries-promoting conditions. A significant increase was observed in the bacterial-infected group ($p < 0.0001$).

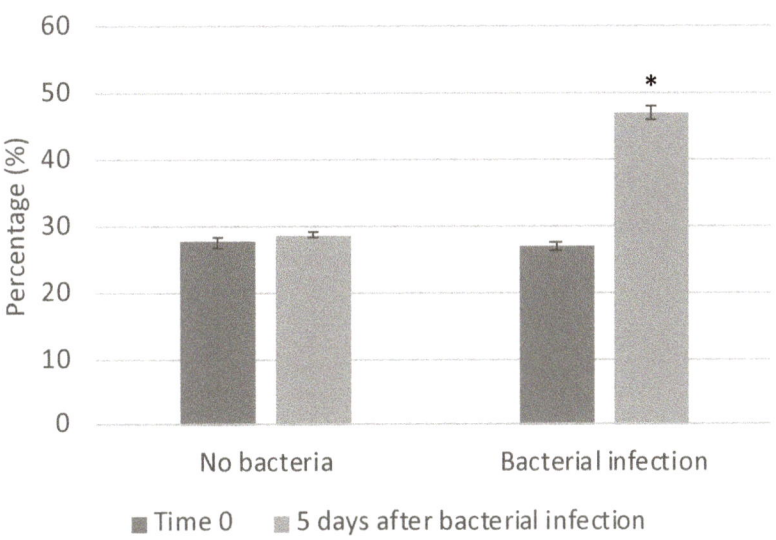

*$p<0.01$

Figure 5. Quantification of demineralization. μCT analysis comparison of volumetric percentage in the pulp and caries representing range (500–1500 mgHA/ccm) before (dark gray) and after (light gray) the experimental period. A significant increase ($p = 0.000069$) in the caries representing range was observed in the *S. mutans UA159* bacterial-infected group.

3.1.3. Bacterial Outgrowth Evaluation

At the end-point of the experiments, bacterial viable count in the bacterial-infected group was around 10^4 CFU/mL, while the control group remained non-contaminated.

3.1.4. Caries Scoring over Hemi-Sectioned Molars

As shown in Figure 6, the caries score over hemi-sectioned molars increased significantly ($p = 0.011$) in the bacterial infected jaws (n = 5) compared to the no bacteria jaws (n = 5). Figure 2a,b show representative images of hemi-sectioned molars from the bacterial-infected group with a caries score equal to 5 (units out of 8).

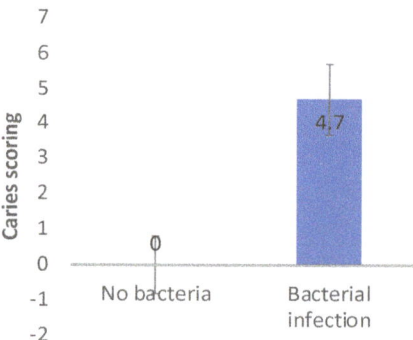

Figure 6. Caries scoring over hemi-sectioned molars after 5 days in caries-promoting conditions. Caries score increased significantly ($p = 0.011$) in the bacterial-infected jaws (n = 5) compared to the no bacteria jaws (n = 5).

3.2. Assessment of Caries Lesions in Jaws from Experimental In Vivo Caries Model in Mice

3.2.1. Clinical Evaluation

Clinical photographs demonstrated carious lesions development in the *UA159* bacterial-infected group, while the teeth in the control and high-sucrose diet groups remained intact. Representative photographs shown in Figure 7a.

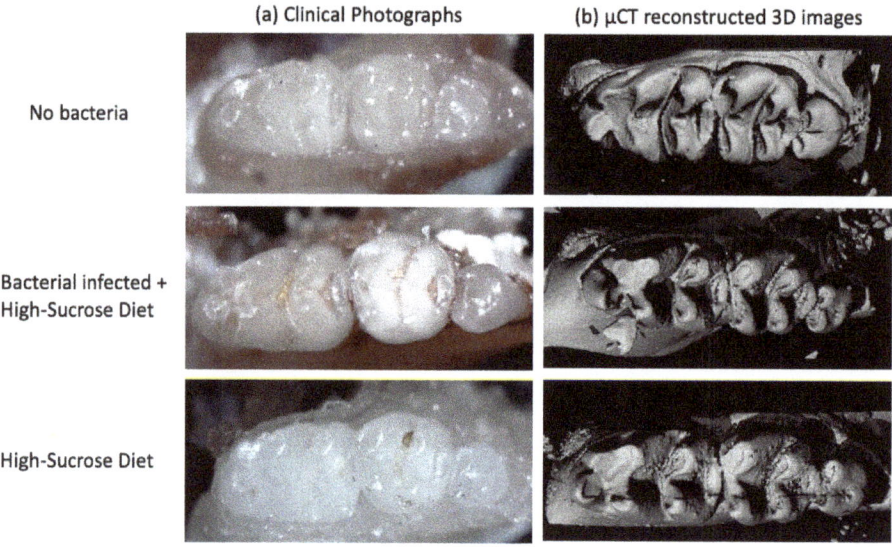

Figure 7. Clinical and radiographic evaluation demonstrates carious lesions development by *S. mutans UA159* bacterial infection and high-sucrose diet. (**a**) Hemi-mandibles were photographed using stereomicroscope. Representative clinical photographs depict extensive carious lesions developed in the *S. mutans UA159* bacterial infected + high-sucrose diet group, no carious lesions were depicted in the control and high-sucrose diet groups. (**b**) Hemi-mandibles were segmented and reconstructed to acquire 3D images by the μCT.

3.2.2. Quantification of Demineralization

μCT radiograph scans demonstrated extensive carious lesions in the *UA159* bacterial-infected group, while for the teeth in the control and high-sucrose diet groups, no demineralization was shown. Representative radiographic images are shown in Figure 8b–d.

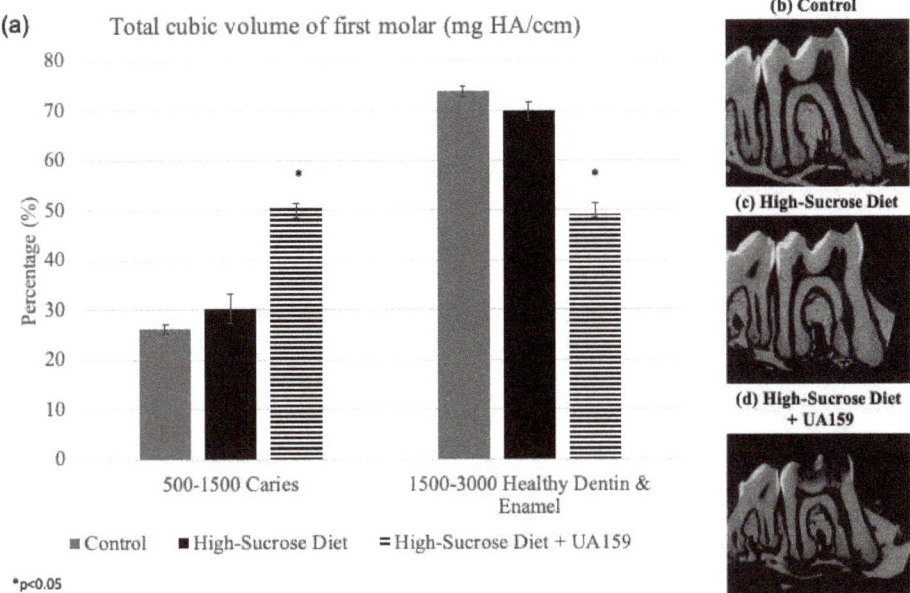

Figure 8. Radiographic μCT analysis shows carious lesions induced by high-sucrose diet and *UA159 S. mutans*. μCT radiographs were analyzed using a dedicated algorithm to divide total crown volume into density ranges. (**a**) Comparison of the volumetric percentage of density ranges by mgHA/ccm (i.e., caries representing range was determined to 500–1500 mgHA/ccm, healthy dentin and enamel representing range was determined to 1500–3000 mgHA/ccm). Mice were divided into three groups: high-sucrose diet (Keyes' #2000 and 10% sucrose containing distilled water) with *UA159* bacterial-infected group (n = 5) (striped column) compared to control (receiving normal diet and distilled water, n = 5) (gray column) and high-sucrose diet (without bacterial infection, n = 5) (black column). Representative radiographic images of the first molar from each group: (**b**) control, (**c**) high-sucrose diet, and (**d**) high-sucrose diet + *UA159*.

When comparing the total cubic volume of the first molar's crown divided into six selected ranges of density (by mgHA/ccm), a significant increase ($p < 0.05$) in the volumetric percentage of the density representing pulp and carious dentin (500–1500 mgHA/ccm) was observed (Figure 8a).

As shown in Figure 7b, μCT radiograph scans were reconstructed by the μCT to acquire 3D images. The 3D reconstructed images demonstrate and emphasize clinical appearance.

3.2.3. *S. Mutans* Dominates Oral Habitat after Infection

After 6 weeks of treatment, cariogenic diet induced an increase of *S. mutans* bacterial load. As expected, higher and significant increase (≈4 log increase) was shown in the bacterial infection group, compared to the control group. Statistical significance was calculated by Student's *t*-test (significance level: $p < 0.05$) compared to the untreated control (n = 5 in every tested group).

Respectively, an Increase in the relative portion of *S. mutans* from total bacteria count was shown in the high-sucrose diet and bacterial-infected group (Figure 9). Total bacteria viable count was evaluated using dilutions plated on BHI agar plate, while *S. mutans* viable count was evaluated using dilutions plated on a mitis–salivarius–bacitracin agar plate. The results are presented as percentages normalized to the total bacteria count in each group.

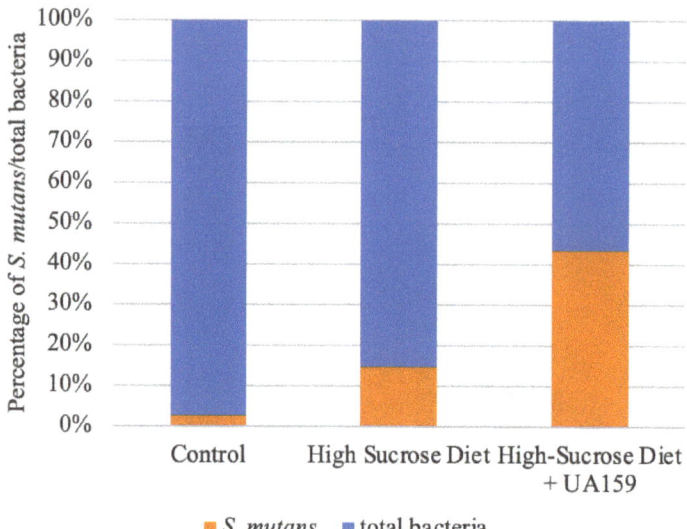

Figure 9. Cariogenic diet and bacterial infection increase the relative percentage of *S. mutans* from total bacterial counts in the mice oral habitat. Cariogenic (high-sucrose) diet and bacterial infections induced a significant increase of *S. mutans* bacterial load. The results are presented as percentages normalized to the total bacterial count in each group. Blue = total bacteria viable count. Orange =*S. mutans* viable count.

4. Discussion

An innovative in vitro caries model was developed herein aiming to decrease unnecessary animal sacrifice. Caries-promoting conditions mimicking in vivo caries models in murine were used to induce reproducible carious lesions within 5 days in extracted jaws of healthy animals sacrificed for other experiments and were no longer needed. To ensure the reliability of the in vitro development process, a resembling in vivo model study was conducted, and carious lesions were compared using qualitative and quantitative methods in both models. In the in vitro model, reproducible caries lesions were induced six times faster than in the in vivo model without compromising the data that can be drawn from the experimental conditions and without additional animal death.

Caries lesions treatment requires the removal of the infected hard dental tissues, and restoring the lost tissues using different types of restorative dental materials, mainly by amalgam, composite resin or glass-ionomer cement. Caries removal was mostly done by traditional low-speed and high-speed rotatory instruments. Recently, several innovative techniques have been suggested for minimal-invasive caries removal: sonic and ultrasonic oscillating devices [22], lasers [23], and chemo-mechanical solutions [24]. Caries modeling is necessary for evaluating innovative restorative and removal materials before clinical trials.

Maske et al. [25] have reviewed in vitro biofilm models to study dental caries. They described the high variability and complexity of in vitro models; numerous models were conducted over human teeth or enamel slabs. Demineralization is very difficult to diagnose and quantify using these models, and it often requires unique equipment with a highly sensitive technique, such as polarized light microscopy [26,27], microhardness [28,29], atomic force microscopy [30], or quantitative light fluorescence (QLF) [31,32].

Numerous caries studies have tried to quantify carious lesions development in vivo. Keyes [14] was the first to describe caries-scoring over hemi-sections rat molars. His scoring method, using murexide dye, is a common method still in use [33–35]. Zhang et al. [34] described the radiographic analysis of caries induced in rats; μCT scans were used to compare the mineral density of rats' molar enamel after calibration with hydroxyapatite standards of appropriate density. To our knowledge, Culp et al. [15] described exclusively the use of

Larson's modification [36] for Keyes' caries scoring method in a murine mice model; all mandibular and maxillary molars were scored for smooth surface and sulcal caries.

The clinical and radiographic demonstrations of the carious lesions evolved in the models described in the present study enables the identification of the lesion, quantification of the demineralization, and characterization in a similarity to the identification of carious lesions by dentists. Furthermore, the methods described require only stereomicroscope and µCT, the analysis is relatively simple, and the results are repeatable.

The demineralization process is dependent on the surface width and morphology. Murine molar teeth morphology contain sulci and fissures [37], which mimics the human molar morphology, but they are smaller, and the dental hard tissues are thinner than humans. Hence, the caries lesion development in the murine teeth is accelerated compared to the process in human teeth or enamel slabs [38]. For example, Park et al. [31] showed initial caries lesions over human molar enamel blocks after 30 days in caries-promoting conditions. The relatively rapid caries production in our model, after 5 days only, allows multiple repetitions, multiple dental materials evaluation, and avoidance of external infections or influences, and therefore provides a superior alternative over other in vitro models. Moreover, the use of extracted jaws from dissected healthy mice allowed us the control of multiple criteria, such as identical genetics, age, diet, growth conditions, and the starting condition of the dental hard tissues. Thus, monitoring multiple factors that may affect outcomes allows the examination and isolation of each factor and better understanding of carious lesions development and means to prevent it.

The mouth is a dynamic environment; salivary flow and its components have a protective role in reducing caries incidence [15,16,39]. The absence of salivary flow in the in vitro caries model may be the reason for more extensive lesion development, in shorter time, compared to the in vivo model. Moreover, clinical and radiographic photos exhibit some differences in the demineralization pattern: in the in vivo model, carious lesions were developed mostly in fissures' depth, while in the vitro model, enamel was detached, and demineralization occurred also in smooth surfaces.

In addition to animal lives, diet, and maintenance cost, the animal model requires a much longer time and effort compared to in vitro modeling. Given that the clinical and µCT analysis in both models are compatible and consistent, the in vitro model may offer many advantages over the in vivo model.

While animal experiments require skilled manpower, time-consuming protocols, and high cost [18], and in vitro acid-generated demineralization does not mimic the bacterial-induction of caries lesions in vivo, compared to other in vitro models, our in vitro model using murine extracted jaws, which mimics a natural caries-inducing environment, serves as a reliable and reproducible in vitro caries model.

5. Conclusions

A novel in vitro model using jaws from euthanized healthy mice was introduced. The present in vitro model allows reproducible extensive carious lesions within 5 days, similar to carious lesions that are induced within 6–7 weeks in vivo. The in vitro model may be beneficial for the evaluation of caries prevention and treatment means. It can be suggested that the model presented here may help reduce and replace animal use for caries research in the future.

Author Contributions: Conceptualization, Y.H.-H. and N.B.; methodology, Y.H.-H. and N.B.; validation, A.W.-Z., Y.H.-H. and N.B.; formal analysis, A.W.-Z.; investigation, A.W.-Z., Y.H.-H. and N.B.; resources, Y.H.-H. and N.B.; data curation, A.W.-Z., Y.H.-H. and N.B.; writing—original draft preparation, A.W.-Z.; writing—review and editing, A.W.-Z., Y.H.-H. and N.B.; visualization, Y.H.-H. and N.B.; supervision, Y.H.-H. and N.B.; project administration, Y.H.-H. and N.B.; funding acquisition, Y.H.-H. and N.B. All authors have read and agreed to the published version of the manuscript.

Funding: The research was supported from a grant from The Israel Science Foundation (ISF), grant number 986/16.

Institutional Review Board Statement: The study was conducted according to the guidelines of the Declaration of Helsinki and approved by the authorized by the institutional ethics committee #HMO-0706-16. All animal experimental procedures were reviewed and approved by the IACUC of the Hadassah—Hebrew University Medical Center (MD-17-15315-3).

Informed Consent Statement: Informed consent was obtained from all subjects involved in saliva collection for the study.

Acknowledgments: We would like to thank all those who contributed to this research, including Judith Goldstein, Yael Feinstein-Rotkopf from the Light Microscopy Laboratory of the intradepartmental unit of the Hebrew University, Raphael lieber for helping with μCT. In addition, we would like to thank David Polak and Joseph Tam for their help with euthanized healthy mice.

Conflicts of Interest: The authors declare no conflict of interest. The funders had no role in the design of the study; in the collection, analyses, or interpretation of data; in the writing of the manuscript, or in the decision to publish the results.

References

1. Featherstone, J.D. Modeling the caries-inhibitory effects of dental materials. *Dent. Mater.* **1996**, *12*, 194–197. [CrossRef]
2. Beighton, D. The complex oral microflora of high-risk individuals and groups and its role in the caries process. *Community Dent. Oral Epidemiol.* **2005**, *33*, 248–255. [CrossRef] [PubMed]
3. Wolff, D.; Frese, C.; Maier-Kraus, T.; Krueger, T.; Wolff, B. Bacterial biofilm composition in caries and caries-free subjects. *Caries Res.* **2013**, *47*, 69–77. [CrossRef]
4. Choi, E.J.; Lee, S.H.; Kim, Y.J. Quantitative real-time polymerase chain reaction for *Streptococcus mutans* and Streptococcus sobrinus in dental plaque samples and its association with early childhood caries. *Int. J. Paediatr. Dent.* **2009**, *19*, 141–147. [CrossRef]
5. Loesche, W.J. Role of *Streptococcus mutans* in human dental decay. *Microbiol. Rev.* **1986**, *50*, 353–380. [CrossRef]
6. Li, F.; Wang, P.; Weir, M.D.; Fouad, A.F.; Xu, H.H. Evaluation of antibacterial and remineralizing nanocomposite and adhesive in rat tooth cavity model. *Acta Biomater.* **2014**, *10*, 2804–2813. [CrossRef]
7. Salli, K.M.; Ouwehand, A.C. The use of in vitro model systems to study dental biofilms associated with caries: A short review. *J. Oral Microbiol.* **2015**, *7*, 26149. [CrossRef]
8. Ccahuana-Vásquez, R.A.; Cury, J.A.S. mutans biofilm model to evaluate antimicrobial substances and enamel demineralization. *Braz. Oral Res.* **2010**, *24*, 135–141. [CrossRef]
9. Giacaman, R.A.; Campos, P.; Munoz-Sandoval, C.; Castro, R.J. Cariogenic potential of commercial sweeteners in an experimental biofilm caries model on enamel. *Arch. Oral Biol.* **2013**, *58*, 1116–1122. [CrossRef] [PubMed]
10. Velusamy, S.K.; Markowitz, K.; Fine, D.H.; Velliyagounder, K. Human lactoferrin protects against *Streptococcus mutans*-induced caries in mice. *Oral Dis.* **2016**, *22*, 148–154. [CrossRef]
11. Bowen, W.H. Rodent model in caries research. *Odontology* **2013**, *101*, 9–14. [CrossRef]
12. Culp, D.J.; Quivey, R.Q.; Bowen, W.H.; Fallon, M.A.; Pearson, S.K.; Faustoferri, R. A mouse caries model and evaluation of aqp5−/− knockout mice. *Caries Res.* **2005**, *39*, 448–454. [CrossRef]
13. Keyes, P.H. Dental caries in the molar teeth of rats. I. Distribution of lesions induced by high-carbohydrate low-fat diets. *J. Dent. Res.* **1958**, *37*, 1077–1087. [CrossRef] [PubMed]
14. Keyes, P.H. Dental caries in the molar teeth of rats. II. A method for diagnosing and scoring several types of lesions simultaneously. *J. Dent. Res.* **1958**, *37*, 1088–1099. [CrossRef]
15. Culp, D.J.; Robinson, B.; Cash, M.N. Murine Salivary Amylase Protects Against. *Front. Physiol.* **2021**, *12*, 699104. [CrossRef]
16. Culp, D.J.; Robinson, B.; Cash, M.N.; Bhattacharyya, I.; Stewart, C.; Cuadra-Saenz, G. Salivary mucin 19 glycoproteins: Innate immune functions in *Streptococcus mutans*-induced caries in mice and evidence for expression in human saliva. *J. Biol. Chem.* **2015**, *290*, 2993–3008. [CrossRef]
17. Yang, H.; Bi, Y.; Shang, X.; Wang, M.; Linden, S.B.; Li, Y.; Li, Y.; Nelson, D.C.; Wei, H. Antibiofilm Activities of a Novel Chimeolysin against *Streptococcus mutans* under Physiological and Cariogenic Conditions. *Antimicrob. Agents Chemother.* **2016**, *60*, 7436–7443. [CrossRef] [PubMed]
18. Doke, S.K.; Dhawale, S.C. Alternatives to animal testing: A review. *Saudi Pharm. J.* **2015**, *23*, 223–229. [CrossRef]
19. Rai, J.; Kaushik, K. Reduction of Animal Sacrifice in Biomedical Science & Research through Alternative Design of Animal Experiments. *Saudi Pharm. J.* **2018**, *26*, 896–902. [CrossRef]
20. Kalfas, S.; Rundegren, J. Biological qualities of saliva sterilized by filtration or ethylene oxide treatment. *Oral Microbiol. Immunol.* **1991**, *6*, 182–186. [CrossRef] [PubMed]
21. Goldman, E.; Reich, E.; Abramovitz, I.; Klutstein, M. Inducing Apical Periodontitis in Mice. *J. Vis. Exp.* **2019**. [CrossRef]
22. Cianetti, S.; Abraha, I.; Pagano, S.; Lupatelli, E.; Lombardo, G. Sonic and ultrasonic oscillating devices for the management of pain and dental fear in children or adolescents that require caries removal: A systematic review. *BMJ Open* **2018**, *8*, e020840. [CrossRef]

23. Montedori, A.; Abraha, I.; Orso, M.; D'Errico, P.G.; Pagano, S.; Lombardo, G. Lasers for caries removal in deciduous and permanent teeth. *Cochrane Database Syst. Rev.* **2016**, *9*, CD010229. [CrossRef]
24. Cardoso, M.; Coelho, A.; Lima, R.; Amaro, I.; Paula, A.; Marto, C.M.; Sousa, J.; Spagnuolo, G.; Marques Ferreira, M.; Carrilho, E. Efficacy and Patient's Acceptance of Alternative Methods for Caries Removal-a Systematic Review. *J. Clin. Med.* **2020**, *9*, 3407. [CrossRef]
25. Maske, T.T.; Van de Sande, F.H.; Arthur, R.A.; Huysmans, M.C.D.N.J.M.; Cenci, M.S. In vitro biofilm models to study dental caries: A systematic review. *Biofouling* **2017**, *33*, 661–675. [CrossRef]
26. Sabel, N.; Robertson, A.; Nietzsche, S.; Norén, J.G. Demineralization of enamel in primary second molars related to properties of the enamel. *Sci. World J.* **2012**, *2012*, 587254. [CrossRef]
27. Montasser, M.A.; El-Wassefy, N.A.; Taha, M. In vitro study of the potential protection of sound enamel against demineralization. *Prog. Orthod.* **2015**, *16*, 12. [CrossRef]
28. Premaraj, T.S.; Rohani, N.; Covey, D.; Premaraj, S. In vitro evaluation of surface properties of Pro Seal((R)) and Opal((R)) Seal(TM) in preventing white spot lesions. *Orthod Craniofac. Res.* **2017**, *20* (Suppl. 1), 134–138. [CrossRef]
29. Almeida, L.F.; Marín, L.M.; Martínez-Mier, E.A.; Cury, J.A. Fluoride Dentifrice Overcomes the Lower Resistance of Fluorotic Enamel to Demineralization. *Caries Res.* **2019**, *53*, 567–575. [CrossRef]
30. Caldeira, E.M.; Telles, V.; Mattos, C.T.; Nojima, M.D.C.G. Surface morphologic evaluation of orthodontic bonding systems under conditions of cariogenic challenge. *Braz. Oral. Res.* **2019**, *33*, e029. [CrossRef]
31. Park, K.J.; Kroker, T.; Groß, U.; Zimmermann, O.; Krause, F.; Haak, R.; Ziebolz, D. Effectiveness of caries-preventing agents on initial carious lesions within the scope of orthodontic therapy. *Korean J. Orthod.* **2019**, *49*, 246–253. [CrossRef]
32. Paulos, R.S.; Seino, P.Y.; Fukushima, K.A.; Marques, M.M.; de Almeida, F.C.S.; Ramalho, K.M.; de Freitas, P.M.; Brugnera, A.; Moreira, M.S. Effect of Nd:YAG and CO. *Photomed. Laser Surg.* **2017**, *35*, 282–286. [CrossRef]
33. Luo, J.; Feng, Z.; Jiang, W.; Jiang, X.; Chen, Y.; Lv, X.; Zhang, L. Novel lactotransferrin-derived synthetic peptides suppress cariogenic bacteria. *J. Oral Microbiol.* **2021**, *13*, 1943999. [CrossRef]
34. Zhang, Q.; Qin, S.; Xu, X.; Zhao, J.; Zhang, H.; Liu, Z.; Chen, W. Inhibitory Effect of Lactobacillus planetarium CCFM8724 towards *Streptococcus mutans*- and Candida albicans—Induced Caries in Rats. *Oxid. Med. Cell Longev.* **2020**, *2020*, 4345804. [CrossRef]
35. Liang, J.; Liang, D.; Liang, Y.; He, J.; Zuo, S.; Zhao, W. Effects of a derivative of reutericin 6 and gassericin A on the biofilm of *Streptococcus mutans* in vitro and caries prevention in vivo. *Odontology* **2021**, *109*, 53–66. [CrossRef] [PubMed]
36. Larson, R.H. Merits and modifications of scoring rat dental caries by Keyes' method. In *Proceedings of "Symposium on Animal Models in Cariology", Spl. Supp. Microbiology Abstracts*; CiNii: Tokyo, Japan, 1981; pp. 195–203.
37. Lazzari, V.; Tafforeau, P.; Aguilar, J.P.; Michaux, J. Topographic maps applied to comparative molar morphology: The case of murine and cricetine dental plans (Rodentia, Muroidea). *Paleobiology* **2016**, *34*, 46–64. [CrossRef]
38. Hartles, R.L. Experimental dental caries in the rat. *Proc. R Soc. Med.* **1960**, *53*, 528–531. [CrossRef]
39. Wang, K.; Wang, Y.; Wang, X.; Ren, Q.; Han, S.; Ding, L.; Li, Z.; Zhou, X.; Li, W.; Zhang, L. Comparative salivary proteomics analysis of children with and without dental caries using the iTRAQ/MRM approach. *J. Transl. Med.* **2018**, *16*, 11. [CrossRef]

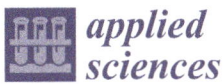

Article

Influencing Factors on Aesthetics: Highly Controlled Study Based on Eye Movement and the Forensic Aspects in Computer-Based Assessment of Visual Appeal in Upper Front Teeth

Monika Bjelopavlovic [1,*], Michael Weyhrauch [2], Christina Erbe [3], Franziska Burkard [4], Katja Petrowski [5] and Karl Martin Lehmann [1]

1 Department of Prosthetic Dentistry, University Medical Center of the Johannes Gutenberg-University Mainz, Augustusplatz 2, 55131 Mainz, Germany; karl.lehmann@unimedizin-mainz.de
2 Private Practice, Fliednerweg 8, 64367 Mühltal, Germany; michiweyhrauch@googlemail.com
3 Department of Orthodontics, University Medical Center of the Johannes Gutenberg-University Mainz, Augustusplatz 2, 55131 Mainz, Germany; erbe@uni-mainz.de
4 Private Practice, Am Houiller Platz2, 61381 Friedrichsdorf, Germany; f.burkard@gmx.de
5 Department of Medical Psychology and Medical Sociology, University Medical Center of the Johannes Gutenberg-University Mainz, Duesbergweg 6, 55131 Mainz, Germany; kpetrows@uni-mainz.de
* Correspondence: monika.bjelopavlovic@unimedizin-mainz.de; Tel.: +49-6131-17-5263; Fax: +49-6131-17-5517

Abstract: First impressions are formed by the external appearance and, in this respect, essentially by an examination of the face. In the literature, the teeth, especially the maxillary front, are among an eye-catching and sensitive area that plays a significant role in the overall evaluation of appearance. In this study, the first eye fixation of 60 subjects with different levels of dental training (layperson, trained layperson, dental student, and dentist) is recorded using an eye-tracking system, and their subsequent evaluation of the images is recorded. Ten unedited original photographs of different maxillary anterior teeth and ten subsequently edited photographs will be used to evaluate forensic aspects such as the effect of symmetry and color on the overall evaluation. The results will be used to determine which areas of the maxillary anterior are demonstrably viewed and whether knowledge of dental esthetics influences evaluation and viewing.

Keywords: eye-tracking; aesthetics; golden ratio; forensics

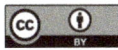

1. Introduction

Aesthetics is an outstanding topic in dentistry and sometimes determines essential aspects of therapy, as patients often desire an optical benefit from a dental intervention. Therefore, the selection of tooth color and shape, as well as the correction of tooth position plays a major role. To follow the light-colored and straight teeth, particularly in the anterior region [1]. This is performed by teeth whitening-bleaching-and, for example, by veneers, which are thin shells bonded to the enamel and can correct discoloration, surface irregularities, but also slight tooth misalignments and asymmetries. Another growing area of the (aesthetic dentistry) industry is the treatment of misaligned teeth with orthodontic aligner therapies. Crowns or modifications of the anterior teeth out of cosmetic aesthetics, are treatments of choice for patients who want to optimize their external appearance through dental therapy. Since the introduction of aligner therapy in 1997, there has been an increased demand for this non fixed treatment in cosmetic dentistry [2–4]. The empirical literature tries to determine criteria associated with beauty and searches for the therapy of a perfect smile. In this context, the assessment of the most frequently exposed teeth in smiling, maxillary anterior teeth region 13–23, is outstanding in the literature [1,5–7]. Hereby, the central incisor plays the dominant role for an esthetic smile. The ideal relationship between the central incisor and the lateral incisor is discussed widely in the literature. The lateral incisor should be 1.5 mm longer, and the height of the gingival margin should be 0.5 mm below that of the canine [5]. Furthermore, the condition of the gum, the symmetrical course and the color of the gingiva are included in the assessment of an attractive external appearance, since conclusions can be drawn about the health status of the oral cavity [7]. Based on the literature another dominant criteria is the tooth color [8]. A self-report based study among young adults showed that tooth color is the decisive factor in the subjective perception of their oral health [9]. This also corelates with the increased demand for dental aesthetic corrections such as bleaching and veneer treatment. Over 77% of general practitioner's patients demanded tooth whitening and over 54% wanted a veneer treatment in recent years due to the media influence. In addition, both the color correction by a bleaching procedure and the correction by ceramic shells adhesively bonded to the natural enamel have become very popular [10]. The influence of appearance by exposing the maxillary anterior teeth during social interaction leads to an evaluation of the person vis-à-vis. Hereby, the maxillary anterior teeth give rise to an overall impression, which has been highly investigated both from a sociological as well as population-based point of view [11–13]. These results highlight the importance of oral health in terms of external appearance and potential stigma and association with social status, for example, in the case of missing teeth [8,14,15]. In order to be able to respond to the needs of the patient, generally valid criteria are sought that are perceptible to the environment and are perceived as beautiful. In this context, the assessment of a beautiful smile by laypersons, i.e., the environment of a patient, is decisive and the subject of the literature. In a systematic review of 6032 studies laypeople's assessment of smile aesthetics was analyzed to identify the most important criteria. Hereby, the central incisor and the canine were again identified as the most important teeth for an esthetic smile [16–18]. Important aspects such as symmetry and tooth positions were also noted, which, with slight deviations, nevertheless resulted in an overall positive evaluation [1,19]. The assessments of the gingiva by laypersons were inconsistent, however a high smile line with a so-called "Gummy Smile" tended to score worse [20,21]. Which regions thereby fell first into the field of vision of the laymen and which characteristics of a smiling person were crucial "in the eye fall" was not reported nor worked out in these studies.

Therefore, the aim, of the present investigation deals with the question of whether dentists, trained laypersons and laypersons have different ways of looking at teeth and, accordingly, view and evaluate the 20 images of smiling patients in different ways. It is further investigated whether a predictability of the look is possible, since the assumption is made that the expert degree has substantial influence on the way of looking and evaluating a smile. Therefore, it can be hypothesized that dentists see the problem zones that have to be treated first, whereas laypersons always look at the center.

2. Materials and Methods

2.1. Subject Group

The study included a group of sixty adults containing 15 laymen, 15 trained laymen, 15 dental students in the clinical study section and 15 dentists/experts. The group of laypersons did not show any dental reference in the professional profile.

In a 12-page power point presentation, the trained laypersons were shown basics of dental esthetics regarding gingiva, proportions and size relationships. The dental students were all at the clinical study stage and had clinical experience. The group of experts consisted of dentists who were licensed to practice dentistry.

2.2. Design

Twenty images were available for viewing and evaluation by the subjects. They were composed as follows (Figure 1):

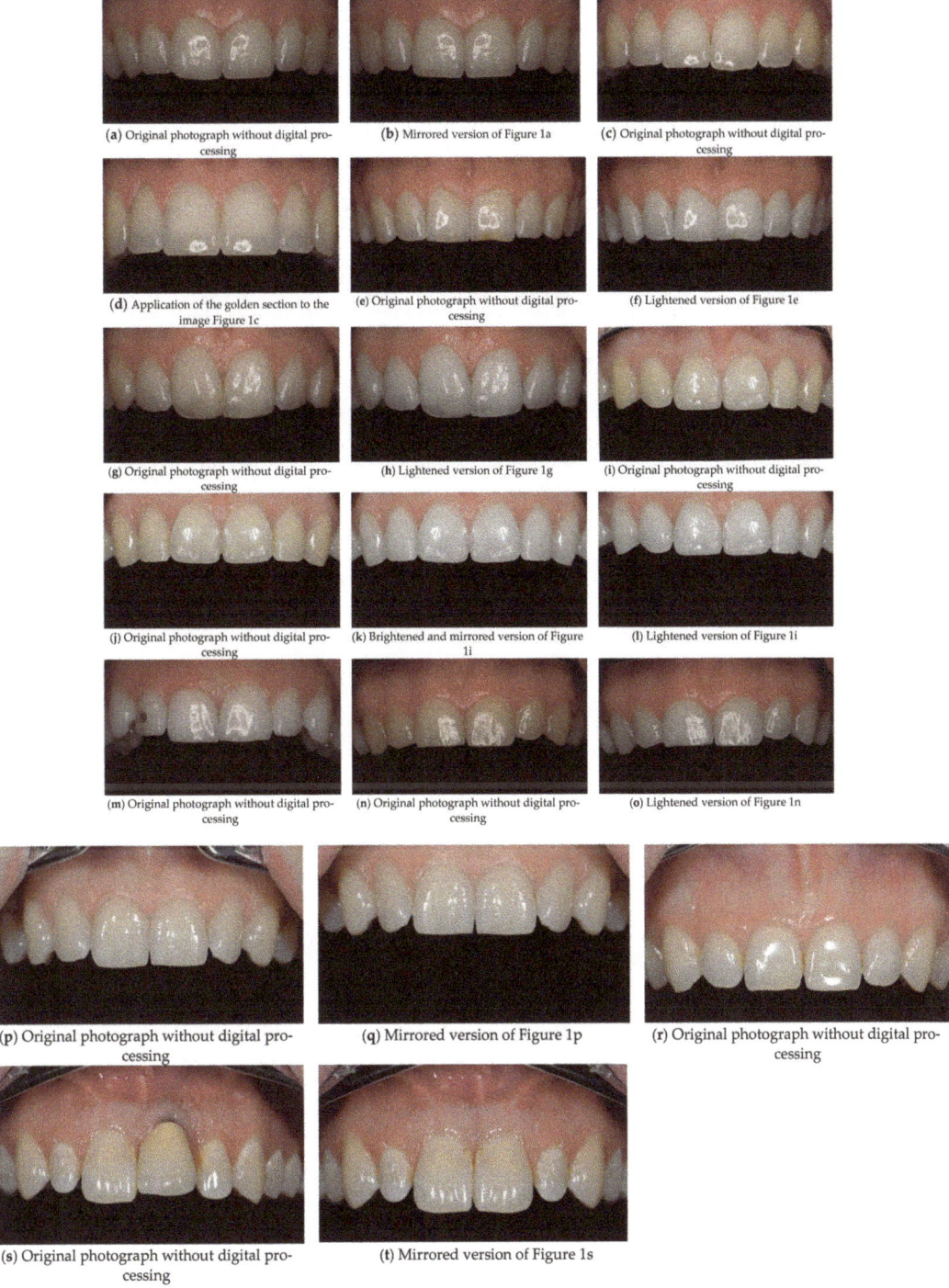

Figure 1. Images for viewing and evaluation by the subjects.

Eleven unedited original photos of persons who had agreed to have their anterior teeth photographed were used. In each case, the region 13–23 including the gingiva was depicted and recognizable. The photos were taken using a cheek retractor, contrastor, camera (Nikon D5200, micro Nikkor Lens 105 mm, Nikon®, Tokyo, Japan) and macro flash (R1C1).

Nine edited photos: b,d,f,h,k,l,o,q,t. Picture b,j,k,q,t mirrored photos from original images a,i,p,f,h,k,l,o and and brightened photos from original images e,g,l,n (yellow saturation: 70% yellow brightness: +50%, general brightening: +5); picture d = golden section from original images c,k,o brightened and mirrored from original image n.

Each subject was placed individually and with the help of a chinrest in a fixed position in front of the viewing monitor. Calibration of the Eye Tracking System (NYAN 2.0 Eye Tracking Data Analysis Suit, LC Technologies, Inc., Fairfax, VA, USA) was performed for 15 s at a time. After a successful detection of eye movements and pupil recognition, the image sequence started automatically. The sequence always showed the unedited photo first.

Each image was projected for 8 s and the subjects' viewing patterns were recorded. Subsequently, the subjects were presented with an evaluation form containing a rating from 0–10 (VAS–visual analog scale), where 0 stood for very bad and 10 for very good. The images were played again in the same order but without a time limit for evaluation. The analysis program of the eye tracking system evaluated the first fixation point of each subject. Four points were defined (1 = central incisor, 2 = lateral incisor, 3 = canine, 4 = gum and 0 = outside the regions).

Consequently, 1200 initial fixation points and 1200 evaluations of the images were created.

2.3. Statistical Analysis

The analysis was performed with SPSS 27 (IBM, Munich, Germany) and after descriptive statistics with Kendall's tau, a regression calculation was applied to be able to determine the predictability of the first eye fixation depending on expert level, age and gender.

3. Results

3.1. Descriptive Analysis

In the group of dentists and dental students, as among laypersons, the rating 7 was given most frequently. Overall, this rating was given 243 times out of 1200 evaluations (20.3%). The trained laypersons most frequently assigned the rating 6. This rating was the second most frequent overall (201 times, 16.8%). The group of trained laypersons showed the most stringent evaluation and chose the evaluation between 0 and 4 with 25% most frequently in the overall comparison. Only 14.3% of the dental students chose to rate the photos in the score range of 0–4, and overall, they most frequently rated the photos with above-average points (mean 6.42).

The top score of 10 was given most frequently by dental students (10 times) and least frequently by laypersons and dentists (8 times). All four groups considered image s to be the worst aesthetically (eight times 0, twelve times 1) and image o to be the most beautiful (ten times 10, nineteen times 9) with dental students giving the best rating to image number a (three times 10, two times 9). For further detail see Figures 2–4. However, no significant differences in the evaluation between the individual groups could be determined ($p = 0.013$, see Table 1). Likewise, no gender-specific significances were found. In the group of dental students and dentists, a tendency towards a better rating was found among the women; in the group of untrained laypersons, there was a reverse tendency (see Table 1).

Appl. Sci. **2021**, *11*, 6797

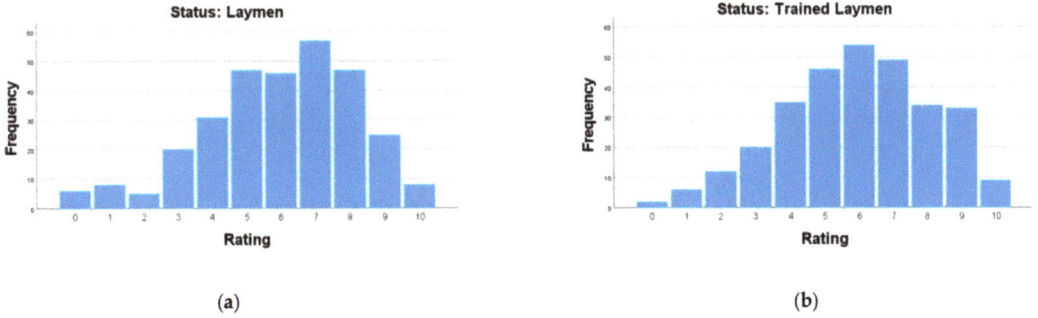

Figure 2. Evaluation of (**a**) laymen and (**b**) trained laymen.

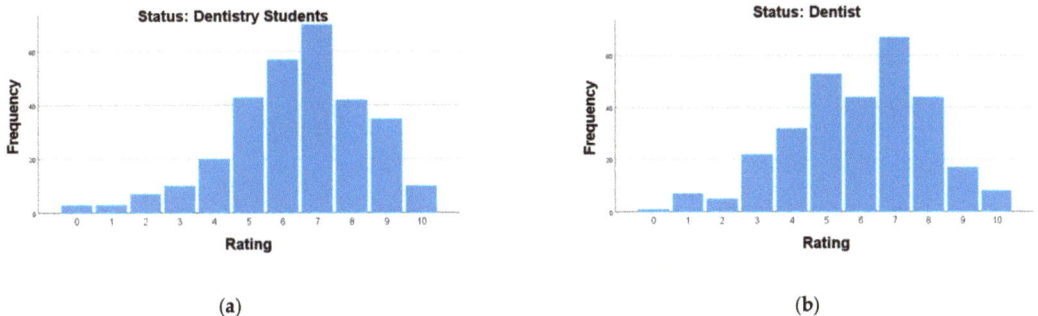

Figure 3. Evaluation of (**a**) dental students and (**b**) dentists.

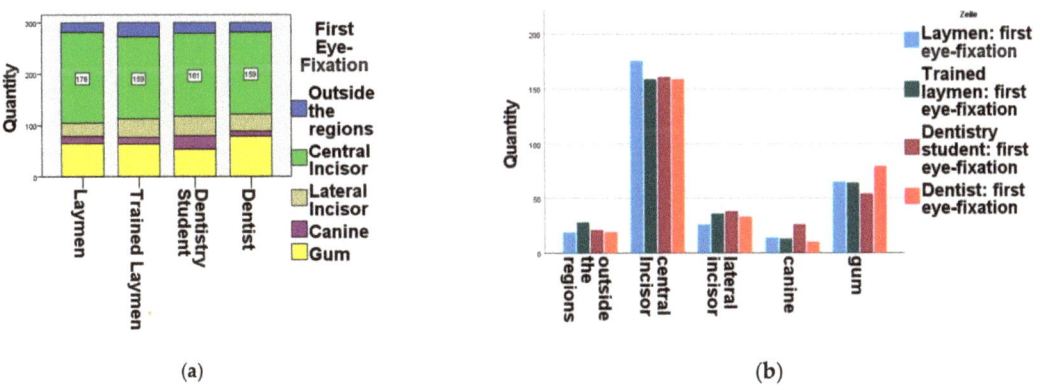

Figure 4. Quantity of first eye fixation illustrated in (**a**) expert level group (*x*-axis) and (**b**) first eye-fixation point (*x*-axis).

Table 1. Kendall tau correlation.

			Correlations				
			Rating	Gender	Status	Age	First_Eyefixation
Kendall-Tau-b	Rating	Correlation coefficient Sig. (two-sided) N	1000 - 1200	−0.006 0.815 1200	0.013 0.57 1200	* −0.069 0.003 1200	* −0.069 0.003 1200
	Gender	Correlation coefficient Sig. (two-sided) N	−0.006 0.815 1200	1000 - 1200	* 0.226 <0.001 1200	* 0.212 <0.001 1200	0.023 0.391 1200
	Status	Correlation coefficient Sig. (two-sided) N	0.013 0.57 1200	* 0.226 <0.001 1200	1000 - 1200	* −0.27 <0.001 1200	0.033 0.173 1200
	Age	Correlation coefficient Sig. (two-sided) N	* −0.069 0.003 1200	* 0.212 <0.001 1200	* −0.27 <0.001 1200	1000 - 1200	−0.028 0.266 1200
	First_Eyefixation	Correlation coefficient Sig. (two-sided) N	* −0.069 0.003 1200	0.023 0.391 1200	0.033 0.173 1200	−0.028 0.266 1200	1000 - 1200

* The correlation on level 0.01 is significant (two-sided).

3.2. Ordinal Regression

The ordinal regression should provide information on how the variables behave depending on the first point of view. Therefore, a step wise regression model was performed. The first fixation point as the dependent variable was compared with the independent variables, gender, age and status. The regression model is not significant ($p = 0.076$) and thus the null hypothesis cannot be rejected (Table 2). The corrected R-squared is R = 0.003, and only age shows significance with negative correlation ($p = 0.03$). Consequently, older subjects predictably looked more often at the regions outside the displayed structures (=0).

Table 2. Regression.

	Non-Standardized Coefficients		Standardized Coefficients			95.0% Confidence Intervals for B	
	Reg. Coefficient B	Std.-Mistake	Beta	T	Sig.	Lower Limit	Upper Limit
Constant	1.875	0.172	-	10.874	<0.001	1.537	2.213
Gender	0.117	0.085	0.043	1.379	0.168	−0.05	0.284
Status	−0.013	0.041	−0.011	−0.302	0.763	−0.094	0.069
Age	−0.067	0.031	−0.075	−2.176	0.03	−0.128	−0.007

Dependent variable: First_Eyefixation.

4. Discussion

This study investigated the first point of view of the four groups of subjects in order to identify a possible difference in the approach and definition of aesthetics between laypersons and experts in this field. The methodology used was the eye-tracker described in the literature, which is non-invasive and harmless to the health of the subjects due to corneal reflection using infrared light [22,23]. In the study by Yamamoto et al. [24], 47 laypersons were shown intraoral images of teeth with and without restorations and the gaze points and duration of each were evaluated with an eye-tracker. The restorations were subsequently inserted into photographs of the mouth-closed and mouth-opened condition using an editing program. This was done only on one side in each of the four quadrants and did not fit aesthetically into the overall image. Consequently, a sequence of images was created, showing unprocessed photos and photos with non-aesthetic restorations. The first fixation point in the images shown with restorations was significantly more often detectable first on the restoration and the viewing of the restoration was additionally of longer duration. No difference in viewing time was observed in the photos without non-esthetic restorations [24]. In contrast in the present study design, also the identification of the difference between laypersons and experts, who could have different approaches to the observation due to their level of experience, should be performed. The hypothesis that experts pay more attention to the "problem area" and laypersons primarily look at the central incisor cannot be confirmed.

The literature, on the other hand, shows a clear tendency for the dominant viewpoint, regardless of gender and age, to be the anterior region, with particular emphasis on the central incisor [25,26]. In our study, the photos did not allow any conclusions to be drawn about the gender of the model, whereas in the study by Baker et al. [23], only male faces, showing the whole face, were provided for the viewing analysis and a difference was found between women and men when viewing. Women were significantly more likely to have viewing points in the eye region, whereas men had viewing points in the mouth region [23]. No gender difference could be identified in the results of the study presented here. In general, the central incisor could be identified as the dominant first consideration point in all four subject groups, which is reflected in the literature [26]. The evaluation of the images also confirmed the literature, which places an emphasis on color in dental esthetics, with white teeth being perceived as significantly more beautiful [5,8]. The highest rated photo, number o, was subsequently lightened. Only the group of dental students also showed outstandingly good ratings for image number a, which was not lightened but corresponded to the unprocessed original. Photo number s, on the other hand, which was rated the worst of all the groups of test subjects, showed a prosthetic restoration in the region of the central incisor in region 21. Compared to tooth 11, this crown appeared incisally shortened and heavily discolored in the area of the crown margin.

Consequently, the literature results are confirmed, which entails an immediate focus of the eye in esthetically restrictive restorations [24]. The overall socio-psychological image of a person is clearly influenced by the oral area and especially the teeth and their aesthetics. Furthermore, teeth play a crucial role in the well-known first impression. The present study was able to show that the assessment and evaluation of aesthetics takes place independently of experience level, gender, or age and no occupational context needs to exist to perceive certain oral characteristics positively or negatively and to fix them visually. The clinical aspect in the treatment of anterior teeth should have a focus on symmetry and color, which is associated with more positive evaluations as proven in our study. The esthetically sensitive facial area of the maxillary anterior region requires special consideration regarding the selection of the restoration and its design.

Both an accomplished expert and laypersons make quick evaluations based on presumed universally valid criteria. An appearance associated with "health" is also proven to be a factor for positive evaluation, reflected in healthy gingiva and a light tooth color. This is also shown in the literature and implies a positive effect considering the first appeal [27]. The dwell time of the eye gaze, as well as a uniform subject selection in gender and age, as well as experience level in the occupational field, would be worth considering for follow-up studies.

5. Conclusions

The evaluation of the data shows that there is no demonstrable difference in the approach and evaluation at different expert levels. The null hypothesis that dentists have a different approach to the evaluation or assessment of their counterpart can therefore not be confirmed. A general focus in the first eye fixation can be detected on the central incisor, which is in line with the existing literature. Overall, a generally valid ideal of beauty can be derived in the evaluation of the 20 images, which places color and symmetry in the foreground, despite differing levels of knowledge depending on the expert level. Lighter and symmetrical anterior teeth tend to be rated better. Individual deviations from the golden ratio are nevertheless perceived as aesthetic and still allow the statement that beauty is in the eye of the beholder.

Author Contributions: Conceptualization, M.W., K.M.L. and M.B.; methodology, C.E.; software, C.E.; validation, K.P., M.B. and K.M.L.; formal analysis, M.W.; investigation, F.B.; resources, M.B.; data curation, M.B.; writing—original draft preparation, M.B.; writing—review and editing, K.P. and K.M.L.; visualization, M.B.; supervision, K.M.L.; project administration, M.B. and M.W.; funding acquisition, C.E. All authors have read and agreed to the published version of the manuscript.

Funding: This research received no external funding.

Institutional Review Board Statement: The study was conducted according to the guidelines of the Declaration of Helsinki, and approved by the Ethics Committee Rheinland-Pfalz.

Informed Consent Statement: Informed consent was obtained from all subjects involved in the study.

Data Availability Statement: The data from this study were part of the dissertation paper from F.B. Data can be seen in Tables 1 and 2.

Conflicts of Interest: The authors declare no conflict of interest.

References

1. Machado, A.W.; Moon, W.; Gandini, L.G., Jr. Influence of maxillary incisor edge asymmetries on the perception of smile esthetics among orthodontists and laypersons. *Am. J. Orthod. Dentofac. Orthop.* **2013**, *143*, 658–664. [CrossRef]
2. Borda, A.F.; Garfinkle, J.S.; Covell, D.A.; Wang, M.; Doyle, L.; Sedgley, C.M. Outcome assessment of orthodontic clear aligner vs fixed appliance treatment in a teenage population with mild malocclusions. *Angle Orthod.* **2020**, *90*, 485–490. [CrossRef]
3. Hennessy, J.; Al-Awadhi, E.A. Clear aligners generations and orthodontic tooth movement. *J. Orthod.* **2016**, *43*, 68–76. [CrossRef]
4. Gu, J.; Tang, J.S.; Skulski, B.; Fields, H.W., Jr.; Beck, F.M.; Firestone, A.R.; Kim, D.-G.; Deguchi, T. Evaluation of Invisalign treatment effectiveness and efficiency compared with conventional fixed appliances using the Peer Assessment Rating index. *Am. J. Orthod. Dentofac. Orthop.* **2017**, *151*, 259–266. [CrossRef]
5. Machado, A.W. 10 commandments of smile esthetics. *Dent. Press J. Orthod.* **2014**, *19*, 136–157. [CrossRef]
6. Liao, P.; Fan, Y.; Nathanson, D. Evaluation of maxillary anterior teeth width: A systematic review. *J. Prosthet. Dent.* **2019**, *122*, 275–281.e7. [CrossRef] [PubMed]
7. Monnet-Corti, V.; Antezack, A.; Pignoly, M. Perfecting smile esthetics: Keep it pink! *Orthod. Fr.* **2018**, *89*, 71–80. [CrossRef]
8. Khalid, A.; Quiñonez, C. Straight, white teeth as a social prerogative. *Sociol. Health Illn.* **2015**, *37*, 782–796. [CrossRef] [PubMed]
9. Daneshvar, M.; Devji, T.F.; Davis, A.B.; White, M.A. Oral health related quality of life: A novel metric targeted to young adults. *J. Public Health Dent.* **2015**, *75*, 298–307. [CrossRef]
10. Theobald, A.H.; Wong, B.K.J.; Quick, A.N.; Thomson, W.M. The impact of the popular media on cosmetic dentistry. *N. Z. Dent. J.* **2006**, *102*, 58–63. [PubMed]
11. Pithon, M.M.; Nascimento, C.C.; Barbosa, G.C.G.; Coqueiro, R.D.S. Do dental esthetics have any influence on finding a job? *Am. J. Orthod. Dentofac. Orthop.* **2014**, *146*, 423–429. [CrossRef]
12. Malkinson, S.; Waldrop, T.C.; Gunsolley, J.C.; Lanning, S.K.; Sabatini, R. The effect of esthetic crown lengthening on perceptions of a patient's attractiveness, friendliness, trustworthiness, intelligence, and self-confidence. *J. Periodontol.* **2013**, *84*, 1126–1133. [CrossRef]
13. Correa, B.D.; Bittencourt, M.A.V.; Machado, A.W. Influence of maxillary canine gingival margin asymmetries on the perception of smile esthetics among orthodontists and laypersons. *Am. J. Orthod. Dentofac. Orthop.* **2014**, *145*, 55–63. [CrossRef] [PubMed]
14. Holden, A.C.L. Consumed by prestige: The mouth, consumerism and the dental profession. *Med. Health Care Philos.* **2019**, *23*, 261–268. [CrossRef] [PubMed]
15. Kleinberger, J.A.; Strickhouser, S.M. Missing Teeth: Reviewing the Sociology of Oral Health and Healthcare. *Sociol. Compass* **2014**, *8*, 1296–1314. [CrossRef]
16. Parrini, S.; Rossini, G.; Castroflorio, T.; Fortini, A.; Deregibus, A.; Debernardi, C. Laypeople's perceptions of frontal smile esthetics: A systematic review. *Am. J. Orthod. Dentofac. Orthop.* **2016**, *150*, 740–750. [CrossRef]
17. Brough, E.; Donaldson, A.N.; Naini, F.B. Canine substitution for missing maxillary lateral incisors: The influence of canine mor-phology, size, and shade on perceptions of smile attractiveness. *Am. J. Orthod. Dentofac. Orthop.* **2010**, *138*, 705.e1–705.e9, discussion-7. [CrossRef]
18. Thomas, M.; Reddy, R.; Reddy, B.J. Perception differences of altered dental esthetics by dental professionals and laypersons. *Indian J. Dent. Res.* **2011**, *22*, 242–247. [CrossRef]
19. Ma, W.; Preston, B.; Asai, Y.; Guan, H.; Guan, G. Perceptions of dental professionals and laypeople to altered maxillary incisor crowding. *Am. J. Orthod. Dentofac. Orthop.* **2014**, *146*, 579–586. [CrossRef]
20. Kaya, B.; Uyar, R. Influence on smile attractiveness of the smile arc in conjunction with gingival display. *Am. J. Orthod. Dentofac. Orthop.* **2013**, *144*, 541–547. [CrossRef]
21. Sarver, D.; Jacobson, R.S. The Aesthetic Dentofacial Analysis. *Clin. Plast. Surg.* **2007**, *34*, 369–394. [CrossRef] [PubMed]

22. Richards, M.R.; Fields, H.W., Jr.; Beck, F.M.; Firestone, A.R.; Walther, D.B.; Rosenstiel, S.; Sacksteder, J.M. Contribution of malocclusion and female facial attractiveness to smile esthetics evaluated by eye tracking. *Am. J. Orthod. Dentofac. Orthop.* **2015**, *147*, 472–482. [CrossRef]
23. Baker, R.S.; Fields, H.W., Jr.; Beck, F.M.; Firestone, A.R.; Rosenstiel, S.F. Objective assessment of the contribution of dental esthetics and facial attractiveness in men via eye tracking. *Am. J. Orthod. Dentofac. Orthop.* **2018**, *153*, 523–533. [CrossRef]
24. Yamamoto, M.; Torii, K.; Sato, M.; Tanaka, J.; Tanaka, M. Analysis of gaze points for mouth images using an eye tracking system. *J. Prosthodont. Res.* **2017**, *61*, 379–386. [CrossRef]
25. Suwa, K.; Furukawa, A.; Matsumoto, T.; Yosue, T. Analyzing the eye movement of dentists during their reading of CT images. *Odontol.* **2001**, *89*, 54–61. [CrossRef] [PubMed]
26. Del Monte, S.; Afrashtehfar, K.I.; Emami, E.; Abi Nader, S.; Tamimi, F. Lay preferences for dentogingival esthetic parameters: A systematic review. *J. Prosthet. Dent.* **2017**, *118*, 717–724. [CrossRef] [PubMed]
27. Joiner, A.; Luo, W. Tooth colour and whiteness: A review. *J. Dent.* **2017**, *67*, S3–S10. [CrossRef]

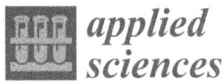

Review

Comparison of CAD/CAM and Conventional Denture Base Resins: A Systematic Review

Cindy Batisse [1,2,*] and Emmanuel Nicolas [1,2]

1. UFR d'Odontologie, Université Clermont Auvergne, CROC, F-63000 Clermont-Ferrand, France; emmanuel.nicolas@uca.fr
2. CHU Clermont-Ferrand, Service d'Odontologie, F-63003 Clermont-Ferrand, France
* Correspondence: cindy.lance@uca.fr

Abstract: At present, complete dentures (CDs) remain the only treatment available for the majority of edentulous patients. CDs are primarily fabricated using a conventional method using polymethylmethacrylate (PMMA) resin. The steps involved in PMMA polymerisation directly affect the quality of the resin prosthetic base and any error reduces retention and occlusal accuracy of CDs. Furthermore, when using the conventional technique, the residual monomer alters the resin mechanical properties and may cause mucosal reactions. Recently, computer aided design and computer aided manufacture (CAD/CAM) techniques were increasingly used to fabricate CDs by machining resin discs that have been manufactured under high pressure and temperature. This systematic review compares CAD/CAM and conventional CDs according to their mechanical, physical and chemical characteristics, as well as the clinical impact of any differences between them. A review was conducted according to the preferred reporting items for systematic reviews and meta-analyses checklist on 392 publications from both PubMed and backward research. Fifteen studies have been included. Results showed that CAD/CAM resins had globally better physical and mechanical properties than conventional resins. The use of machined resin could improve the clinical performance, maintenance and longevity of CDs. Further studies in clinical use would be required to complement these results.

Keywords: denture base; complete denture; acrylic resin; CAD-CAM; milling resin

1. Introduction

Due to anatomical, physiological or financial restrictions, complete dentures (CDs) still represent the only treatment available for the majority of edentulous patients. Since the 1950s, complete dentures have been primarily designed and fabricated by hand, using conventional methods that follow well-defined clinical protocols and laboratory techniques. To produce a set of complete dentures, edentulous patients must have at least five clinical appointments with their dentist to (1) make preliminary and (2) final impressions to make a replica of the oral tissues (gypsum cast), (3) record the maxillomandibular relationship and select the appropriate denture teeth, (4) test the trial wax prostheses and (5) insert the complete prostheses. Once the trial wax dentures are deemed appropriate, the laboratory steps to make the final prostheses begin. The gypsum cast and the trial wax replica are flasked in more gypsum to produce the external surface form. Once all the gypsum is solidified, the trial wax is removed using hot water, producing a mold cavity. The resin to fabricate the final denture is then introduced into the mold cavity within the flask by either pressure or injection. Each technique has advantages and disadvantages. The quality of the prosthetic resin material obtained is strongly influenced by the steps involved in handling the resin.

To date, acrylic resin polymethylmethacrylate (PMMA) is the most popular denture base material [1]. PMMA resin best meets all the specifications for an ideal denture base material. Its advantages range from easy repair to good appearance and reasonable cost. It has simple handling characteristics and polymerization is initiated by mixing polymethyl methacrylate (polymer) and methyl methacrylate (monomer) [2]. The polymerization of this type of PMMA resin is completed by application of heat. When this resin is used for dental prostheses, it shows linear distortions by contraction with a theoretical shrinkage of 6%. When using the conventional technique, internal stresses are created during the final heat application during polymerization. These stresses are released when the prosthesis is removed from the gypsum mold and flask, resulting in twisting, bending and dimensional variations of the denture bases compared to the cast. Clinically, these deformations result in a loss of accuracy and retention of the complete dentures.

There is also a loss of precision in the occlusal relationship as compared to the wax trial prosthesis [3]. Furthermore, the chemical reaction between the monomer and the polymer is never complete. The residual monomer that remains after the polymerization process can alter the mechanical properties of the resin [4]. The released monomer is also suspected of being responsible for allergic or irritating chemical reactions such as burning sensations in the mouth, stomatitis, edema or ulceration of the oral mucosa [5].

With the development of digital technology, computer aided design and manufacture (CAD/CAM) techniques are increasingly popular in dentistry. Thirty years after the first articles on digital removable prostheses, many systems now exist to both reduce the number of patient appointments needed and the laboratory time needed for prothesis fabrication [6–9]. The process of manufacturing CDs with computer-assisted technology involves the acquisition of clinical information and the digital design of prostheses on computer software. CDs can be produced using an additive (3D printing) or subtractive (milling) process. The most commonly used method at present is the subtractive method [10–13]. In the subtractive method, the prostheses are milled from proprietary resin discs that are polymerized under high pressure and high temperature [14]. CAD/CAM techniques for denture fabrication have many clinical and laboratory advantages [15–18]. The computer-aided design and manufacture of complete prostheses simplifies the laboratory protocol, stores data and reduces the number of appointments required. A literature review by Wang et al. [19] studied the impact of this manufacturing process on the adaptation of CDs and occlusion. Their review showed that all prostheses tested had a clinically acceptable fit. The CAD/CAM CDs showed a similar adaptation to conventional prostheses, sometimes even better. Recently, Baba et al. [20] reviewed currently available techniques to manufacture CAD/CAM complete dentures and concluded that their physical properties were improved over those fabricated by conventional laboratory techniques. With these results in mind, the present literature review is aimed at expanding the evaluation of CAD/CAM dentures by comparing their mechanical, physical and chemical characteristics with those of conventional dentures. For the first time, the clinical repercussions of the CAD/CAM machining process were assessed and discussed.

2. Materials and Methods

A thorough search of the literature was conducted using the Medline database (via PubMed). A search strategy developed for Medline via PubMed was employed using the following keywords: (CAD/CAM complete denture base); (CAD/CAM complete denture) NOT (implant); (CAD/CAM complete denture base) AND (resin properties). A systematic review according to the PRISMA checklist was applied. A manual search of the included articles was also performed to identify further eligible studies not detected by keyword search and this strategy is outlined in Figure 1. In January 2021, 392 titles listed in PubMed were identified. After screening the initial articles and backward searching, some publications were excluded based on the following criteria: papers not written in English, animal and in vivo studies, case reports, systematic reviews and when only abstracts were available.

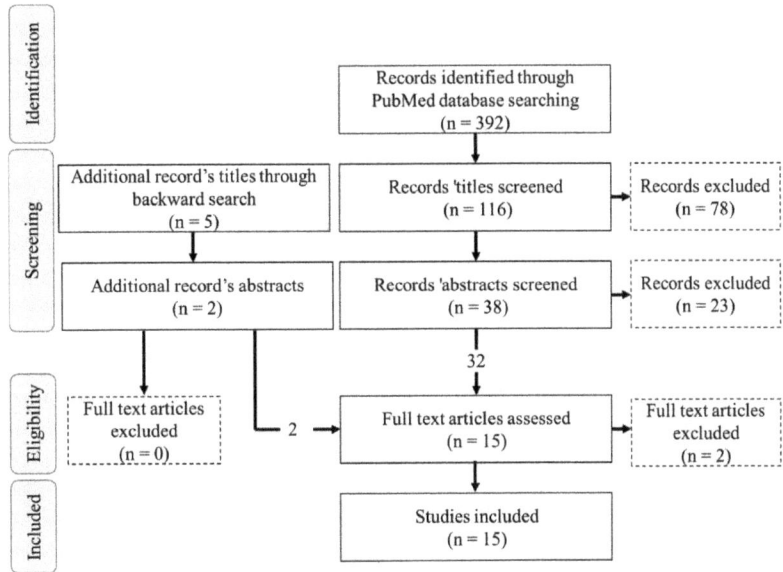

Figure 1. PRISMA flow chart of records based on initial PubMed database searches and backward searching.

Studies comparing the properties of CD resins manufactured conventionally to those manufactured digitally by milling were targeted. Articles dealing with CDs digitally manufactured by 3D printing methods were excluded, leaving only the manufacturing process by machining for comparison to the conventional manufacturing method. Studies comparing the manufacturing techniques of complete removable prostheses based on criteria other than the properties of resins were also excluded, as well as studies on implant-supported prostheses, immediate dentures, or partial removable prostheses.

Full-text analysis was performed independently by two reviewers. Finally, fifteen articles were included.

3. Results

Three hundred and ninety-two titles were identified from the PubMed electronic search. The PRISMA selection methodology resulted in the inclusion of fifteen studies is summarized in Table 1.

The objective of this literature review was to compare the characteristics of manufactured CAD/CAM PMMA resins with those of PMMA resins produced by conventional laboratory techniques. For this purpose, the results are presented according to the mechanical, physical and chemical properties of the resins. In all the studies, the conventional resins were produced using clamping pressure or injection techniques, followed by polymerization by heat using common dental laboratory techniques. The CAD/CAM resins were obtained from industrially manufactured resin discs that were polymerized under high pressure and high temperature.

Table 1. Included articles (HP: Heat_polymerising; IM: Injected molding).

Year	Title	Authors	Conventional Resins	CAD/CAM Resins	Samples of Studied Resins	Studied Characteristics	Properties
2017	Adherence of Candida to Complete Denture Surfaces in vitro: A Comparison of Conventional and CAD/CAM Complete Dentures [28]	Al-Fouzan et al.	HP resin (Major dental)	Wieland Digital Dentures (Ivoclar Vivadent)	Resin discs (10 × 3 mm)	Surface roughness Adherence of *Candida albicans*	Physical
2017	Do CAD/CAM dentures really release less monomer than conventional dentures? [14]	Steinmassl et al.	HP resin (Candulor)	Baltic denture System (Merz dental GmbH) Vita VIONIC (Vita Zahnfabrik) Whole You Nexteeth (Whole You Inc.) Wieland Digital Dentures (Ivoclar Vivadent)	Dentures	Residual monomer content	Chemical
2017	The residual monomer content and mechanical properties of CAD\CAM resins used in the fabrication of complete dentures as compared to heat cured resins [21]	Ayman et al.	HP resin (Vertex RS)	Polident (Polident d.o.o)	Resin bar specimens (65 × 10 × 3 mm)	Flexural strength, Hardness, Residual monomer content	Mechanical Chemical
2018	In Vitro Analysis of the Fracture Resistance of CAD/CAM Denture Base Resins [29]	Steinmassl et al.	HP resin (Candulor) Autopolymerising resin (Candulor)	AvaDent (Global Dental Science) Baltic denture System (Merz dental GmbH) Vita VIONIC (Vita Zahnfabrik) Wieland Digital Dentures (Ivoclar Vivadent) Whole You Nexteeth (Whole You Inc.)	Resin bar specimens (39 × 8 × 4 mm)	Toughness, Elastic modulus, Surface roughness	Mechanical Physical
2018	Influence of CAD/CAM fabrication on denture surface properties [30]	Steinmassl et al.	HP resin (Candulor)	AvaDent (AvaDent Global Dental) Baltic dental denture System (Merz dental GmbH) Vita VIONIC (Vita Zahnfabrik) Whole You Nexteeth (Whole You Inc.) Wieland Digital Dentures (Ivoclar Vivadent)	Dentures Resin bar specimens (39×8×4 mm)	Surface roughness, Hydrophobicity	Physical

Table 1. *Cont.*

Year	Authors	Title	Conventional Resins	CAD/CAM Resins	Samples of Studied Resins	Studied Characteristics	Properties
2018	Srinivasan et al.	CAD/CAM milled complete removable dental prostheses: An in vitro evaluation of biocompatibility, mechanical properties, and surface roughness [24]	HP resin (Candulor)	AvaDent (Global Dental Science)	Resin coupon specimens ($11 \times 11 \times 2$ mm) Resin bar specimens ($65 \times 10 \times 3$ mm) Resin bar specimens ($20 \times 20 \times 1.5$ mm)	Elastic modulus, Hardness, Toughness, Surface roughness	Mechanical Physical
2018	Arslan et al.	Evaluation of Flexural Strength and Surface Properties of Prepolymerized CAD/CAM PMMA-based Polymers Used for Digital 3D Complete Dentures [31]	HP resin (Promolux)	M-PM Disc (Merz Dental GmbH) AvaDent (AvaDent Global Dental) Polident (Polident d.o.o)	Resin bar specimens ($64 \times 10 \times 3.3$ mm)	Flexural strength, Hydrophobicity, Surface roughness	Mechanical Physical
2019	Murat et al.	In vitro evaluation of Adhesion of *Candida albicans* on CAD/CAM PMMA-Based Polymers [32]	HP resin	M-PM Disc (Merz Dental GmbH) AvaDent (AvaDent Global Dental) Pink CAD/CAM disc	Resin discs (10×2 mm)	Hydrophobicity, Surface roughness, Adherence of *Candida albicans*	Physical
2019	Al-Dwairi et al.	A Comparison of the Surface Properties of CAD/CAM and Conventional Polymethylmethacrylate (PMMA) [22]	HP resin (Meliodent)	AvaDent (Global Dental Science) Tizian Blank PMMA (Schütz Dental)	Resin coupon specimens ($25 \times 25 \times 3$ mm)	Hardness, Hydrophobicity, Surface roughness	Mechanical Physical
2019	Pacquet et al.	Mechanical Properties of CAD/CAM Denture Base Resins [25]	Conventional heat-activated pack en press PMMA (Probase Hot) (PRO) IM resin (Ivocap)(CAP)	Wieland Digital Dentures (Ivoclar Vivadent): Ivobase (DD)	Resin bar specimens ($65 \times 10 \times 2.5$ mm) (DD, PRO) and Resin bar specimens ($40 \times 4 \times 2$ mm) (CAP) Resin bar specimens ($39 \times 8 \times 4$ mm)	Flexural strength Fracture toughness Hardness	Mechanical

Table 1. *Cont.*

Year	Authors	Title	Conventional Resins	CAD/CAM Resins	Samples of Studied Resins	Studied Characteristics	Properties
2020	Aguirre et al.	Flexural strength of denture base acrylic resins processed by conventional and CAD-CAM methods [33]	Compressed molding resin (Microstone) IM resin (Microstone)	AvaDent (Global Dental Science)	Resin bar specimens (64 × 10 × 3.3 mm)	Flexural strength, Flexural modulus	Mechanical
2020	Al-Dwairi et al.	A Comparison of the Flexural and Impact Strengths and Flexural Modulus of CAD/CAM and Conventional Heat-Cured Polymethyl Methacrylate (PMMA) [34]	HP resin (Meliodent)	AvaDent (Global Dental Science) Tizian Blank PMMA (Schütz Dental)	Resin bar specimens (65 × 10 × 3 mm)	Flexural strength, Flexural modulus, impact strength	Mechanical
2020	Prpić et al.	Comparison of Mechanical Properties of 3D-Printed, CAD/CAM, and Conventional Denture Base Materials [23]	HP resin (ProBase Hot, Paladon 65, Interacryl Hot)	Interdent (Interdent d.o.o) Polident (Polident d.o.o) Wieland Digital Dentures (Ivoclar Vivadent)	Resin bar specimens (64 × 10 × 3.3 mm)	Flexural strength Hardness	Mechanical
2021	Becerra et al.	Influence of High-Pressure Polymerization on Mechanical Properties of Denture Base Resins [26]	HP resin (ProBase Hot) ± high pressure	Wieland Digital Dentures (Ivoclar Vivadent)	Resin bar specimens (65 × 10 × 3.3 mm)	Flexural strength, Elastic modulus Hardness	Mechanical
2021	Perea-Lowery et al.	Assessment of CAD-CAM polymers for digitally fabricated complete dentures [27]	HP resin (Paladon 65) Autopolymerizing resin (Palapress)	Degos Dental L-Temp (Degos Dental) Zirkonzahn Temp Basic Tissue (Zirkonzahn SRL) Wieland Digital Dentures (Ivoclar Vivadent)	Resin bar specimens (65 × 10 × 3.2 mm) Resin coupon specimens (10 × 10 × 2 mm)	Flexural strength, Microhardness, Nanohardness, Elastic modulus	Mechanical

3.1. Mechanical Properties

Seven articles have focused on the surface hardness of the PMMA resins. Hardness is a measure of the resistance of a material to plastic deformation, induced by either abrasion or mechanical indentation. The data are presented in Table 2. Two studies have shown that resins for CAD/CAM prostheses have a higher microhardness than conventional resins [21–23]. Others studies showed no significant difference in hardness between the two types of resins when tested for nano-hardness [24,25]. Recently, however, one study showed that the hardness of CAD/CAM resin was significantly lower than that of hot-pressed conventional resin [26]. Perea–Lowery [27] revealed differences in material-related hardness and microhardness between CAD/CAM and conventional resins

Table 2. Hardness test results.

	Average Hardness (±Standard Deviation) of Conventional Resin	Average Hardness (±Standard Deviation) of CAD/CAM Resin
Al-Dwairi et al. (2019) [22] (in mPa)	18.09 (±0.31)	T: 19.80 (±1.08) *,a A: 20.60 (±0.33) *,b
Ayman et al. (2017) [21] (in mPa)	13.22 (±0.88)	P: 22.41 (±1.50) ***
Becerra et al. (2021) [26] (in HVN)	23.1 (±1.9)	18.7 (±1.7)
Pacquet et al. (2019) [25] (in mPa)	19.46 (±0.4)	19.31 (±1.48)
Perea-Lowery et al. (2021) [27] (in mPa)	NC	NC
Prpić et al. (2020) [23] (in mPa)	NC	NC
Srinivasan et al. (2018) [24] (in mPa) (nano-hardness)	232 (±15)	A: 221 (±14)

CAD/CAM resin discs: A: Avadent; P: Polident; T: Tizian-Schütz; NC: Graphic data: precise values not communicated. * Statistically significant difference compared to conventional resin ($p < 0.05$); *** Statistically significant difference compared to conventional resin ($p < 0.001$); a and b indicate a statistical difference between CAD/CAM resins.

The resistance to deformation was studied by three-point bending tests in nine studies [21,23,24,26,27,29,31,33,34]. Results showed that CAD/CAM resins have superior mechanical properties; higher elastic moduli [21,24,26,29,33], flexural strength [23,24,26,31,33,34], impact strength [34] and yield strength [24,25] as compared to conventional resins. However, two studies [21,27] revealed that the mechanical properties of CAD/CAM resins were not always superior to that of conventional resins. Arslan et al. showed that the flexural strength of all the resins tested was significantly lower after thermocycling [31]. Most CAD/CAM resins have a higher toughness than conventional resins [24,29].

Only one study focused on the analysis of the load at fracture of resins using a 3-point bending test on rectangular resin samples (4 mm-thick). The maximum load at fracture of six CAD/CAM resins was then compared with that of conventional heat-cured and self-curing resins [29]. Table 3 shows the results of the fracture tests. The fracture resistance of CAD/CAM resins was not always superior to that of conventional heat-cured or self-curing resins. Indeed, fracture resistance is highly variable within CAD/CAM resins. The average breaking loads ranged from 40.27 N ± 3.40 to 82.49 N ± 7.47 for CAD/CAM resins. Of the six CAD/CAM resins tested, only the Wieland digital dentures (WWD) resin had significantly higher values than conventional resins. This study also showed that there was a positive correlation between fracture surface roughness and the maximum load at fracture of the resin. For example, the WDD CAD/CAM resin had the roughest fracture surface with the highest maximum breaking load.

Table 3. Breaking load test results.

	Mean Load at Fracture (±Standard Deviation) of Conventional Resin (N)	Mean Load at Fracture (±Standard Deviation) of CAD/CAM Resin (N)
Steinmassl et al. (2018) [29]	Conventional heat-cured resin: 61.66 (±5.60)	A: 50.26 (±4.02) **
	Self-curing resin: 53.51 (±4.07)	BDS: 49.37 (±4.91) ** VV: 40.27 (±3.40) ** DD: 82.49 (±7.47) ** WNu: 62.35 (±2.44) ** WNc: 63.44 (±4.91) **

CAD/CAM resin discs: A: Avadent; BDS: Baltic denture system; DD: Wieland digital denture; VV: Vita Vionic; WNu: Whole You Nexteeth, dentures without the customary full surface coating, WNc: Whole You Nexteeth, dentures with the customary full surface coating; ** Statistically significant difference compared to conventional resin ($p < 0.01$); The different subscript letters indicate a statistical difference between CAD/CAM resins.

The study by Steinmassl et al. [29] highlighted the differences in mechanical properties between CAD/CAM resins.

3.2. Physical Properties

Seven studies compared the surface roughness of CAD/CAM and conventional resins [22,24,28–32]. Surface roughness was measured using laser or contact profilometers. Three of the seven studies showed that conventional resins had significantly higher surface roughness than CAD/CAM resins [22,28,32]. Another study also showed that conventional resins had a higher roughness, except for one brand of CAD/CAM resin that showed a slightly lower roughness that was not statistically significant [30]. The study by Steinmassl et al. showed that two of the five CAD/CAM resins tested had lower roughness than conventional resins [29]. One study showed that surface roughness was significantly higher for CAD/CAM resins [24]. The study by Arslan et al. showed that the resins did not exhibit different roughness values before and after thermal cycling [31]. The data are summarized in Table 4.

Four studies have focused on the hydrophobicity of resins using the sessile drop technique with calculation of the contact angle [22,30–32]. The results of the studies are presented in Table 5. Two studies showed that most CAD/CAM resins were more hydrophobic than conventional resins [22,31], while another study showed a higher hydrophobicity rate for conventional resins [30]. All the studies highlighted variations in hydrophobicity according to the CAD/CAM resin used [22,30–32].

One study used thermocycling to simulate the clinical aging process and found that conventional resins become more hydrophobic and CAD/CAM resins become more hydrophilic after aging [31].

3.3. Chemical Properties

Two studies have investigated the content of residual monomer in industrially polymerized CAD/CAM resins [14,21]. The results are presented in Table 6. Steinmassl et al. showed that CAD/CAM resins release very little free monomer after milling. However, their residual monomer content was not statistically lower than that of conventional laboratory-polymerized resins, regardless of the CAD/CAM process tested (BalticDenture, Whole You Nexteeth, Wieland Digital Dentures or Vita) for the manufacture of CDs. Another study showed lower free monomer content in industrially polymerized resin specimens, compared to conventionally polymerized resins [21].

Table 4. Surface roughness test results.

	Average Surface Roughness (±Standard Deviation) of Conventional Resin (μm)	Average Surface Roughness (±Standard Deviation) of CAD/CAM Resin (μm)
Al-Dwairi et al. (2019) [22]	0.22 (±0.07)	A: 0.16 (±0.03) **[a] T: 0.12 (±0.02) ***[b]
Al-Fouzan et al. (2017) [28]	0.073 (±0.015)	WDD: 0.037 (±0.001) *
Arslan et al. (2018) [31]	Without thermocycling: 0.22 (±0.07) [a] With thermocycling: 0.29 (±0.09) [b]	Without thermocycling: A: 0.22 (±0.06) [a] M: 0.21 (±0.07) [b] P: 0.26 (±0.09) [a] With thermocycling: A: 0.24 (±0.04) [c] M: 0.18 (±0.04) [d] P: 0.32 (±0.08) [c]
Murat et al. (2018) [32]	0.34 (±0.06)	M: 0.18 (±0.04) *,[a] P: 0.21 (±0.04) *,[a] A: 0.20 (±0.05) *,[a]
Srinivasan et al. (2018) [24]	0.12 (±0.29)	0.37 (±0.03) ***
Steinmassl et al. (2018) [29]	Conventional heat-cured resin: 3.47 (±0.10) Self-curing resin: 2.42 (±0.79)	A: 1.11 (±0.38) * BDS: 2.04 (±0.42) VV: 3.23 (±0.31) WDD: 6.25 (±2.74) WN: 0.65 (±0.11)
Steinmassl et al. (2017) [14]	0.55 (±0.14)	A: 0.28 (±0.16) ** BDS: 0.44 (±0.13) VV: 0.28 (±0.07) ** WN: 0.04 (±0.01) ** DD: 0.30 (±0.10) **

CAD/CAM resin discs: A: Avadent; BDS: Baltic denture system; DD: Wieland digital denture; M: M-PM; P: Polident; T: Tizian-Schütz; VV: Vita Vionic; WN: Whole You Nexteeth; * Statistically significant difference compared to conventional resin ($p < 0.05$); ** Statistically significant difference compared to conventional resin ($p < 0.01$); *** Statistically significant difference compared to conventional resin ($p < 0.001$). a, b, c, d indicate a statistical difference between CAD/CAM resins.

Table 5. Hydrophobicity test results.

	Average Contact Angle (±Standard Deviation) of Conventional Resin (°)	Average Contact Angle (±Standard Deviation) of CAD/CAM Resin (°)
Arslan et al. (2018) [31]	Without thermocycling: 73.97 (±3.53) With thermocycling: 83.35 (±4.37)	Without thermocycling: A: 92.95 (±2.65) ***,[a] M: 81.03 (±3.29) ***,[b] P: 82.39 (±3) ***,[b] Without thermocycling: A: 83.52 (±2.6) [c] M: 77.21 (±3.01) ***,[d] P: 76.16 (±3.3) ***,[d]
Al-Dwairi et al. (2019) [22]	65.97 (±4.67°)	A: 72.87 (±4.83°) *** T: 69.53 (±3.87°)
Murat et al. (2018) [32]	Without saliva: 73.43 (±17.82) With saliva: 86.51 (±11.07)	Without saliva: A: 69.72 (±10.57) *,[a] M: 71.31 (±6.94) *,[a] P: 69.63 (±4.85) *,[a] With saliva: A: 74.98 (±4.28) *,[b] M: 79.56 (±5.06) *,[c] P: 86.19 (±5.82) [d]

Table 5. Cont.

	Average Contact Angle (±Standard Deviation) of Conventional Resin (°)	Average Contact Angle (±Standard Deviation) of CAD/CAM Resin (°)
Steinmassl et al.(2018) [30]	82.50 (±3.44)	A: 70.35 (±8.99)* BDS: 75 (±5.42) * VV: 74.4 (±2.32)*** WN: 77.7 (±9.87) DD: 77.5 (±3.34)

CAD/CAM resin discs: A: Avadent; BDS: Baltic Denture System; DD: Wieland Digital denture; M: M-PM; P: Polident; T: Tizian-Schütz; VV: Vita Vionic; WN: Whole You Nexteeth; * Statistically significant difference compared to conventional resin ($p < 0.05$); *** Statistically significant difference compared to conventional resin ($p < 0.001$); a, b, c, d indicate a statistical difference between CAD/CAM resins.

Table 6. Residual monomer content test results.

	Average Residual Monomer (±SD) of Conventional Resin (ppm)	Average Residual Monomer (±SD) of CAD/CAM Resin (ppm)
Ayman et al. (2017) [21]	At baseline: 17.10 (±0.38) At two-day: 16.04 (±0.13) At seven-day: 13.54 (±0.46)	At baseline: P: 1.61 (±0.05) *** At two-day: P: 1.03 (±0.06) *** At seven-day: P: 0.90 (±0.01) ***
Steinmassl et al. (2017) [14]	1.5 (±1.6)	BDS: 0.6 (±0.4) WN: 6 (±2.7) **

CAD/CAM resin discs: BDS: Baltic denture system; P: Polident; WN: Whole You Nexteeth; ** Statistically significant difference compared to conventional resin ($p < 0.01$); *** Statistically significant difference compared to conventional resin ($p < 0.001$).

4. Discussion

The objective of this literature review was to compare the characteristics of CAD/CAM resins with those of conventional resins in order to assess the impact of CAD/CAM resins on the CDs' clinical performance and durability. Results showed that switching to digital technology for the manufacturing process of resins led to different properties between conventional and CAD/CAM resins. Throughout this discussion, the effect of the physical property differences of these resins on the success of clinical denture treatment will be highlighted.

4.1. Retention of Denture Bases

The clinical performance of CDs is partly determined by their retention within the oral cavity. Lack of retention and instability are two of the main complaints from people wearing CDs. Retention refers to the amount of vertical force needed to resist the dislodgement of the prosthesis away from its supporting structures, similar to the force needed to remove a suction cup. As with a suction cup, wettability of the resins influences the prostheses' retention to the supporting mucosa and has to be taken into account in the manufacturing process. Wettability indicates whether saliva is able to spread more or less easily on a surface and reflects whether fluids aid retention of the denture surface to oral mucosa, thus affecting retention. CDs with good wettability therefore optimize retention. The wettability of a material is defined by observing the angle of contact between the material and a drop of water: the greater the angle, the lower the wettability and therefore, the more hydrophobic the material will be. In the studies included in the review, hydrophobicity varied according to the type of resin used and could be explained by several hypotheses. Hydrophobicity could be correlated with the rate of monomer released by the resins during polymerization [31]. Another hypothesis could call into question the additives contained in the resins. Indeed, dentures are not made of pure PMMA. They contain numerous additives such as polymerization initiators, cross-linking agents, fillers and dyes, which can all influence the hydrophobicity of the resins [31]. The origin of these variations in hydrophobicity value in dental resins, as well as the effect of aging on resin hydrophobicity, should be investigated.

On the one hand, these results on hydrophobicity do not clearly explain why some studies show that digital CDs are more retentive than conventional CDs. On the other hand, one study has shown through adhesion tests that the retention of digital CDs is better [35]. If the resins' physical properties do not play a major role in CAD/CAM denture retention, then the manufacturing process itself could favor the precision of adaptation and the adhesion of digital CDs. Still, the precision of the manufacturing process of these resins favors adaptation and the adhesion of digital CDs and has shown that the retention of digital CDs is better than that of conventional prostheses [35]. The review by Wang et al. [19] on the accuracy of digital full dentures showed that digital CDs have a similar or better fit than conventionally manufactured CDs. The manufacture of CDs using digital techniques helps to meet the three biomechanical requirements to ensure CD success; namely retention, stability and support (accuracy of fit to the oral tissues) as defined in Housset's triad.

4.2. Resistance to Deformation and Breakage

When worn, complete dentures are subjected to high stresses during chewing. This creates cyclic deformation of the denture polymer, which in turn can lead to crack formation and possible fatigue fracture of the denture [36]. Therefore, good resistance of the resins to deformation is very important. The results of this literature review showed that CAD/CAM resins have superior mechanical properties to conventional resins.

First of all, conventional resins had a lower modulus of elasticity than CAD/CAM resins. The elastic modulus is an important property in characterizing the material's rigidity. Resins with a higher modulus of elasticity will be more resistant to elastic deformation. A high elastic modulus may make it possible to fabricate prostheses with reduced thickness without compromising the mechanical properties, an important attribute for patient comfort and acceptance of the prosthesis. In addition, a deformation-resistant prosthesis will have a more stable occlusion. These differences in rigidity between CAD/CAM and conventional resins are probably due to the manufacturing process. The modulus of elasticity would be related to the residual monomer content. It has been shown that a high monomer content reduces the glass transition temperature, making the resin more flexible. The high-temperature, high-pressure polymerization of CAD/CAM resins leads to higher monomer conversion with lower residual monomer values, thus resulting in a more rigid resin. High-pressure and high-temperature polymerization also allows a different arrangement of the polymer chains. Previous studies had shown that the use of high pressure during polymerization increased crosslinks between polymer chains [15,37].

Secondly, fracture resistance characterizes the maximum stress a material can withstand before breaking. Results have shown that fracture resistance varied within CAD/CAM resins. For example, in the study by Steinmassl et al. [29], the Wieland digital denture (WDD) resin exhibited higher loads to fracture but had a lower elastic modulus than the others. Thus, it had lower rigidity and more susceptible to plastic deformation. It would therefore be preferable not to reduce the bases thickness too much to compensate for the risk of plastic deformation. Of the six CAD/CAM resins tested, only the WWD resin had significantly higher yield strength values compared to conventional resins. WDD also exhibited the roughest fracture surface. It was the only resin with fine grains on the fracture surface. This difference in resin surfaces is thought to be due to the geometry, size and distribution of the polymer powders used to make the resins. In the study by Steinmassl et al. [29] the measured maximum breaking loads were all greater than 40 N. However, the maximum bite force was reduced to 40 N in complete prosthesis wearers with high resorption of the mandibular alveolar bone [38]. Based on these results, some manufacturers encourage the fabrication of full dentures with reduced resin thickness. It is imperative to remain skeptical regarding this commercial argument, especially since in the study, the tests were performed on 4 mm thick resin samples, which is much thicker than a prosthetic base. Furthermore, CDs are subjected to much more complex stresses in the mouth, involving different types of forces in different directions (such as chewing). For a valid prediction of clinical fatigue resistance, further studies on cyclic loading behavior and fracture toughness are necessary.

The results highlighted differences in mechanical properties between CAD/CAM resins. More information on the composition and manufacturing processes of CAD/CAM resins would help to better understand some of the results.

4.3. Adhesion of Microorganisms

Preventing the adhesion of microorganisms to dentures helps preserve the health of tissues in the oral cavity. The prevalence of denture stomatitis among denture wearers has been shown average around 28% [39]. Microorganisms can cause pathology in the mucosa supporting the prosthesis, such as candidiasis (induced mainly by *Candida albicans*). Microorganisms accumulate more easily on prostheses than on natural tissue. The surfaces of removable maxillary prostheses are the main reservoir of *Candida albicans* [40,41]. The physical properties of the prosthetic resin influence this adhesion, including surface roughness and hardness. The results of this literature review showed that CAD/CAM machined resins had globally more advantageous physical properties than conventional resins.

Surface roughness is the most important factor for *Candida albicans'* adhesion to the prosthesis surface. Optical and electron microscopy studies revealed that initial adhesion of microorganisms usually begins in the microscopic pits and cracks of rough surfaces. This surface roughness provides protection against removal (shear) forces and gives time for microbes to irreversibly adhere to the surface [42–45]. A smoother surface might reduce *Candida albicans* adhesion, which ultimately lowers the risk of prosthetic stomatitis. It has been demonstrated that CAD/CAM resins have significantly lower surface roughness than conventional resins [22,28,29,32]. The polishing technique and the operator's ability to polish both affect the roughness of the resins' cameo (external) surface [46]. However, the prosthetic intaglio (internal surface in contact with the supporting mucosa) is never polished, and only the polymerization of the resins would determine surface roughness. Therefore, irregularities in conventionally fabricated dentures would be due to the evaporation of monomers during polymerization. This can be avoided by applying high-pressure polymerization, as seen when utilizing proprietary CAD/CAM resins [32]. In case of conventional resin polymerization, the amount of pressure applied is limited to avoid fracturing the gypsum mold in which resins are polymerized. Conversely, machined resins for CAD/CAM prosthetics are made from resin discs that are polymerized at very high pressure, which could explain their lower roughness [30]. Furthermore, in order to avoid the accumulation and colonization of microorganisms on the prostheses' surface, roughness of the resins should not exceed 0.2 µm [47]. In this review, most of the resins had roughness above 0.2 µm. This characteristic should be improved in the future, taking into consideration that the surface profile of the prosthetic intaglio surface always exhibits striations due to milling process used for CAD/CAM resins.

In addition to the biofilm adhesion onto the resins, surface roughness also tends to induce halitosis and mucosal inflammation [48], and reduces patient comfort. Thus, milling resins could reduce these nuisances and facilitate denture maintenance.

Hardness is another factor influencing bacterial adhesion to the prostheses over time. Surface hardness is defined as the ability of the material to resist penetration or permanent indentation related to the wear and scratches appearing as the dentures are worn and cleaned. A prosthesis should have a hard surface to reduce denture deterioration and therefore limit the adhesion of microorganisms [37,49]. Included studies focused on the microhardness as well as the nanohardness of resins. For the most part, surface microhardness was higher in CAD/CAM prosthetic resin blocks and no significant difference was found between nanohardness values. These results could be related to the polymerization process because the polymerization conditions of the CAD/CAM resin discs (high temperature and pressure) and the addition of inorganic substances promote the formation of longer polymer chains and limit the dimensional shrinkage of polymerization [50]. This high-temperature, high-pressure polymerization leads to higher monomer conversion, minimizing the plasticizing effect of the residual monomer [51,52]. Thus, CAD/CAM resins seem to be harder than conventional resins, which could help prevent bacterial adhesion and therefore increase the long-term comfort of the dentures.

4.4. Residual Monomer Content

The residual monomer alters the resins' mechanical properties. It is also suspected of being responsible for allergic or irritating chemical reactions such as burning sensations in the mouth, stomatitis, edema or ulcerations of the oral mucosa. A certain amount of residual monomer is unavoidable due to the monomer-polymer balance required for the radical polymerization of resins [53]. Although the ISO 20795-1 norm (2013) allows a maximum residual monomer content of 2.2% by weight [54], the presence of residual monomer in the denture base resins should be reduced to a least amount possible.

In the study by Steinmassl et al. [14], the amount of residual monomer in industrially-polymerized and then machined CAD/CAM resins was not statistically different from that of conventional resins. Four CAD/CAM resins were tested (BalticDenture, Whole You Nexteeth, Wieland digital dentures and Vita). The BalticDenture process exhibited the least residual monomer of the resins tested. In the BalticDenture system, the prosthetic teeth are incorporated into the base during polymerization. In the other systems, the prosthetic teeth are bonded separately to the base after milling, using a PMMA bonding agent. These results suggest that the bonding agents used to attach the teeth to the milled resin base are a source of methacrylate monomer release. Thus, industrially polymerized resins would contain less residual monomer than laboratory-cured resins [21]. PMMA discs are polymerized industrially at high temperature and high pressure. This type of polymerization promotes the formation of longer polymer chains and would therefore lead to a higher level of monomer conversion with lower residual monomer values [37]. Assembling the prosthetic teeth to the machined bases during the CD manufacturing process would explain why the residual monomer content of some machined CDs is not that different from that of conventional CDs. Further studies need to be conducted to confirm this hypothesis, using, for example, Ivotion (Ivoclar's newest monolithic CD material).

5. Conclusions

This review showed that CAD/CAM resins have similar or even superior characteristics to conventional resins, particularly in terms of mechanical properties. However, it should be noted that the variabilities of the characteristics are not only due to the manufacturing techniques but could also be due to the composition of resins. This entails that manufacturers should provide more complete information in terms of resin composition, and their manufacturing process, as it often remains confidential. CAD/CAM resins exhibit properties that can improve patient satisfaction and clinical success of CDs. The longevity of CDs should also be investigated in future studies in clinical use by investigating the resins' aging process and fatigue resistance.

Using digital techniques to manufacture CDs would help meet the three biomechanical requirements to ensure CDs balance, namely retention, stability and support (Housset's triad). Ultimately, this literature review is encouraging for more frequent utilization of CAD/CAM resins in the future, to become the new standard protocol.

Author Contributions: Conceptualization, C.B. and E.N.; methodology, C.B.; validation, C.B. and E.N.; formal analysis, C.B.; investigation, C.B.; original draft preparation, C.B.; writing—review and editing, C.B and E.N. All authors have read and agreed to the published version of the manuscript.

Funding: This research received no external funding.

Institutional Review Board Statement: Not applicable.

Informed Consent Statement: Not applicable.

Data Availability Statement: Not applicable.

Acknowledgments: The authors thank Caroline Eschevins for her valuable technical support, Isabelle Denry and Julie A Holloway for their help in revising the manuscript.

Conflicts of Interest: The authors declare no conflict of interest.

References

1. Gharechahi, J.; Asadzadeh, N.; Shahabian, F.; Gharechahi, M. Dimensional Changes of Acrylic Resin Denture Bases: Conventional versus Injection-Molding Technique. *J. Dent. Tehran Iran* **2014**, *11*, 398–405.
2. Takamata, T.; Setcos, J.C. Resin Denture Bases: Review of Accuracy and Methods of Polymerization. *Int. J. Prosthodont.* **1989**, *2*, 555–562.
3. Keenan, P.L.J.; Radford, D.R.; Clark, R.K.F. Dimensional Change in Complete Dentures Fabricated by Injection Molding and Microwave Processing. *J. Prosthet. Dent.* **2003**, *89*, 37–44. [CrossRef]
4. Kalipçilar, B.; Karaağaçlioğlu, L.; Hasanreisoğlu, U. Evaluation of the Level of Residual Monomer in Acrylic Denture Base Materials Having Different Polymerization Properties. *J. Oral Rehabil.* **1991**, *18*, 399–401. [CrossRef]
5. Lee, H.-J.; Kim, C.-W.; Kim, Y.-S. The Level of Residual Monomer in Injection Molded Denture Base Materials. *J. Korean Acad. Prosthodont.* **2003**, *41*, 360–368.
6. Kattadiyil, M.T.; AlHelal, A. An Update on Computer-Engineered Complete Dentures: A Systematic Review on Clinical Outcomes. *J. Prosthet. Dent.* **2017**, *117*, 478–485. [CrossRef]
7. Steinmassl, P.-A.; Klaunzer, F.; Steinmassl, O.; Dumfahrt, H.; Grunert, I. Evaluation of Currently Available CAD/CAM Denture Systems. *Int. J. Prosthodont.* **2017**, *30*, 116–122. [CrossRef]
8. Kattadiyil, M.T.; Goodacre, C.J.; Baba, N.Z. CAD/CAM Complete Dentures: A Review of Two Commercial Fabrication Systems. *J. Calif. Dent. Assoc.* **2013**, *41*, 407–416.
9. Schwindling, F.S.; Stober, T. A Comparison of Two Digital Techniques for the Fabrication of Complete Removable Dental Prostheses: A Pilot Clinical Study. *J. Prosthet. Dent.* **2016**, *116*, 756–763. [CrossRef]
10. Kalberer, N.; Mehl, A.; Schimmel, M.; Müller, F.; Srinivasan, M. CAD-CAM Milled versus Rapidly Prototyped (3D-Printed) Complete Dentures: An in Vitro Evaluation of Trueness. *J. Prosthet. Dent.* **2019**, *121*, 637–643. [CrossRef]
11. Takeda, Y.; Lau, J.; Nouh, H.; Hirayama, H. A 3D Printing Replication Technique for Fabricating Digital Dentures. *J. Prosthet. Dent.* **2020**, *124*, 251–256. [CrossRef] [PubMed]
12. Bilgin, M.S.; Baytaroğlu, E.N.; Erdem, A.; Dilber, E. A Review of Computer-Aided Design/Computer-Aided Manufacture Techniques for Removable Denture Fabrication. *Eur. J. Dent.* **2016**, *10*, 286–291. [CrossRef] [PubMed]
13. Janeva, N.M.; Kovacevska, G.; Elencevski, S.; Panchevska, S.; Mijoska, A.; Lazarevska, B. Advantages of CAD/CAM versus Conventional Complete Dentures-A Review. *Open Access Maced. J. Med. Sci.* **2018**, *6*, 1498–1502. [CrossRef] [PubMed]
14. Steinmassl, P.-A.; Wiedemair, V.; Huck, C.; Klaunzer, F.; Steinmassl, O.; Grunert, I.; Dumfahrt, H. Do CAD/CAM Dentures Really Release Less Monomer than Conventional Dentures? *Clin. Oral Investig.* **2017**, *21*, 1697–1705. [CrossRef]
15. Bidra, A.S.; Taylor, T.D.; Agar, J.R. Computer-Aided Technology for Fabricating Complete Dentures: Systematic Review of Historical Background, Current Status, and Future Perspectives. *J. Prosthet. Dent.* **2013**, *109*, 361–366. [CrossRef]
16. Infante, L.; Yilmaz, B.; McGlumphy, E.; Finger, I. Fabricating Complete Dentures with CAD/CAM Technology. *J. Prosthet. Dent.* **2014**, *111*, 351–355. [CrossRef] [PubMed]
17. Saponaro, P.C.; Yilmaz, B.; Heshmati, R.H.; McGlumphy, E.A. Clinical Performance of CAD-CAM-Fabricated Complete Dentures: A Cross-Sectional Study. *J. Prosthet. Dent.* **2016**, *116*, 431–435. [CrossRef]
18. Goodacre, C.J.; Garbacea, A.; Naylor, W.P.; Daher, T.; Marchack, C.B.; Lowry, J. CAD/CAM Fabricated Complete Dentures: Concepts and Clinical Methods of Obtaining Required Morphological Data. *J. Prosthet. Dent.* **2012**, *107*, 34–46. [CrossRef]
19. Wang, C.; Shi, Y.-F.; Xie, P.-J.; Wu, J.-H. Accuracy of Digital Complete Dentures: A Systematic Review of in Vitro Studies. *J. Prosthet. Dent.* **2021**. [CrossRef]
20. Baba, N.Z. CAD/CAM Complete Denture Systems and Physical Properties: A Review of the Literature. *J. Prosthodont.* **2021**, *30*, 113–124. [CrossRef] [PubMed]
21. Ayman, A.-D. The Residual Monomer Content and Mechanical Properties of CAD\CAM Resins Used in the Fabrication of Complete Dentures as Compared to Heat Cured Resins. *Electron. Physician* **2017**, *9*, 4766–4772. [CrossRef]
22. Al-Dwairi, Z.N.; Tahboub, K.Y.; Baba, N.Z.; Goodacre, C.J.; Özcan, M. A Comparison of the Surface Properties of CAD/CAM and Conventional Polymethylmethacrylate (PMMA). *J. Prosthodont.* **2019**, *28*, 452–457. [CrossRef]
23. Prpić, V.; Schauperl, Z.; Ćatić, A.; Dulčić, N.; Čimić, S. Comparison of Mechanical Properties of 3D-Printed, CAD/CAM, and Conventional Denture Base Materials. *J. Prosthodont.* **2020**, *29*, 524–528. [CrossRef] [PubMed]
24. Srinivasan, M.; Gjengedal, H.; Cattani-Lorente, M.; Moussa, M.; Durual, S.; Schimmel, M.; Müller, F. CAD/CAM Milled Complete Removable Dental Prostheses: An in Vitro Evaluation of Biocompatibility, Mechanical Properties, and Surface Roughness. *Dent. Mater. J.* **2018**, *37*, 526–533. [CrossRef] [PubMed]
25. Pacquet, W.; Benoit, A.; Hatège-Kimana, C.; Wulfman, C. Mechanical Properties of CAD/CAM Denture Base Resins. *Int. J. Prosthodont.* **2019**, *32*, 104–106. [CrossRef]
26. Becerra, J.; Mainjot, A.; Hüe, O.; Sadoun, M.; Nguyen, J.-F. Influence of High-Pressure Polymerization on Mechanical Properties of Denture Base Resins. *J. Prosthodont.* **2021**, *30*, 128–134. [CrossRef]
27. Perea-Lowery, L.; Minja, I.K.; Lassila, L.; Ramakrishnaiah, R.; Vallittu, P.K. Assessment of CAD-CAM Polymers for Digitally Fabricated Complete Dentures. *J. Prosthet. Dent.* **2021**, *125*, 175–181. [CrossRef] [PubMed]

28. Al-Fouzan, A.F.; Al-mejrad, L.A.; Albarrag, A.M. Adherence of Candida to Complete Denture Surfaces in Vitro: A Comparison of Conventional and CAD/CAM Complete Dentures. *J. Adv. Prosthodont.* **2017**, *9*, 402–408. [CrossRef]
29. Steinmassl, O.; Offermanns, V.; Stöckl, W.; Dumfahrt, H.; Grunert, I.; Steinmassl, P.-A. In Vitro Analysis of the Fracture Resistance of CAD/CAM Denture Base Resins. *Mater. Basel Switz.* **2018**, *11*, 401. [CrossRef]
30. Steinmassl, O.; Dumfahrt, H.; Grunert, I.; Steinmassl, P.-A. Influence of CAD/CAM Fabrication on Denture Surface Properties. *J. Oral Rehabil.* **2018**, *45*, 406–413. [CrossRef] [PubMed]
31. Arslan, M.; Murat, S.; Alp, G.; Zaimoglu, A. Evaluation of Flexural Strength and Surface Properties of Prepolymerized CAD/CAM PMMA-Based Polymers Used for Digital 3D Complete Dentures. *Int. J. Comput. Dent.* **2018**, *21*, 31–40.
32. Murat, S.; Alp, G.; Alatalı, C.; Uzun, M. In Vitro Evaluation of Adhesion of Candida Albicans on CAD/CAM PMMA-Based Polymers. *J. Prosthodont.* **2019**, *28*, e873–e879. [CrossRef]
33. Aguirre, B.C.; Chen, J.-H.; Kontogiorgos, E.D.; Murchison, D.F.; Nagy, W.W. Flexural Strength of Denture Base Acrylic Resins Processed by Conventional and CAD-CAM Methods. *J. Prosthet. Dent.* **2020**, *123*, 641–646. [CrossRef]
34. Al-Dwairi, Z.N.; Tahboub, K.Y.; Baba, N.Z.; Goodacre, C.J. A Comparison of the Flexural and Impact Strengths and Flexural Modulus of CAD/CAM and Conventional Heat-Cured Polymethyl Methacrylate (PMMA). *J. Prosthodont.* **2020**, *29*, 341–349. [CrossRef] [PubMed]
35. AlRumaih, H.S.; AlHelal, A.; Baba, N.Z.; Goodacre, C.J.; Al-Qahtani, A.; Kattadiyil, M.T. Effects of Denture Adhesive on the Retention of Milled and Heat-Activated Maxillary Denture Bases: A Clinical Study. *J. Prosthet. Dent.* **2018**, *120*, 361–366. [CrossRef]
36. Takamiya, A.S.; Monteiro, D.R.; Marra, J.; Compagnoni, M.A.; Barbosa, D.B. Complete Denture Wearing and Fractures among Edentulous Patients Treated in University Clinics. *Gerodontology* **2012**, *29*, e728–e734. [CrossRef] [PubMed]
37. Murakami, N.; Wakabayashi, N.; Matsushima, R.; Kishida, A.; Igarashi, Y. Effect of High-Pressure Polymerization on Mechanical Properties of PMMA Denture Base Resin. *J. Mech. Behav. Biomed. Mater.* **2013**, *20*, 98–104. [CrossRef]
38. Fontijn-Tekamp, F.A.; Slagter, A.P.; Van Der Bilt, A.; Van 'T Hof, M.A.; Witter, D.J.; Kalk, W.; Jansen, J.A. Biting and Chewing in Overdentures, Full Dentures, and Natural Dentitions. *J. Dent. Res.* **2000**, *79*, 1519–1524. [CrossRef]
39. Shulman, J.D.; Rivera-Hidalgo, F.; Beach, M.M. Risk Factors Associated with Denture Stomatitis in the United States. *J. Oral Pathol. Med.* **2005**, *34*, 340–346. [CrossRef]
40. Coco, B.J.; Bagg, J.; Cross, L.J.; Jose, A.; Cross, J.; Ramage, G. Mixed Candida Albicans and Candida Glabrata Populations Associated with the Pathogenesis of Denture Stomatitis. *Oral Microbiol. Immunol.* **2008**, *23*, 377–383. [CrossRef]
41. Gleiznys, A.; Zdanavičienė, E.; Žilinskas, J. Candida Albicans Importance to Denture Wearers. A Literature Review. *Stomatologija* **2015**, *17*, 54–66.
42. Radford, D.R.; Sweet, S.P.; Challacombe, S.J.; Walter, J.D. Adherence of Candida Albicans to Denture-Base Materials with Different Surface Finishes. *J. Dent.* **1998**, *26*, 577–583. [CrossRef]
43. da Silva, W.J.; Leal, C.M.B.; Viu, F.C.; Gonçalves, L.M.; Barbosa, C.M.R.; Del Bel Cury, A.A. Influence of Surface Free Energy of Denture Base and Liner Materials on Candida Albicans Biofilms. *J. Investig. Clin. Dent.* **2015**, *6*, 141–146. [CrossRef] [PubMed]
44. Satpathy, A.; Dhakshaini, M.R.; Gujjari, A.K. An Evaluation of the Adherence of Candida Albicans on the Surface of Heat Cure Denture Base Material Subjected to Different Stages of Polishing. *J. Clin. Diagn. Res. JCDR* **2013**, *7*, 2360–2363. [CrossRef] [PubMed]
45. Pereira-Cenci, T.; Pereira, T.; Cury, A.A.D.B.; Cenci, M.S.; Rodrigues-Garcia, R.C.M. In Vitro Candida Colonization on Acrylic Resins and Denture Liners: Influence of Surface Free Energy, Roughness, Saliva, and Adhering Bacteria. *Int. J. Prosthodont.* **2007**, *20*, 308–310.
46. Kuhar, M.; Funduk, N. Effects of Polishing Techniques on the Surface Roughness of Acrylic Denture Base Resins. *J. Prosthet. Dent.* **2005**, *93*, 76–85. [CrossRef]
47. Bollenl, C.M.L.; Lambrechts, P.; Quirynen, M. Comparison of Surface Roughness of Oral Hard Materials to the Threshold Surface Roughness for Bacterial Plaque Retention: A Review of the Literature. *Dent. Mater.* **1997**, *13*, 258–269. [CrossRef]
48. Harrison, Z.; Johnson, A.; Douglas, C.W.I. An in Vitro Study into the Effect of a Limited Range of Denture Cleaners on Surface Roughness and Removal of Candida Albicans from Conventional Heat-Cured Acrylic Resin Denture Base Material. *J. Oral Rehabil.* **2004**, *31*, 460–467. [CrossRef]
49. Susewind, S.; Lang, R.; Hahnel, S. Biofilm Formation and Candida Albicans Morphology on the Surface of Denture Base Materials. *Mycoses* **2015**, *58*, 719–727. [CrossRef]
50. Consani, R.L.X.; Pucciarelli, M.G.R.; Mesquita, M.F.; Nogueira, M.C.F.; Barão, V.A.R. Polymerization Cycles on Hardness and Surface Gloss of Denture Bases. *Int. J. Contemp. Dent. Med. Rev.* **2014**, *2014*, ID041114.
51. Farina, A.P.; Cecchin, D.; Soares, R.G.; Botelho, A.L.; Takahashi, J.M.F.K.; Mazzetto, M.O.; Mesquita, M.F. Evaluation of Vickers Hardness of Different Types of Acrylic Denture Base Resins with and without Glass Fibre Reinforcement. *Gerodontology* **2012**, *29*, e155–e160. [CrossRef]
52. Azevedo, A.; Machado, A.L.; Vergani, C.E.; Giampaolo, E.T.; Pavarina, A.C. Hardness of Denture Base and Hard Chair-Side Reline Acrylic Resins. *J. Appl. Oral Sci.* **2005**, *13*, 291–295. [CrossRef]
53. Lung, C.Y.K.; Darvell, B.W. Minimization of the Inevitable Residual Monomer in Denture Base Acrylic. *Dent. Mater.* **2005**, *21*, 1119–1128. [CrossRef]
54. International Organization for Standardization. *Dentistry-Base Polymers Part I: Denture Base Polymers*; ISO 20795-1; ISO: Geneva, Switzerland, 2013; p. 35.